ECG from Basics to Essentials

Step by Step

Roland X. Stroobandt
MD, PhD, FHRS

Professor Emeritus of Medicine
Heart Center, Ghent University Hospital
Ghent, Belgium

S. Serge Barold
MD, FRACP, FACP, FACC, FESC, FHRS

Clinical Professor of Medicine Emeritus
Department of Medicine
University of Rochester School of Medicine and Dentistry
Rochester, New York, USA

Alfons F. Sinnaeve
Ing. MSc

Professor Emeritus of Electronic Engineering
KUL – Campus Vives Oostende, Department of Electronics
Oostende, Belgium

WILEY Blackwell

This edition first published 2016 © 2016 by John Wiley & Sons, Ltd.

Registered office: John Wiley & Sons, Ltd, The Atrium, Southern Gate, Chichester, West Sussex, PO19 8SQ, UK

Editorial offices: 9600 Garsington Road, Oxford, OX4 2DQ, UK
The Atrium, Southern Gate, Chichester, West Sussex, PO19 8SQ, UK
111 River Street, Hoboken, NJ 07030-5774, USA

For details of our global editorial offices, for customer services and for information about how to apply for permission to reuse the copyright material in this book please see our website at www.wiley.com/wiley-blackwell

Library of Congress Cataloging-in-Publication Data are available

ISBN 9781119066415

A catalogue record for this book is available from the British Library.

Wiley also publishes its books in a variety of electronic formats. Some content that appears in print may not be available in electronic books.

Cover image: Courtesy of Alfons F. Sinnaeve
Set in 9/10 Helvetica LT Std by Aptara

Printed and bound by CPI Group (UK) Ltd, Croydon, CR0 4YY

C9781119066415_061023

ECG from Basics to Essentials

Step by Step

Contents

Preface

Before deciding to write this book, we examined many of the multitude of books on electrocardiography to determine whether there was a need for a new book with a different approach focusing on graphics. In our experience the success of our "step by step" books on cardiac pacemakers and implanted cardioverter-defibrillators was largely due to the extensive use of graphics according to feedback we received from many readers. Consequently in this book we used the same approach with the liberal use of graphics. This format distinguishes the book from all the other publications. In this way, the book can be considered as a companion to our previous "step by step" books. The publisher offers a large number of PowerPoint slides obtainable on the Internet.

Based on a number of suggestions an accompanying set of test ECG tracings is also provided on the Internet. We are confident that our different approach to the teaching of electrocardiography will facilitate understanding by the student and help the teacher, the latter by using the richly illustrated work.

The authors would also like to thank Garant Publishers, Antwerp, Belgium /Apeldoorn, The Netherlands for authorizing the use of figures from the Dutch ECG book, *ECG: Uit of in het Hoofd*, 2006 edition, by E. Andries, R. Stroobandt, N. De Cock, F. Sinnaeve and F. Verdonck,

Roland X. Stroobandt
S. Serge Barold
Alfons F. Sinnaeve

About the companion website

This book is accompanied by a companion website, containing all the figures from the book for you to download: www.wiley.com/go/stroobandt/ecg

CHAPTER 1

ANATOMY AND BASIC PHYSIOLOGY

* What is an ECG?
* Blood circulation – the heart in action
* The conduction system of the heart
* Myocardial electrophysiology
    ◦ About cardiac cells
    ◦ Depolarization of a myocardial fiber
    ◦ Distribution of current in myocardium
* Recording a voltage by external electrodes
* The resultant heart vector during ventricular depolarization

ECG from Basics to Essentials: Step by Step. First Edition. Roland X. Stroobandt, S. Serge Barold and Alfons F. Sinnaeve.
Published 2016 © 2016 by John Wiley & Sons, Ltd. Companion Website: www.wiley.com/go/stroobandt/ecg

WHAT IS AN ECG?

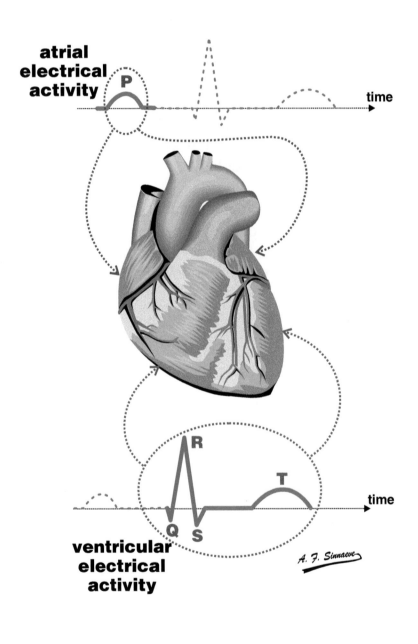

atrial electrical activity

P

time

ventricular electrical activity

R

Q S

T

time

A. F. Sinnaeve

The *electrocardiogram (ECG)* is the recording of the electrical activity generated during and after activation of the various parts of the heart. It is detected by electrodes attached to the skin.

The ECG provides information on:

* the heart rate or cardiac rhythm
* position of the heart inside the body
* the thickness of the heart muscle or dilatation of heart cavities
* origin and propagation of the electrical activity and its possible aberrations
* cardiac rhythm disorders due to congenital anomalies of the heart
* injuries due to insufficient blood supply (ischemia, infarction, ...)
* malfunction of the heart due to electrolyte disturbances or drugs

History

The Dutch physiologist Willem Einthoven was one of the pioneers of electrocardiography and developer of the first useful string galvonometer. He labelled the various parts of the electro-cardiogram using P, Q, R, S and T in a classic article published in 1903. Professor Einthoven received the Nobel prize for medicine in 1924.

BLOOD CIRCULATION – THE HEART IN ACTION

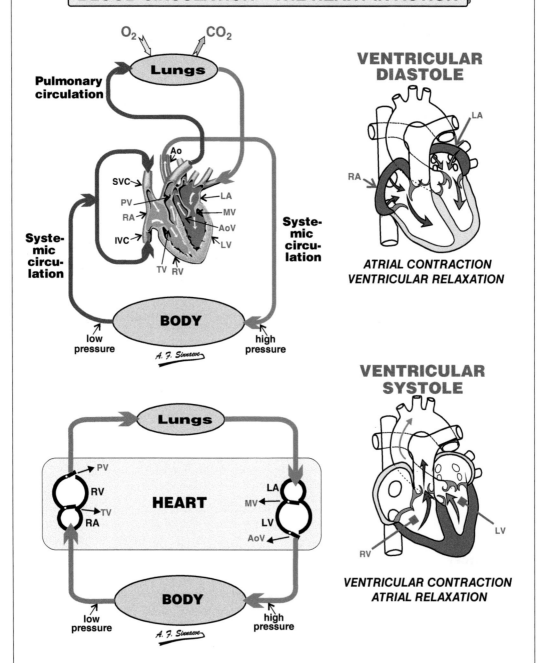

VENTRICULAR DIASTOLE

ATRIAL CONTRACTION
VENTRICULAR RELAXATION

VENTRICULAR SYSTOLE

VENTRICULAR CONTRACTION
ATRIAL RELAXATION

Abbreviations : Ao = aorta ; AoV = aortic valve ; LA = left atrium ; LV = left ventricle ; MV = mitral valve ; PV = pulmonary valve ; RA = right atrium ; RV = right ventricle ; TV = tricuspid valve ; IVC = inferior vena cava ; SVC = superior vena cava ; O_2 = oxygen ; CO_2 = carbon dioxide

The heart is a muscle consisting of four hollow chambers. It is a double pump: the left part works at a higher pressure, while the right part works on a lower pressure.

The right heart pumps blood into the *pulmonary circulation* (i.e. the lungs). The left heart drives blood through the *systemic circulation* (i.e. the rest of the body).

The *right atrium* (RA) receives deoxygenated blood from the body via two large veins, the superior and the inferior vena cava, and from the heart itself by way of the coronary sinus. The blood is transferred to the *right ventricle* (RV) via the *tricuspid valve* (TV). The right ventricle then pumps the deoxygenated blood via the *pulmonary valve* (PV) to the lungs where it releases excess carbon dioxide and picks up new oxygen.

The *left atrium* (LA) accepts the newly oxygenated blood from the lungs via the pulmonary veins and delivers it to the *left ventricle* (LV) through the *mitral valve* (MV). The oxygenated blood is pumped by the left ventricle through the *aortic valve* (AoV) into the aorta (Ao), the largest artery in the body.

The blood flowing into the aorta is further distributed throughout the body where it releases oxygen to the cells and collects carbon dioxide from them.

The cardiac cycle consists of two primary phases:
1. VENTRICULAR DIASTOLE is a period of myocardial relaxation when the ventricles are filled with blood.
2. VENTRICULAR SYSTOLE is the period of contraction when the blood is forced out of the ventricles into the arterial tree.

At rest, this cycle is normally repeated at a rate of approximately 70–75 times/minute and slower during sleep.

6

THE CONDUCTION SYSTEM OF THE HEART

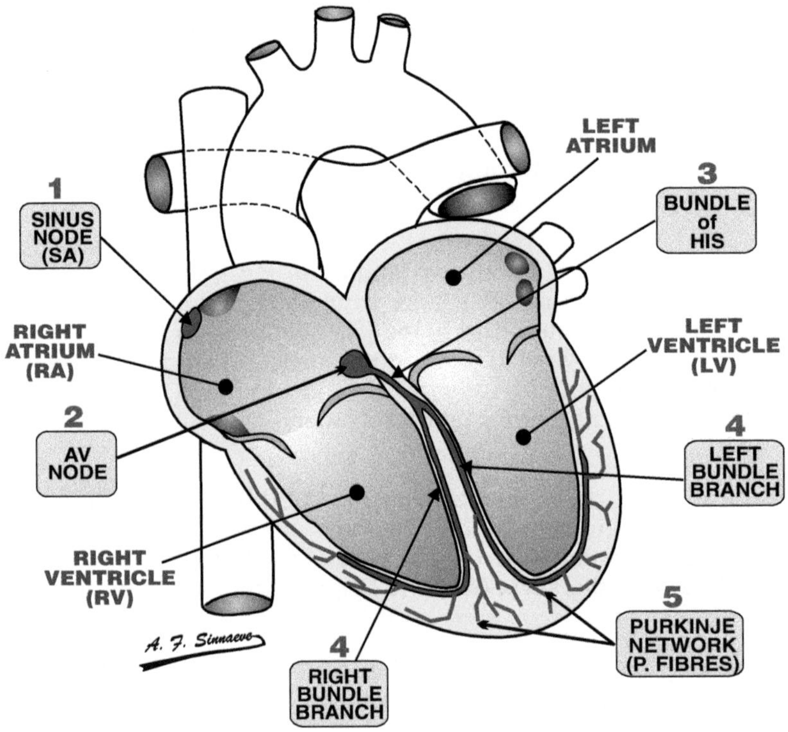

LEFT ATRIUM

1 SINUS NODE (SA)

3 BUNDLE of HIS

RIGHT ATRIUM (RA)

2 AV NODE

LEFT VENTRICLE (LV)

4 LEFT BUNDLE BRANCH

RIGHT VENTRICLE (RV)

4 RIGHT BUNDLE BRANCH

5 PURKINJE NETWORK (P. FIBRES)

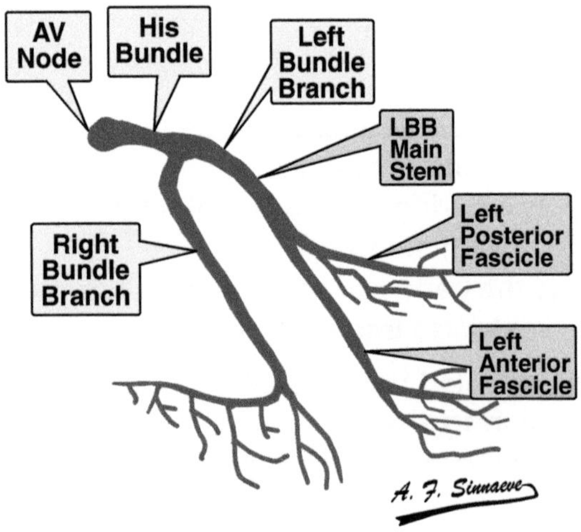

A. F. Sinnaeve

AV Node

His Bundle

Left Bundle Branch

LBB Main Stem

Left Posterior Fascicle

Right Bundle Branch

Left Anterior Fascicle

A. F. Sinnaeve

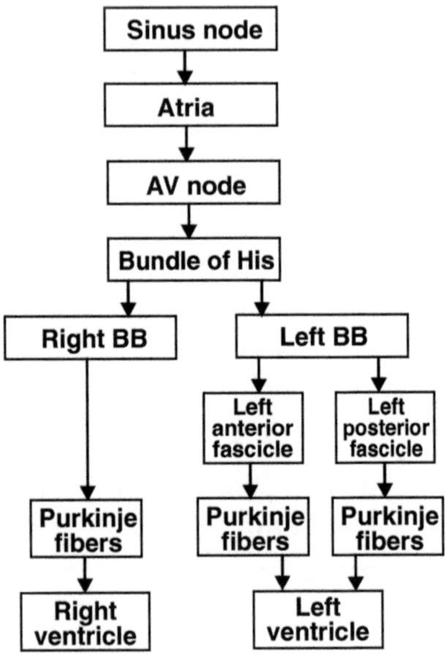

Sinus node → Atria → AV node → Bundle of His

Right BB → Purkinje fibers → Right ventricle

Left BB → Left anterior fascicle → Purkinje fibers → Left ventricle

Left posterior fascicle → Purkinje fibers → Left ventricle

The contractions of the various parts of the heart have to be carefully synchronized. It is the prime function of the electrical conduction system to ensure this synchronization. The atria should contract first to fill the ventricles before the ventricles pump the blood in the circulation.

1. The excitation starts in the sinus node consisting of special pacemaker cells. The electrical impulses spread over the right and left atria.

2. The AV node is normally the only electrical connection between the atria and the ventricles. The impulses slow down as they travel through the AV node to reach the bundle of His.

3. The bundle of His, the distal part of the AV junction, conducts the impulses rapidly to the bundle branches.

4. The fast conducting right and left bundle branches subdivide into smaller and smaller branches, the smallest ones connecting to the Purkinje fibers.

5. The Purkinje fibers spread out all over the ventricles beneath the endocardium and they bring the electrical impulses very fast to the myocardial cells.

All in all it takes the electrical impulses less than 200 ms to travel from the sinus node to the myocardial cells in the ventricles.

ABOUT CARDIAC CELLS 1

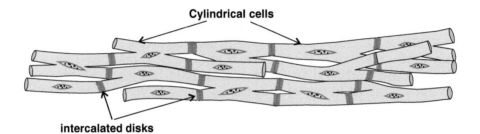

Cylindrical cells

intercalated disks

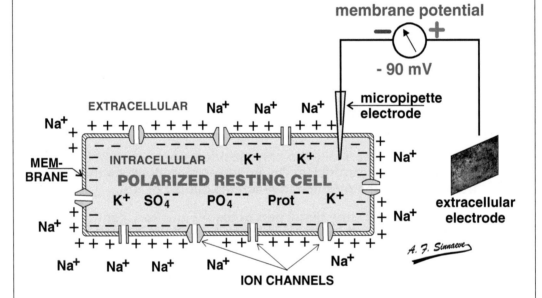

membrane potential

$-$ 90 mV

micropipette electrode

EXTRACELLULAR   Na$^+$ Na$^+$ Na$^+$

Na$^+$ $+ + +$ $+ + + +$ $+ + +$ $+ + +$

MEM-
BRANE

INTRACELLULAR   K$^+$ K$^+$ Na$^+$

POLARIZED RESTING CELL

K$^+$ SO$_4^{--}$ PO$_4^{---}$ Prot^{--} K$^+$ Na$^+$

Na$^+$ $+ + +$ $+ + + +$ $+ + +$ $+ + +$ Na$^+$

Na$^+$ Na$^+$ Na$^+$ Na$^+$ Na$^+$

extracellular electrode

A. F. Sinnaeve

ION CHANNELS

ION	[ion]$_e$ Extracellular concentration in mmol/liter, mM	[ion]$_i$ Intracellular concentration in mmol/liter, mM
K$^+$	4	150
Na$^+$	145	10
Ca^{++}	1.8	10^{-4}
Cl$^-$	120	20

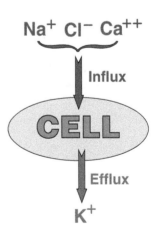

Na$^+$ Cl$^-$ Ca^{++}

Influx

CELL

Efflux

K$^+$

Cardiac muscle cells are more or less cylindrical. At their ends they may partially divide into two or more branches, connecting with the branches of adjacent cells and forming an anastomosing network of cells called a *syncytium*. At the interconnections between cells there are specialized membranes (*intercalated disks*) with a very low electrical resistance. These *"gap-junctions"* allow a very rapid conduction from one cell to another.

All cardiac cells are enclosed in a *semipermeable membrane* which allows certain charged chemical particles to flow in and out of the cells through very *specific channels*. These charged particles are *ions* (positive if they have lost one or more electrons, such as sodium Na^+, potassium K^+ or calcium Ca^{++} and negative if they have a surplus of an electron, e.g. Cl^-).

The ion channels are very selective. Larger ions such as phos-phate ions (PO_4^{---}), sulfate ions (SO_4^{--}) and protein ions are unable to pass through the channels and stay in the inside making the inside of the cell negative. A voltmeter between an intracellular and an extracellular electrode will indicate a potential difference. This voltage is called the *resting membrane potential* (normally about −90 millivolts).

In the resting state, a high concentration of positively charged sodium ions (Na^+) is present outside the cell while a high concentration of positive potassium ions (K^+) and a mixture of the large negatively charged ions (PO_4^{---}, SO_4^{--}, $Prot^{--}$) are found inside the cell.

There is a continuous leakage of the small ions decreasing the resting membrane potential. Consequently other processes have to restore the phenomenon. The Na^+/K^+ pump, located in the cell membrane, maintains the negative resting potential inside the cell by bringing K^+ into the cell while taking Na^+ out of the cell. This process requires energy and therefore it uses adenosine triphosphate (ATP). The pump can be blocked by digitalis. If the Na^+/K^+ pump is inhibited, Na^+ ions are still removed from the inside by the Na^+/Ca^{++} exchange process. This process increases the intracellular Ca^{++} and ameliorates the contractility of the muscle cells.

ABOUT CARDIAC CELLS 2

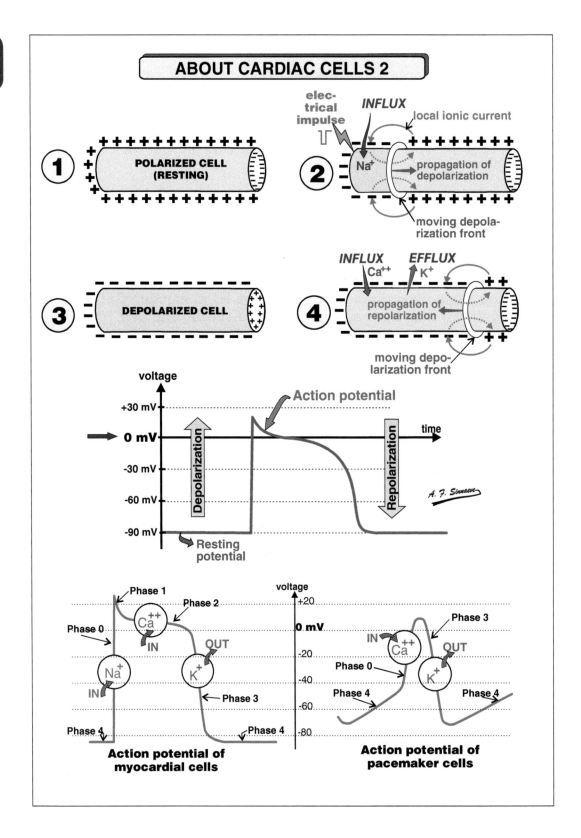

An external negative electric impulse that converts the outside of a myocardial cell from positive to negative, makes the membrane permeable to Na^+. The influx of Na^+ ions makes the inside of the cell less negative. When the membrane voltage reaches a certain value(called the threshold), some fast sodium channels in the membrane open momentarily, resulting in a sudden larger influx of Na^+. Consequently, a part of the cell depolarizes, i.e. its exterior becomes negative with respect to its interior that becomes positive. Due to the difference in concentration of the Na^+ ions, a local ionic current arises between the depolarized part of the cell and its still resting part. These local electric currents give rise to a depolarization front that moves on until the whole cell becomes depolarized.

As soon as the depolarization starts, K^+ ions flow out from the cell trying to restore the initial resting potential. In the meantime, some Ca^{++} ions flow inwards through slow calcium channels. At first, these ion movements and the decreasing Na^+ influx nearly balance each other resulting in a slowly varying membrane potential. Next the Ca^{++} channels are inhibited as are the Na^+ channels while the open K^+ channels together with the Na^+/K^+ pump repolarize the cell. Again local currents are generated and a repolarization front propagates until the whole cell is repolarized.

> **The action potential depicts the changes of the membrane potential during the depolarization and the subsequent repolarization of the cell. The intracellular environment is negative at rest (resting potential) and becomes positive with respect to the outside when the cell is activated and depolarized.**

The cells of the sinus node and the AV junction do not have fast sodium channels. Instead they have slow calcium channels and potassium channels that open when the membrane potential is depolarized to about −50 mV.

ABOUT CARDIAC CELLS 3

Action potential of a sinus node cell

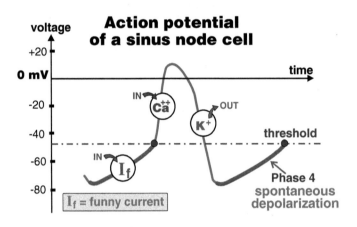

voltage

+20
0 mV
−20
−40
−60
−80

time

IN
Ca^{++}

OUT
K$^+$

threshold

IN
I$_f$

Phase 4
spontaneous
depolarization

I$_f$ = funny current

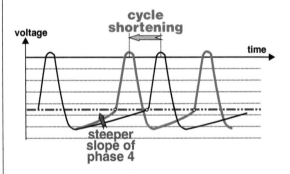

voltage

cycle
shortening

time

steeper
slope of
phase 4

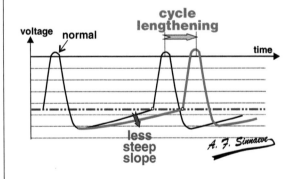

voltage

normal

cycle
lengthening

time

less
steep
slope

A. F. Sinnaeve

Dominant Pacemaker
Sinus Node (SAN)
60–80 /min

**Latent or Escape
Pacemakers**

AV Junction including
the His Bundle
40–60 /min

Right and Left
Bundle Branches
30–40 /min

Purkinje Fibers
20–40 /min

> **Common myocardial cells only depolarize if they are triggered by an external event or by adjacent cells.**
> **However, cells within the sinoatrial node (SAN) exhibit a completely different behavior. During the diastolic phase (phase 4 of their action potential) a** spontaneous depolarization **takes place.**

The major determinant for the diastolic depolarization is the so-called "funny current" I_f. This particularly unusual current consists of an influx of a mix of sodium and potassium ions that makes the inside of the cells more positive.

When the action potential reaches a threshold potential (about –50/–40mV), a faster depolarization by the Ca^{++} ions starts the systolic phase. As soon as the action potential becomes positive, some potassium channels open and the resulting outflow of K^+ ions repolarizes the cells. The moment the repolarization reaches its most negative potential (–60/–70mV), the funny current starts again and the whole cycle starts all over.

> **The funny current I_f is most prominently expressed in the sinoatrial node (SAN), making this node the** natural pacemaker **of the heart that determines the rhythm of the heart beat. Hence I_f is sometimes called the "pacemaker current".**

Spontaneous depolarization may be modulated by changing the slope of the spontaneous depolarization (mostly by influencing the I_f channels). The slope is controlled by the autonomic nervous system.

Increase in sympathetic activity and administration of catecholamines (epinephrine, norepinephrine, dopamine) increases the slope of the phase 4 depolarization. This results in a higher firing rate of the pacemaker cells and a shorter cardiac cycle. Administration of certain drugs decreases the slope of the phase 4 depolarization, reducing the firing rate and lengthening the cardiac cycle.

Spontaneous depolarization is not only present in the sinoatrial node (SAN) but, to a lesser extent, also in the other parts of the conduction system. The intrinsic pacemaker activity of the secondary pacemakers situated in the atrioventricular junction and the His-Purkinje system is normally quiescent by a mechanism termed overdrive suppression. If the sinus node (SAN) becomes depressed, or its action potentials fail to reach secondary pace-makers, a slower rhythm takes over.

> **Secondary pacemakers provide a backup if the activity of the SAN fails**

Overdrive suppression occurs when cells with a higher intrinsic rate (e.g. the dominant pace-maker) continually depolarize or overdrive potential automatic foci with a lower intrinsic rate thereby suppressing their emergence.

Should the highest pacemaking center fail, a lower automatic focus previously inactive because of overdrive suppression emerges or "escapes" from the next highest level.
The new site becomes the dominant pacemaker at its inherent rate and in turn suppresses all automatic foci below it.

DEPOLARIZATION OF A MYOCARDIAL FIBER

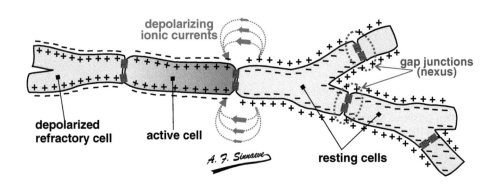

depolarizing
ionic currents

gap junctions
(nexus)

depolarized
refractory cell

active cell

resting cells

A. F. Sinnaeve

DISTRIBUTION OF CURRENT IN MYOCARDIUM
AND RAPID SPREAD OF ELECTRICAL ACTIVITY

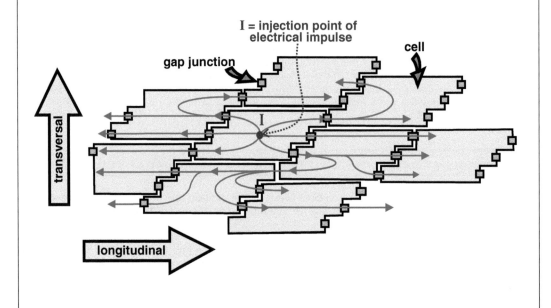

I = injection point of
electrical impulse

gap junction

cell

transversal

I

longitudinal

A depolarization front can propagate through the fibers of the heart muscle in the same way as the depolarization front moves through a single cylindrical cell. Local ionic currents between active cells and resting cells depolarize the resting cells and activate them.

> ✿ **Very rapid conduction of electrical impulses from one cell to another is due to** *"gap junctions"* **with a low electrical resistance between the cylindrical cells.**
>
> ✿ **Cardiac cells partially divide at their ends, forming an anastomosing network or** "syncytium" **causing fast depolarization of the whole myo-cardium.**

Due to the intercalated disks with their gap junctions, a depolarizing electrical impulse spreads out rapidly in all directions. However, the gap junctions with their very low electrical resistance are only present at the short ends of the myocardial cells. Hence, depolarization propagates very fast in the longitudinal direction of the fibers and less fast in the transversal direction.

RECORDING A VOLTAGE BY EXTERNAL ELECTRODES

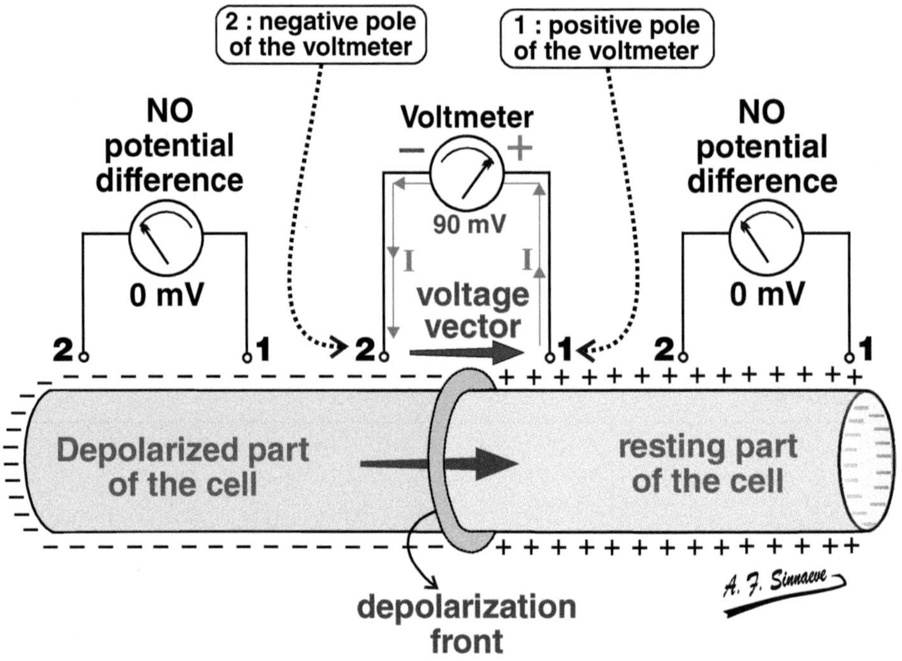

2 : negative pole of the voltmeter

1 : positive pole of the voltmeter

NO potential difference

0 mV

Voltmeter

− +

90 mV

I   I

voltage vector

NO potential difference

0 mV

2   1   2   1   2   1

− − − − − −   + + + + + + + + + +

Depolarized part of the cell   **resting part of the cell**

− − − − − − − −   + + + + + + + + + +

depolarization front

A. F. Sinnaeve

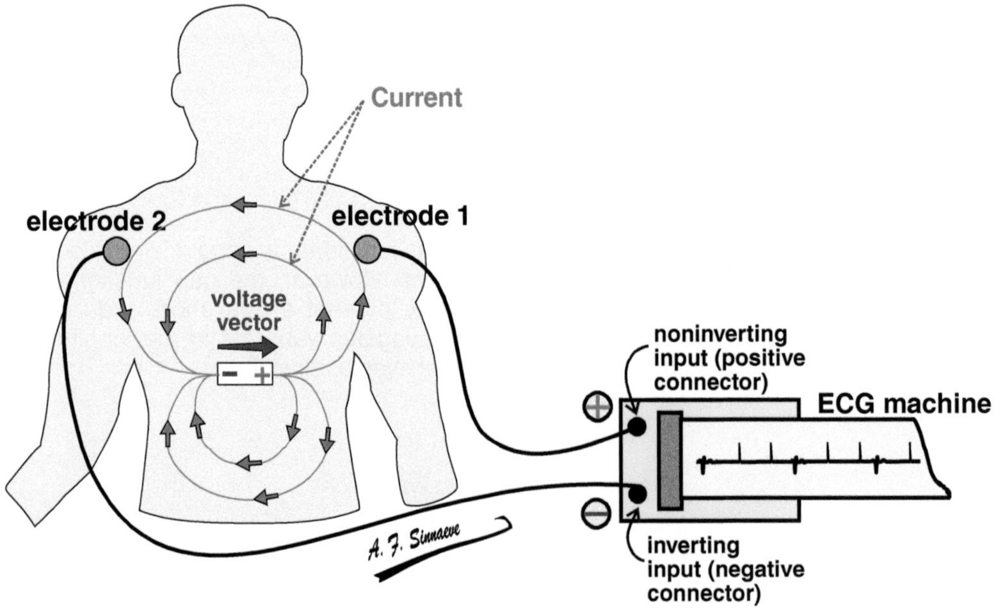

Current

electrode 2   electrode 1

voltage vector

− +

noninverting input (positive connector)

⊕

ECG machine

⊖

inverting input (negative connector)

A. F. Sinnaeve

> ## A voltage is always measured between TWO electrodes.

> **A potential difference or voltage is only caused by a propagating front (either depolarization or repolarization). A resting cell or a depolarized cell does not give rise to a deflection of the voltmeter.**

The voltmeter shows a positive deflection if the voltage vector points towards its positive pole !
A very small current flows through the voltmeter from its positive pole to its negative pole. The internal resistance of the voltmeter has to be extremely high since the small current may not influence the condition of the source, i.e this weak current may not affect the distribution of the ions around the cell.

Due to the high degree of electrical interaction between the branched cells, many cells are depolarizing simultaneously in different regions of the ventricles during the ventricular activation process. The voltage vectors of these many cells may be combined into one resultant vector. When a depolarization front or a repolarization front moves rapidly through a region of the heart it generates a voltage vector and a tiny electrical current flows through the body (which is a good conductor). The ECG recorder acts in the same way as a voltmeter and when the voltage vector points to its positive connector, the ECG registers a positive (+) deflection.

THE RESULTANT HEART VECTOR DURING VENTRICULAR DEPOLARIZATION

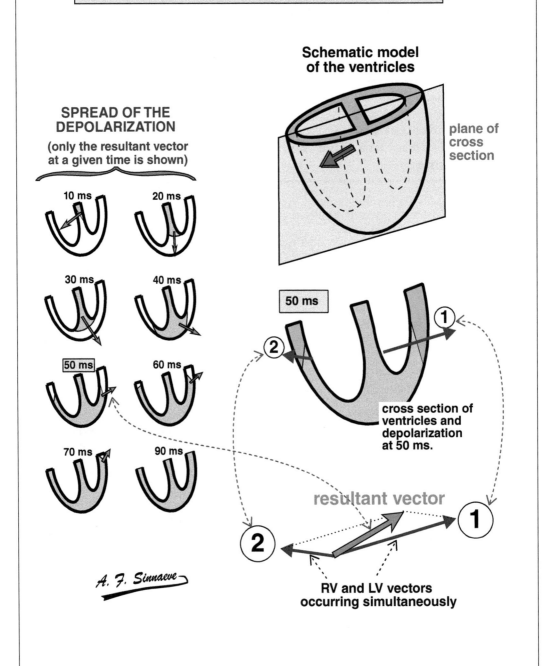

Schematic model of the ventricles

plane of cross section

SPREAD OF THE DEPOLARIZATION

(only the resultant vector at a given time is shown)

10 ms 20 ms

30 ms 40 ms

50 ms 60 ms

70 ms 90 ms

50 ms

cross section of ventricles and depolarization at 50 ms.

resultant vector

RV and LV vectors occurring simultaneously

A. F. Sinnaeve

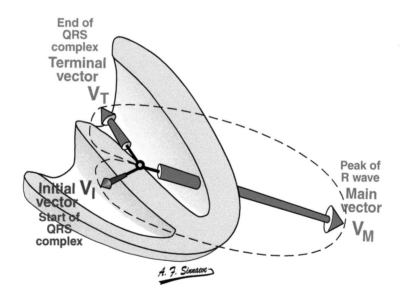

Ventricular activation consists of a series of sequential activation fronts. At each particular time, the vectors of these activation fronts may be combined to form one resultant vector. The resultant vector changes continually as the ventricles are being progressively depolarized. However, at each point in time the multiple activation fronts can be represented by a single resultant vector.

> **THE RESULTANT HEART VECTOR IS NOT CONSTANT**
> *** its direction in space changes continuously**
> *** its magnitude changes all the time**

End of
QRS
complex
**Terminal
vector**
V_T

Peak of
R wave
**Main
vector**
V_M

**Initial V_I
vector**
Start of
QRS
complex

A. J. Sinnaeve

V_I, V_M and V_T occur sequentially

The point of the resultant heart vector traces a closed loop in space. The projection of this path is the vectorcardiogram.

20 **Further Reading**

Barold SS. Willem Einthoven and the birth of clinical electrocardiography a hundred years ago. Card Electrophysiol Rev. 2003;7:99-104.

Hurst JW. Naming of the waves in the ECG, with a brief account of their genesis. Circulation. 1998;98:1937-42.

Janse MJ, Rosen MR. History of arrhythmias. Handb Exp Pharmacol. 2006;171:1-39.

Kligfield P. The centennial of the Einthoven electrocardiogram. J Electrocardiol. 2002;35 Suppl:123-9.

CHAPTER 2

ECG RECORDING
AND
ECG LEADS

* The ECG machine or electrocardiograph
* The ECG grid
* Time interval versus rate
* Registration of an ECG
* Standard leads according to Einthoven
* Wilson central terminal
* Augmented limb leads according to Goldberger
* The precordial leads after Wilson
* How to locate the 4th right and left intercostal spaces
* The 12 leads put together
* Understanding the hexaxial diagram and its importance
* Common errors in recording the ECG from precordial leads
* Lead reversals in frontal plane

ECG from Basics to Essentials: Step by Step. First Edition. Roland X. Stroobandt, S. Serge Barold and Alfons F. Sinnaeve.
Published 2016 © 2016 by John Wiley & Sons, Ltd. Companion Website: www.wiley.com/go/stroobandt/ecg

THE ECG MACHINE OR ELECTROCARDIOGRAPH

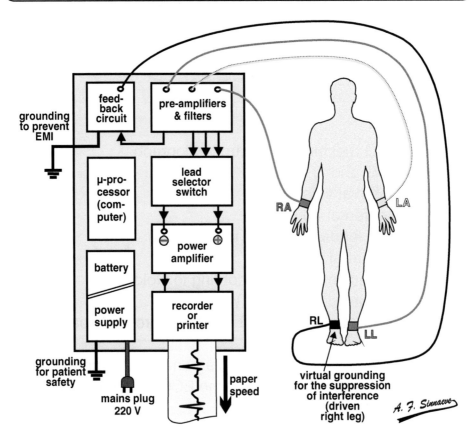

grounding
to prevent
EMI

feed-
back
circuit

pre-amplifiers
& filters

µ-pro-
cessor
(com-
puter)

lead
selector
switch

battery

power
amplifier

power
supply

recorder
or
printer

grounding
for patient
safety

mains plug
220 V

paper
speed

RA

LA

RL

LL

virtual grounding
for the suppression
of interference
(driven
right leg)

A. F. Sinnaeve

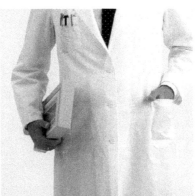

2010
battery powered
and portable

Abbreviations
EMI = electromagnetic interference ; µ = micro (Greek letter mu)
RA = right arm ; LA = left arm ; RL = right leg ; LL = left leg (frontal plane connections)

* A safety grounding prevents electrocution if a fault occurs in the power supply of some ECG machines (class I). This protective wire is normally incorporated in the mains cable. ECG machines with double insulation (class II) do not need such connection. Of course, ECG machines working on a battery and without a connection to the mains are not equipped with a safety ground connection.

* Pre-amplifiers enhance the small signals picked up by the electrodes on the patient. They also provide filters avoiding non-cardiac signals from disturbing the ECG. An AC-filter counteracts 50 or 60 Hz interference (EMI) and another filter cuts down the influence of myopotentials from musculoskeletal sources.

* Contemporary ECG machines may contain an embedded microprocessor (computer) that not only controls the proper functioning of the equipment, but also provides an ECG diagnosis.

* A feed-back circuit combines all spurious signals (noise) of the limb leads and is coupled to the right leg. This eliminates most of the unwanted noise and provides a thin baseline so that small details of the ECG can be observed.

* The power amplifier delivers the necessary power for the movement of the mechanical parts in the recorder or printer which delivers a document on paper.

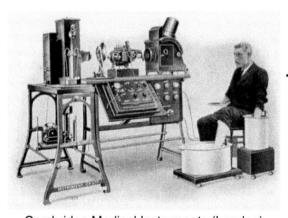

1908
still a long way to go...

Cambridge Medical Instruments (London)

THE ECG GRID

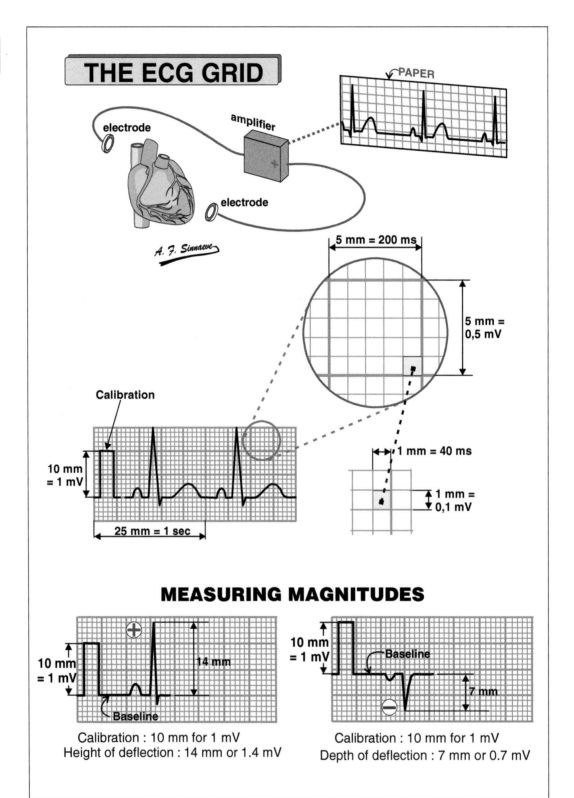

PAPER

electrode

amplifier

electrode

A. F. Sinnaeve

5 mm = 200 ms

5 mm = 0,5 mV

1 mm = 40 ms

1 mm = 0,1 mV

Calibration

10 mm = 1 mV

25 mm = 1 sec

MEASURING MAGNITUDES

10 mm = 1 mV

14 mm

Baseline

Calibration : 10 mm for 1 mV
Height of deflection : 14 mm or 1.4 mV

10 mm = 1 mV

Baseline

7 mm

Calibration : 10 mm for 1 mV
Depth of deflection : 7 mm or 0.7 mV

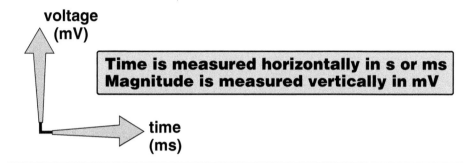

voltage (mV)

time (ms)

**Time is measured horizontally in s or ms
Magnitude is measured vertically in mV**

* Conventionally the sensitivity of the ECG machine is adjusted (i.e. calibrated) so that a 1 millivolt (1 mV) electrical signal produces a 10 mm deflection on the ECG (i.e. two large squares).

* The standard paper speed is 25 mm per second (i.e. 1 s or 1000 ms corresponds to five large squares)

Note:

* If the QRS complexes are too small (low voltage) or too large (tall voltage) the voltage calibration can be doubled or halved accordingly by flipping a switch in the ECG machine.

* The same grid is used in ECG monitoring where the electrical activity of the heart is shown on a display such as on a laptop (or formerly on a cathode-ray tube such as used in older oscilloscopes).

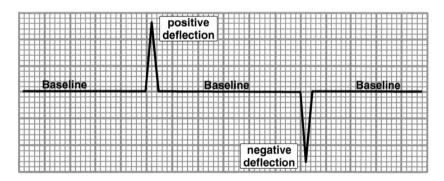

There is no absolute or fixed zero voltage. All measurements of voltages on ECG are relative to the *baseline* or *isoelectric line*.

Upward deflections on an ECG (above the baseline) are called positive. Downward deflections (under the baseline) are called negative.

TIME INTERVAL VS RATE

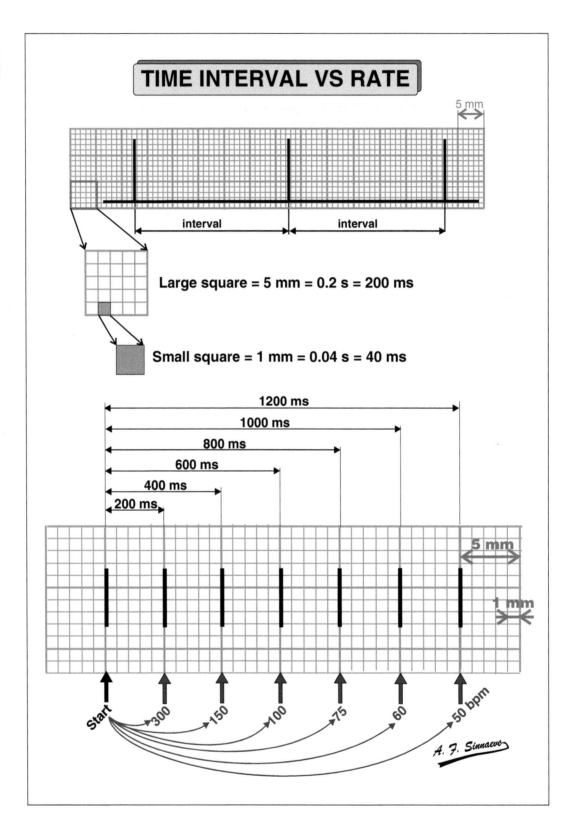

Large square = 5 mm = 0.2 s = 200 ms

Small square = 1 mm = 0.04 s = 40 ms

A. F. Sinnaeve

* The intervals are normally expressed in milliseconds (ms).
* The heart rate or frequency of the heart is expressed in beats per minute (bpm).
* There are 1000 ms in one second and 60 seconds in a minute.
* Hence :

$$\text{Heart Rate (in bpm)} = \frac{60,000}{\text{RR-interval (in ms)}}$$

No calculation needed for a quick estimation of the rate, just count the number of squares between two consecutive R waves !

$$\text{Heart rate (bpm)} = \frac{300}{\text{Number of large squares}}$$

or with more accuracy

$$\text{Heart rate (bpm)} = \frac{1500}{\text{Number of small squares}}$$

For a rapid determination of the rate, memorize the numbers
300 - 150 - 100 - 75 - 60 - 50

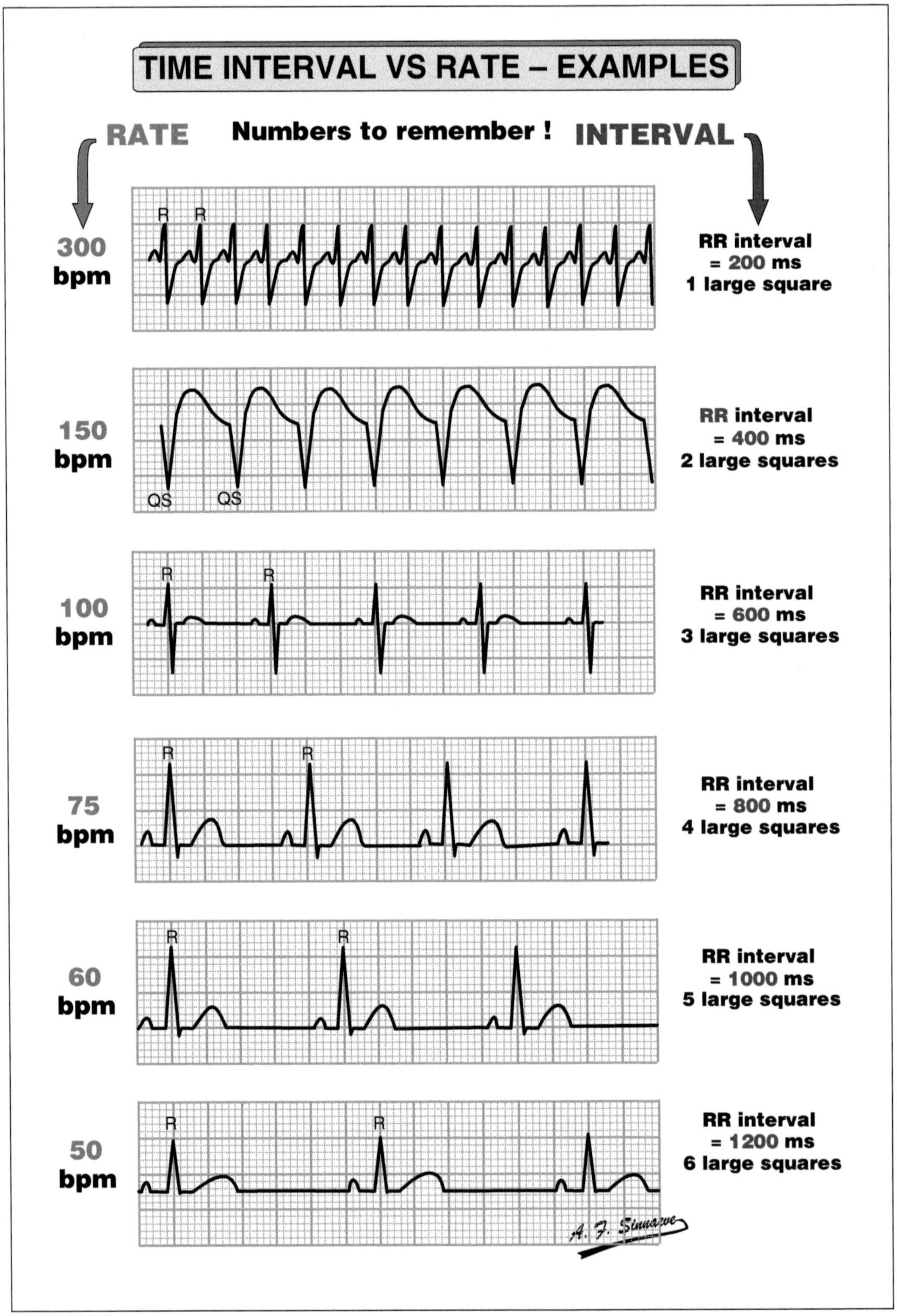
TIME INTERVAL VS RATE – EXAMPLES
RATE
Numbers to remember !
INTERVAL
300 bpm
R R
RR interval = 200 ms 1 large square
150 bpm
QS QS
RR interval = 400 ms 2 large squares
100 bpm
R R
RR interval = 600 ms 3 large squares
75 bpm
R R
RR interval = 800 ms 4 large squares
60 bpm
R R
RR interval = 1000 ms 5 large squares
50 bpm
R R
RR interval = 1200 ms 6 large squares
A. F. Sinnaeve

Methods for determining the heart rate during regular rhythm

1. *Cardiac ruler method*

Place the beginning point of a cardiac ruler over an R wave. Look at the number on which the next R wave falls and read the heart rate.

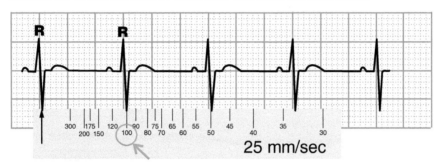

25 mm/sec

2. *The 300 method*

Count the number of large squares (5 mm boxes) between 2 consecutive R waves and divide 300 by that number.

3. *The 1500 method*

Count the number of small squares (1 mm boxes) between 2 consecutive R waves and divide 1500 by that number.

4. *The 6 seconds method*

Obtain a 6 s tracing (30 large squares) and count the number of R waves that appear in that 6 s period and multiply by 10 to obtain the heart rate in bpm.

Methods for determining the heart rate during irregular rhythm

When the heart rate is irregular (e.g. atrial fibrillation), a longer interval should be measured to provide a more precise rate. "1 second time lines" may be used to measure longer intervals. If no "1 s time lines" are marked on the ECG paper, they can be created by counting 5 large squares (5 x 0.2 s = 1 s).

1. *The 6 seconds method*
Heart rate = number of QRS complexes in 6 s multiplied by 10

2. *The 3 seconds method*
Heart rate = number of QRS complexes in 3 s multiplied by 20

Example of the 6 s rule during irregular rhythm

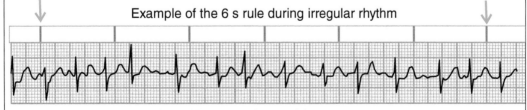

* A 6 s strip is selected between the two blue arrows
* Number of QRS complexes in 6 s is 13
* Mean heart rate is 13 x 10 = 130 bpm

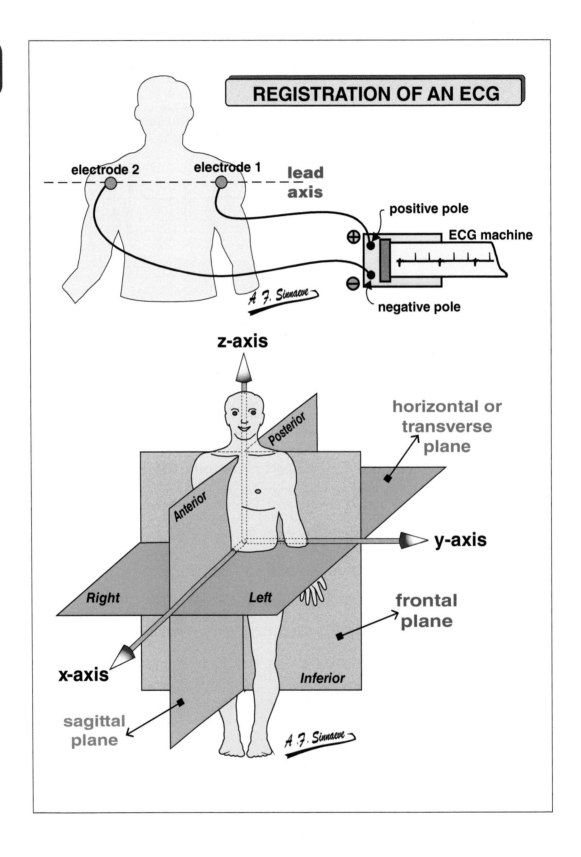

REGISTRATION OF AN ECG

electrode 2

electrode 1

lead axis

positive pole

ECG machine

A. F. Sinnaeve

negative pole

z-axis

Posterior

horizontal or transverse plane

Anterior

y-axis

Right

Left

frontal plane

x-axis

Inferior

sagittal plane

A. F. Sinnaeve

An ECG is the registration of the projection of the resultant heart vector upon the *lead axis*. A lead axis is the hypothetical line joining the two electrodes or poles of that particular lead.

The lead axis of a lead can theoretically be orientated in any direction or plane relative to the heart. Obviously, this will depend upon electrode placement.

Conventionally, however, there are 12 leads which may be divided into two groups on the basis of their orientation. One group is orientated in the frontal plane of the body, the other in the horizontal plane.

In the frontal plane we have:
* 3 standard leads according to Einthoven
* 3 augmented leads according to Goldberger
In the transverse plane are situated:
* 6 precordial leads according to Wilson

STANDARD LEADS ACCORDING TO EINTHOVEN

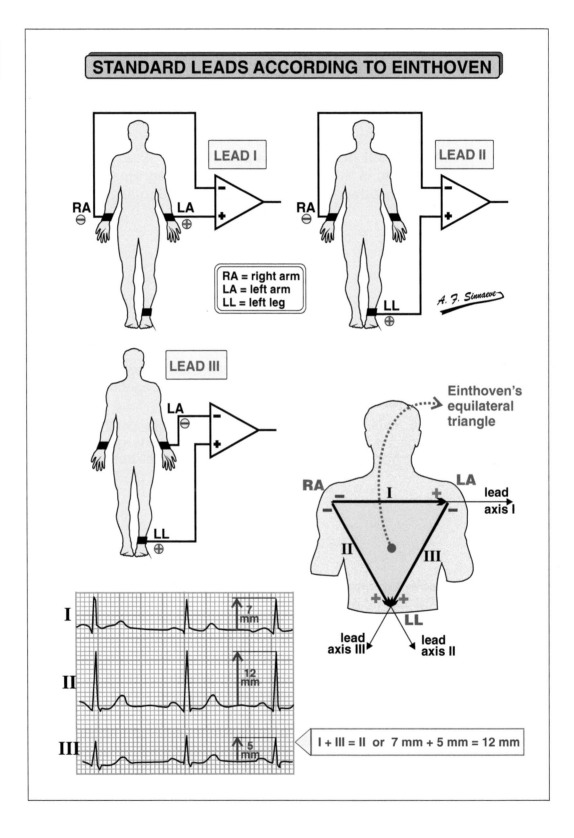

LEAD I

LEAD II

RA = right arm
LA = left arm
LL = left leg

A. F. Sinnaeve

LEAD III

Einthoven's equilateral triangle

RA   I   LA   lead axis I

II   III

LL
lead axis III   lead axis II

I   7 mm

II   12 mm

III   5 mm

I + III = II or 7 mm + 5 mm = 12 mm

The standard leads are :

* **Bipolar leads** since the measurement occurs between two electrodes (+ and –) attached to the body

* **Limb leads** or extremity leads since the electrodes are connected to the extremities

Note : Arms and legs are good electrical conductors, hence the position of the electrodes (hand or shoulder, foot or hip) is not critical.

The positive electrodes (+) of the standard limb leads are electrically at about the same distance from a theoretical zero reference in the heart. Hence, the lead axes form an equilateral triangle with the heart and its zero reference in the center. This triangle is called **Einthoven's triangle**. (Although in reality it is not exactly equilateral, but it is a good approximation.)

Einthoven's law

If : VLA is the potential at the left arm (LA)
VRA is the potential at the right arm (RA)
VLL is the potential at the left leg (LL)

then the potential difference or voltage in the frontal leads is given by :
Lead I = VLA – VRA
Lead II = VLL – VRA
Lead III = VLL – VLA

It follows that (VLA – VRA) + (VLL – VLA) = (VLL – VRA)

or : $\boxed{\text{lead I} + \text{lead III} = \text{lead II}}$

This equation can also be written as :

$$\boxed{\text{lead I} + \text{lead III} - \text{lead II} = 0}$$

which is the well-known form of Einthoven's law!

The relationship between the standard limb leads is such that the sum of the electric voltages recorded in leads I and III equals the electric voltage recorded by lead II.

WILSON CENTRAL TERMINAL

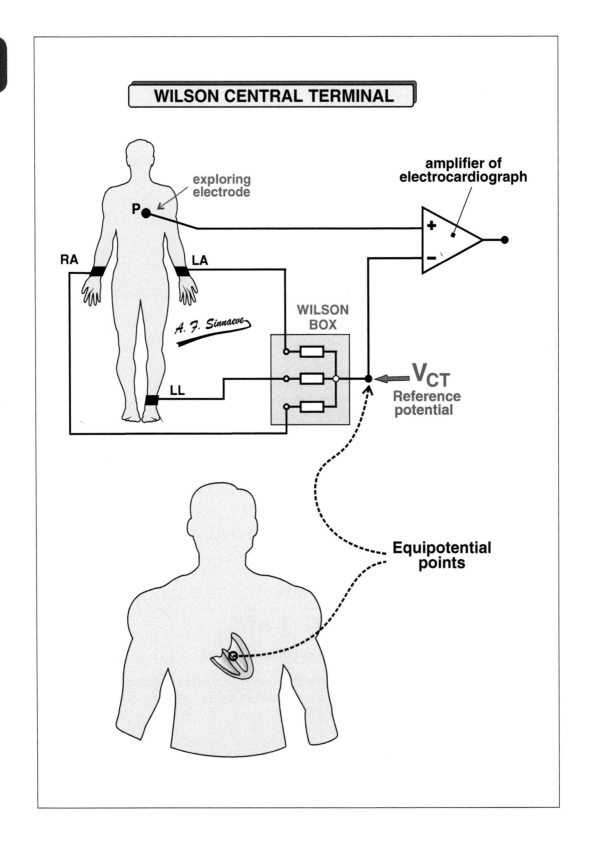

exploring electrode

P

RA

LA

LL

A. F. Sinnaeve

WILSON BOX

amplifier of electrocardiograph

+

−

V_{CT}
Reference potential

Equipotential points

Wilson connected the three standard limb leads through equal-valued resistors to a common point. The potential at this point is the average of the potentials at each limb electrode and is used as a reference potential.

This reference is known as the central terminal potential (VCT) and is used by physicians as zero equivalent.

By linking the three limbs RA, LA and LL through large equal resistors a relatively stable reference potential V_{CT} is created. Although it is technically incorrect to label V_{CT} as the zero potential it may be considered as such because the electrocardiograph only registers variations of voltages and suppresses constant (or DC) voltages.

$$V_{CT} = \frac{V_{RA} + V_{LA} + V_{LL}}{3}$$

Since the potential of the central terminal is essentially constant, the potential difference or voltage recorded by the electrocardiograph only reflects the potential variations at the exploring electrode - hence the term "unipolar lead".

The hypothetical electrical center of the heart, having about the same potential as the reference point in the central terminal (V_{CT}), is located somewhere left of the interventricular septum and below the AV junction.

AUGMENTED LIMB LEADS
ACCORDING TO GOLDBERGER

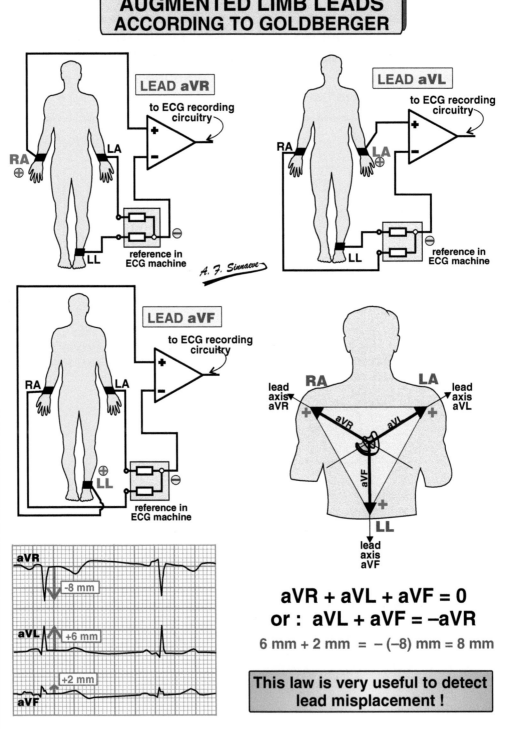

LEAD aVR

to ECG recording circuitry

RA

LA

LL

reference in ECG machine

A. F. Sinnaeve

LEAD aVL

to ECG recording circuitry

RA

LA

LL

reference in ECG machine

LEAD aVF

to ECG recording circuitry

RA

LA

LL

reference in ECG machine

RA

LA

lead axis aVR

lead axis aVL

aVR

aVL

aVF

LL

lead axis aVF

aVR

−8 mm

aVL

+6 mm

+2 mm

aVF

$$aVR + aVL + aVF = 0$$
$$or :\ \ aVL + aVF = -aVR$$

6 mm + 2 mm = − (−8) mm = 8 mm

This law is very useful to detect lead misplacement !

With the Wilson box as a reference potential, additional lead axes were created using one of the three limb electrodes (i.e. RA, LA and LL) as an exploring electrode.

By using only two resistors and omitting the connection between the exploring electrode and the reference point, Dr. Goldberger obtained an amplitude of the deflecton that was 50% larger.

Therefore these leads are called "augmented" hence the letter "a" is applied to the VR, VL and VF leads (aVR, aVL, aVF).

The augmented leads are:

* **Limb leads** because the exploring electrode (+ pole of the ECG machine) is connected to a leg or an arm.

* **Unipolar leads** since only one exploring electrode is used and the negative pole of the ECG machine is connected to the reference point.

* **Frontal plane leads** like leads I, II and III.

> **The lead axis for any particular augmented lead is a straight line drawn between the reference voltage point at the center of the heart and its extremity electrode.**

$$aVR + aVL + aVF = 0$$

For each lead, the potential of the neutral point is the mean of two other limb potentials.

So if: VLA is the potential at the left arm (LA)
VRA is the potential at the right arm (RA)
VLL is the potential at the left leg (LL)

then the voltage of the neutral point for lead aVL is: $Vref = \dfrac{VRA + VLL}{2}$

and lead aVL becomes $aVL = VLA - Vref$ or:

$$aVL = VLA - \frac{VRA + VLL}{2} \quad \text{or} \quad aVL = \frac{2VLA - VRA - VLL}{2}$$

It can be proven in the same way:

$$aVR = \frac{2VRA - VLA - VLL}{2} \quad \text{and} \quad aVF = \frac{2VLL - VRA - VLA}{2}$$

Obviously, the sum of the three augmented leads is aVL + aVR + aVF = 0 beacause:

$$\frac{2VLA - VRA - VLL}{2} + \frac{2VRA - VLA - VLL}{2} + \frac{2VLL - VRA - VLA}{2} =$$

$$\frac{2VLA - VRA - VLL + 2VRA - VLA - VLL + 2VLL - VRA - VLA}{2} = 0$$

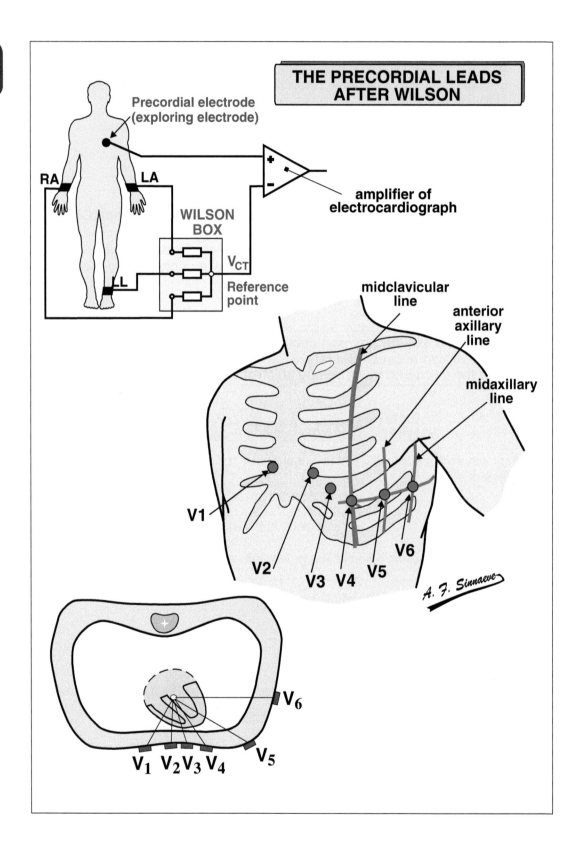

THE PRECORDIAL LEADS AFTER WILSON

Precordial electrode (exploring electrode)

RA   LA

LL

WILSON BOX

V_{CT}

Reference point

amplifier of electrocardiograph

midclavicular line

anterior axillary line

midaxillary line

V1
V2
V3   V4   V5
V6

A. F. Sinnaeve

V_6

V_1 V_2 V_3 V_4 V_5

The Wilson leads are:
* **Unipolar leads** since the measurement occurs with only one exploring or probing electrode (the negative pole of the ECG machine is connected to the central terminal; the reference point V_{CT} acts as a zero potential).
* **Chest leads** or **precordial** leads since the electrodes are placed on the chest around the heart.

Anatomically the RV lies anteriorly and medially but the LV lies laterally and posteriorly. Leads V1 and V2 are situated over the RV, leads V3 and V4 face the interventricular septum and leads V5 and V6 clearly point towards the free lateral wall of the LV. QRS changes emanating from the LV overshadow those from the RV in the absence of a conduction delay involving the RV. Therefore, V1 and V2 reflect the electrical activity of the interventricular septum (pre-dominantly a left-sided structure), leads V3 and V4 point towards the anterior LV, while leads V5 and V6 reflect the lateral LV.

Normal position of precordial electrodes

V1 Right side of the sternum in the fourth intercostal space
V2 Left side of the sternum in the fourth intercostal space
V3 Midway between V2 and V4
V4 Midclavicular line in the fifth intercostal space
V5 Anterior axillary line at the same level as V4
V6 Midaxillary line at the same level as V4

Lead axes in the horizontal plane

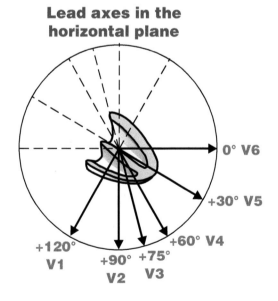

HOW TO LOCATE THE 4TH RIGHT AND LEFT INTERCOSTAL SPACES

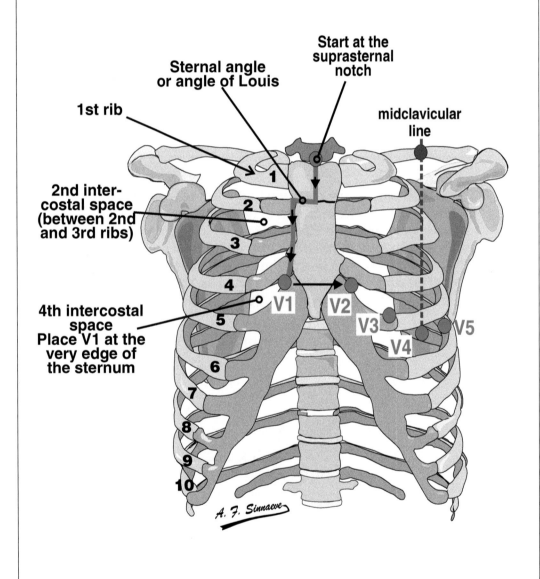

Start at the suprasternal notch

Sternal angle or angle of Louis

1st rib

midclavicular line

2nd inter-costal space (between 2nd and 3rd ribs)

4th intercostal space
Place V1 at the very edge of the sternum

V1 V2 V3 V4 V5

A. F. Sinnaeve

**Locating the 4th intercostal space.
It sounds easy but is not !**

It can be difficult to locate the fourth intercostal space. The best way is to run your fingers from the suprasternal notch starting at the heads of the clavicles down the sternum, until you meet a distinct bony horizontal ridge (the sternal angle or angle of Louis). It is the anterior angle formed by the junction of the manubrium and the body of the sternum. This structure is palpable and easier to find in male patients. The second rib is continuous with the sternal angle. With your finger on this sternal ridge, slide to the patient's right and your finger will drop into an intercostal space which is the second intercostal space, and then move down to the third and then the fourth, where you place V1 at the very edge of the sternum.

Lead V2 is placed in the same way on the other side.

THE 12 LEADS PUT TOGETHER

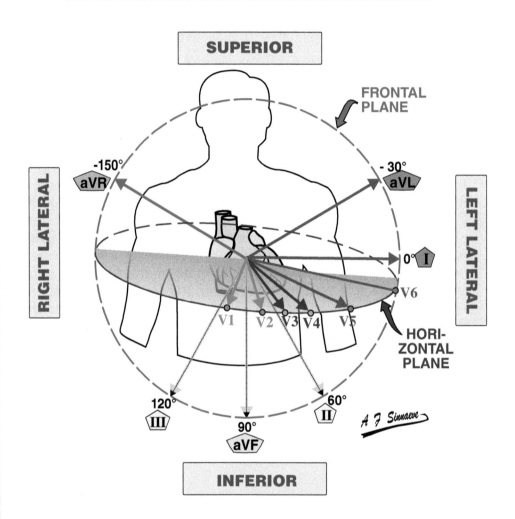

I High Lateral	aVR	V1 Anteroseptal	V4 Anterior
II Inferior	aVL High Lateral	V2 Anteroseptal	V5 Low Lateral
III Inferior	aVF Inferior	V3 Anterior	V6 Low Lateral

WHY DO WE NEED 12 LEADS?

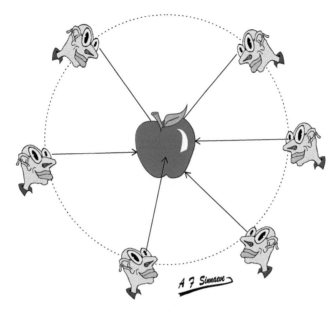

If you want to check the quality of an apple you have to look
for weak spots from many directions !
The same principle applies to the heart !

**The 12-lead ECG provides 12 different views of the electrical
activity of the heart, each view looking from the outside of
the chest toward the reference point within the heart.**

**Lead aVR is directed opposite to that of the other leads and is often
ignored ("the forgotten 12th lead").**

**Lead aVR does not view any single surface of the heart as do other
lead systems. Yet, aVR can be very helpful in diagnosing a number
of different entities. Inverted aVR (or minus aVR) can improve the
diagnosis of inferior and lateral myocardial infarction.**

The deflection on the ECG for a particular lead is proportional to the projection of the resulting heart vector upon that lead axis. The projection of the heart vector on a lead axis, and hence the deflection on the ECG, remains the same when the lead axis is shifted in parallel to its original direction. Therefore, all lead axes can be thought as going through the electrical center of the heart.

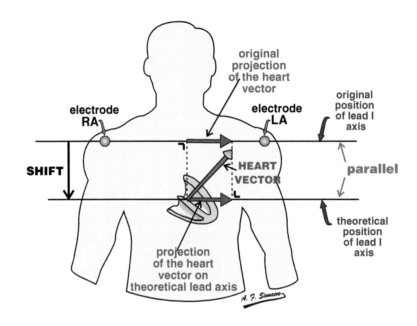

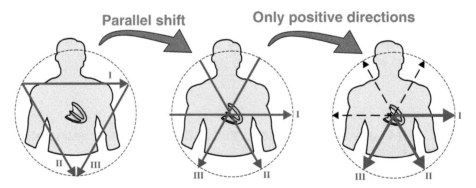

Parallel shift

Only positive directions

Lead I is chosen as the reference direction and (0°). The position of the other leads is expressed by the rotation (angle) from this reference. This rotation is positive in clockwise direction and negative in the counter-clockwise direction.

THE LIMB LEADS IN THE FRONTAL PLANE
(HEXAXIAL REFERENCE FIGURE)

EINTHOVEN

GOLDBERGER

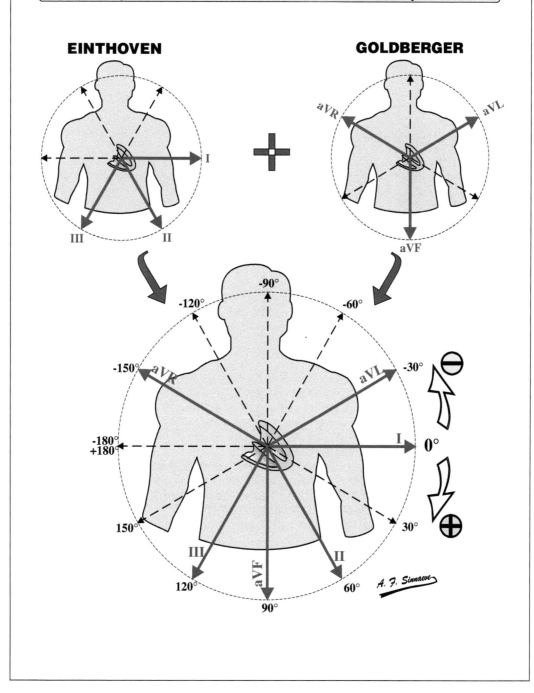

A. F. Sinnaeve

UNDERSTANDING THE HEXAXIAL DIAGRAM AND ITS IMPORTANCE

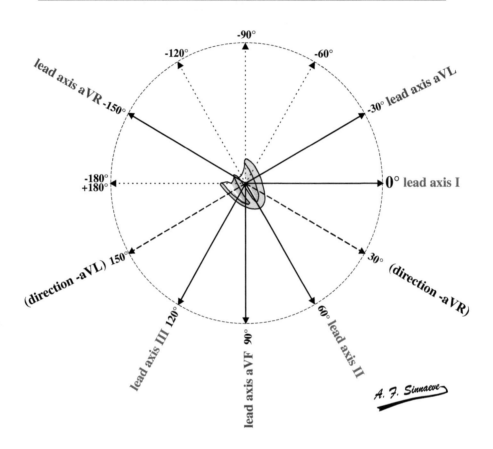

Advantages of the hexaxial diagram:
* Better understanding of the relationships of the various frontal plane leads and their recording sites of myocardial electrical activity. Leads II, III and aVF reflect the inferior surface of the heart, while leads I and aVL reflect the lateral part of the LV.
* Format for the determination and calculation of the mean frontal QRS axis (discussed later).
* Understanding the importance of minus aVR (–aVR)

Note: Lead minus aVL (–aVL) is not used in recording the standard ECG. It is useful in estimating the frontal plane axis and understanding the configuration of the QRS complex. Lead minus aVR (–aVR) is available in relatively few electrocardiographs. It may be used to identify a myocardial infarct (see further on).

A lead axis is selectable. An axis has only a direction and not a magnitude (or amplitude). **Therefore** axes cannot be vectors **and cannot be combined by the parallelogram rule.**

The leads **themselves** are real vector quantities **having magnitude and direction. They may be combined in the classical way.**

All frontal leads are orthogonal projections of the heart vector upon their specific axes (orthogonal means right angles or 90°). By combining these projections, the heart vector can be reconstructed in a continuously changing format. By doing so at many consecutive times a loop in the frontal plane is formed (i.e. the vectocardiogram).

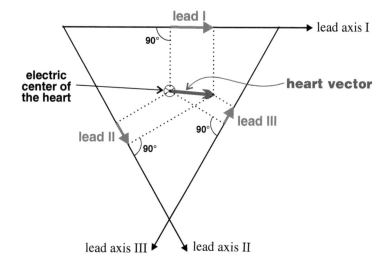

> **Just by looking at the hexaxial diagram with all 6 lead axes originating at the electrical center of the heart, it is quite clear that all frontal limb leads can be considered to function in the same way !**
> **However, it is obvious that they all look at the heart from different directions.**

Since the direction of all lead axes is known, every two leads may be combined by the computer in an ECG machine to find direction and magnitude of the heart vector. Consequently, the resulting heart vector can be decomposed to determine any other lead in the frontal plane. This gives only a good approximation since the human body is not homogeneous and Einthoven's triangle itself is an approximation.

COMMON ERRORS IN RECORDING THE ECG FROM PRECORDIAL LEADS

The precordial electrodes require careful positioning by palpating the bony structures of the chest. Common errors in placement of a chest electrode include:
1. Placing an electrode directly on a rib, rather than on an intercostal space.
2. Placing it on the wrong intercostal space.
3. Placing V1 or V2 directly on the sternum.
4. Placing V1 to the left of the sternum.
5. The right precordial electrodes V1 and V2 are often too high and too far apart.
6. The left precordial electrodes V4 to V6 are commonly placed both too low and too far towards the back for serial ECG recording.

Technicians are commonly trained to place the chest electrodes under the breast of women. The effect of breast tissue on the ECG is smaller than that of misplacement. Therefore it is recommended by some experts to place the electrodes on the breast rather than under the breast to facilitate the precision of electrode placement at the correct horizontal level and at the correct lateral positions. Others believe that there is insufficient evidence to support a switch from traditional sites beneath the left breast to record V4 to V6.

Errors in the placement of the chest electrodes do not influence the morphology of the QRS complex of the limb leads in the frontal plane.

An error in the placement of precordial leads may change the morphology of the ECG and result in inadequate or even wrong diagnosis.

In the example below, the P wave changes from its normal equiphasic appearance to monophasic positive if the electrodes are placed incorrectly too low or monophasic negative if they are placed too high:

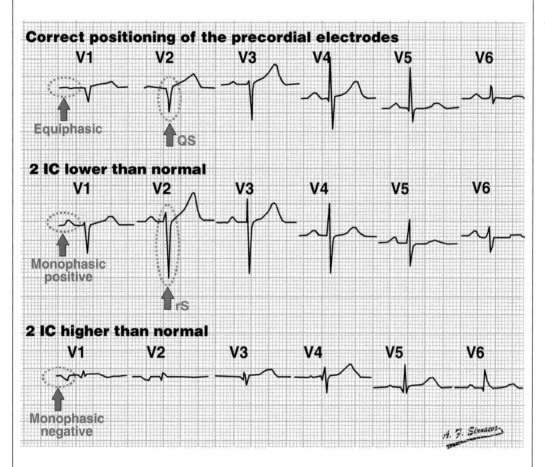

Correct positioning of the precordial electrodes

V1 V2 V3 V4 V5 V6

Equiphasic QS

2 IC lower than normal

V1 V2 V3 V4 V5 V6

Monophasic positive rS

2 IC higher than normal

V1 V2 V3 V4 V5 V6

Monophasic negative

The right precordial leads can be placed deliberately too low in order to make a differential diagnosis between left anterior hemiblock (LAH) and an old anteroseptal infarction.

In the example above, there is a QS pattern in V1 and V2.
If the precordial electrodes are placed 2 intercostal places lower the QS morhology changes to rS indicating LAH.
For an old anteroseptal infarction the QS would persist.

LEAD REVERSALS IN FRONTAL PLANE

Lead switches are a common mistake in ECG recording and can lead to wrong diagnoses. The most common mistake in electrode positioning is reversal of the right and the left arm leads, which occurs in about 3% of ECGs recorded in a hospital setting. Lead I becomes the mirror image of the true lead I so that all deflections (P wave, QRS complex and T wave) are inverted. Lead aVR shows reversed polarity with a positive P wave and QRS complex. Just looking at lead I makes the diagnosis.

Right and left arm lead reversal can be distinguished from the much rarer dextrocardia (where the heart is positioned on the right side) by examination of the precordial R wave progression. This progression is normal with arm lead reversal but is reversed with dextrocardia.

Transposition of the arm and leg electrodes is much less common but quite complex to evaluate, except reversal of the right leg lead with one of the arm leads. In this situation the reversal produces "pseudo-asystole" (a straight line) in either lead II or III because the potential between the two legs is zero. Lead II or III appears "collapsed" (very small voltage), but this sign occurs in only one lead. Consider the switch of the right arm (RA) and the right leg (RL) electrodes. Lead II records the potential difference between the left leg (LL) and RA electrodes (i.e. LL – RA). Now that RA becomes RL as the result of the switch, the electrocardiograph will record lead II with LL – RL which yields an essentially zero potential. The same argument applies to the left arm (LA) and RL switch. Lead III is LL – LA but as LA is now RL, lead III records the difference between LL and RL which is again essentially zero.

> **Always look at lead I to recognize arm lead reversal: P, QRS and T are all inverted.**
> **A straight line in leads II or III suggests arm lead and right leg reversal.**

RA/LA reversal

P, QRS, T negative
in lead I

Normal R wave
progression in
precordial leads

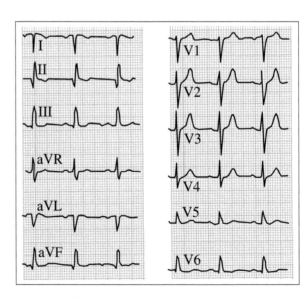

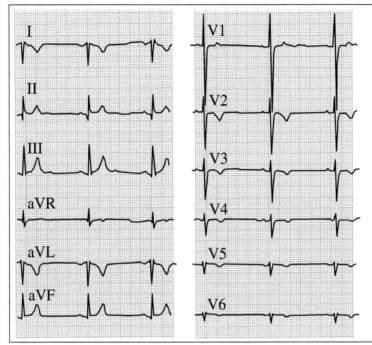

Dextrocardia

P, QRS, T negative
in lead I

Reversed R wave
progression in
precordial leads

LA/RL reversal

**Pseudo-asystole
in lead III**

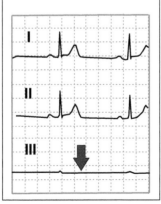

RA/RL reversal

**Pseudo-asystole
in lead II**

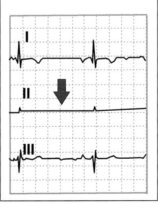

RA/RL and LA/LL reversal

**Zero potential
in lead I**

Both arm leads are on
the legs and both leg
leads are on the arms.

Lead I = LA − RA but
with reversal of arm
and leg electrodes
lead I now becomes
LL − RL = 0

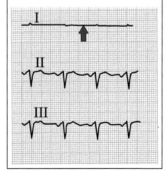

Braun K, Cohen AM. A comparison of unipolar leads obtained with the methods of Wilson and Goldberger. Br Heart J. 1952;14:462-4.

Burch GE. History of precordial leads in electrocardiography. Eur J Cardiol. 1978;8:207-36.

Goldberger E. Recent advances in the use of augmented unipolar extremity leads. Med Clin North Am. 1950;34:857-67.

Goldberger E. The relations of augmented unipolar extremity leads (aVL, aVR VF) to ordinary unipolar extremity leads (VL, VR, VF). Arch Inst Cardiol Mex. 1948;18:68-72.

Herrmann GR, Heitmancik MR, Kopeck JW. The superiority of the Wilson leads and the value of unipolar limb and precordial derivations in clinical electrocardiography. Am Heart J. 1950;40:680-95.

Wilson FN, Johnston FD, Rosenbaum FF, Barker PS. On Einthoven's triangle, the theory of unipolar electrocardiographic leads, and the interpretation of the precordial electrocardiogram. Am Heart J. 1946;32:277-310.

CHAPTER 3

THE NORMAL ECG
AND
THE FRONTAL PLANE
QRS AXIS

* The origin of the ECG – projection of the heart vector
* Neutral plane and hemisphere concept
* The origin of the ECG – normal QRS complex
* Normal QRS complex in the frontal plane
* Summary of the frontal plane for a normal heart
* Summary of the precordial plane for a normal heart
* Rotation of the heart
* Mean frontal plane electrical QRS axis
* Determination of the mean QRS axis in the frontal plane

ECG from Basics to Essentials: Step by Step. First Edition. Roland X. Stroobandt, S. Serge Barold and Alfons F. Sinnaeve.
Published 2016 © 2016 by John Wiley & Sons, Ltd. Companion Website: www.wiley.com/go/stroobandt/ecg

THE ORIGIN OF THE ECG

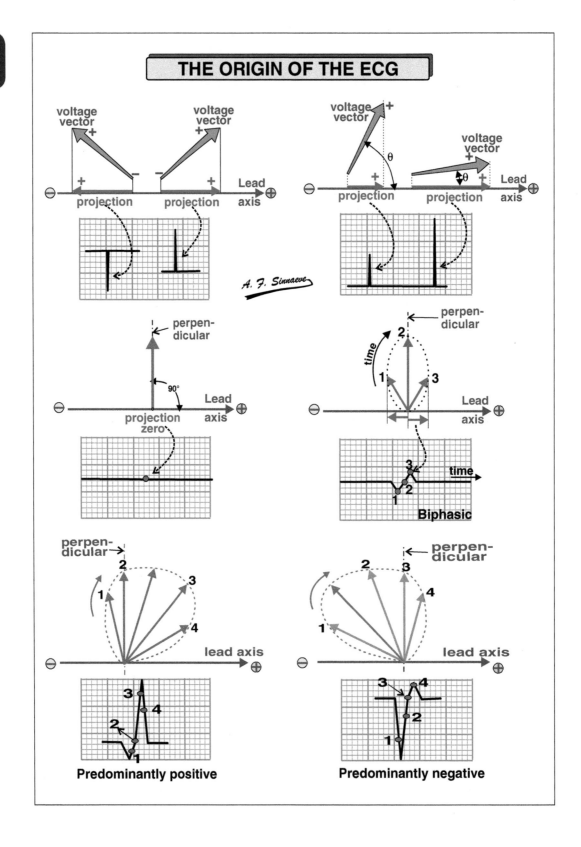

A. F. Sinnaeve

Biphasic

Predominantly positive

Predominantly negative

> The ECG records the electrical activity of the heart.
>
> Potential differences or voltages are created by depolarization and repolarization wavefronts in the heart.
>
> Voltages can be represented by vectors having a direction and a magnitude.
>
> The magnitude of the voltage vector is to a large extent determined by the amount of myocardium that depolarizes simultaneously. Therefore, the thick wall of the left ventricle is electrically dominant.
>
> The deflection on the ECG paper corresponds to the projection of the voltage vector on the lead axis.
>
> The lead axis refers to one of the traditional 12 leads or any special leads.

The deflection on the ECG will be positive if the projection of the voltage vector points to the positive pole of the lead axis. The deflection on the ECG will be negative if the projection of the voltage vector points to the negative pole of the lead axis.

The magnitude of the deflection on the ECG is determined by the angle between the voltage vector and the lead axis.

The resultant voltage vector of the heart is continuously changing during the heart cycle causing ECG deflections to vary with the passage of time. The tip of the resultant voltage vector describes a closed loop in space.

No deflection is produced when the resultant heart vector is perpendicular to the axis of a lead.

When the heart vector fluctuates at both sides of the perpendicular (partly pointing towards the positive pole and partly towards the negative pole) a *biphasic deflection* on the ECG is produced.
If the positive and negative deflections are equal in magnitude, an *equiphasic deflection* is present and the sum of the deflections is *zero*.

The perpendicular to an axis of a lead serves as a boundary between the predominantly positive and the predominantly negative deflections in any given lead.

NEUTRAL PLANE AND HEMISPHERE CONCEPT

No ECG deflection is produced when the resultant heart vector is perpendicular to the axis of a lead: the perpendicular to the lead axis is a *"neutral line"*, it is the boundary between the positive and the negative deflections for any given lead.

When the perpendicular to a lead axis is rotated around that lead axis, a neutral plane is created. Each heart vector lying in that plane is projected on the axis as a single point and does not generate a deflection on the ECG.

The neutral plane divides the space around the heart into two halves. The half along the positive side of the lead axis is the positive hemisphere. Any resultant heart vector in that hemisphere has a positive projection upon the lead axis and causes a positive deflection on the ECG.

Obviously, there is a positive hemisphere for each lead, i.e. six hemispheres for the frontal plane leads: aVL, I, II, aVF, III, aVR. The same concept also applies to the horizontal plane.

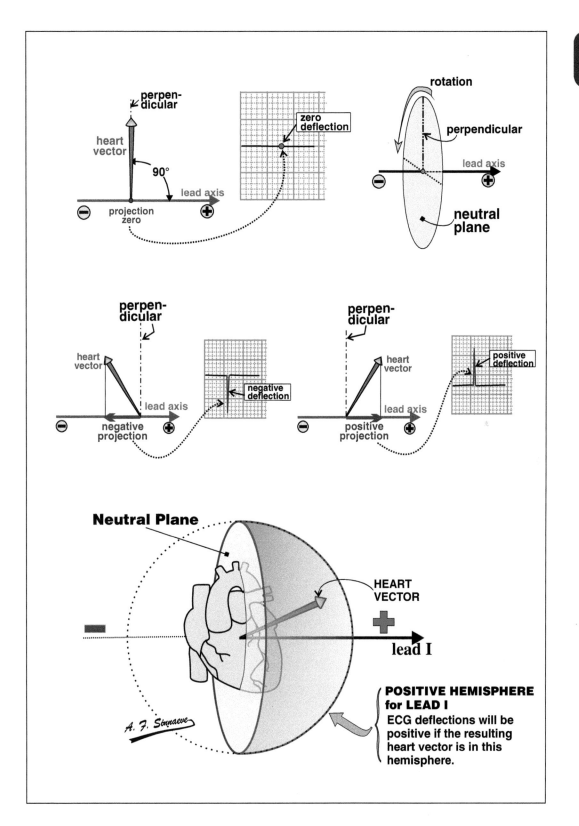

THE ORIGIN OF THE ECG

NORMAL QRS COMPLEX

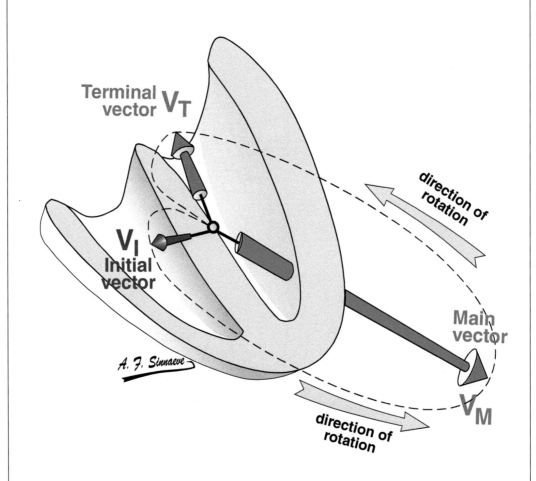

TO REMEMBER !

During the initial phase, depolarization takes place in the inter-ventricular septum, the paraseptal and anteroseptal zones of the left and right ventricles. The initial heart vector V_I is directed to the right, anteriorly and slightly superiorly or inferiorly.

During the main phase ventricular depolarization occurs in the anterolateral and slightly later in the posterolateral regions. The main heart vector V_M is directed to the left, posteriorly and inferiorly.

Ventricular depolarization ends in the posterobasal zone of the left ventricle, the upper part of the interventricular septum and finally the outflow tract of the right ventricle. The terminal heart vector V_T is directed backwards and upwards and may be directed to the left or to the right.a

NORMAL QRS COMPLEX
IN THE FRONTAL PLANE

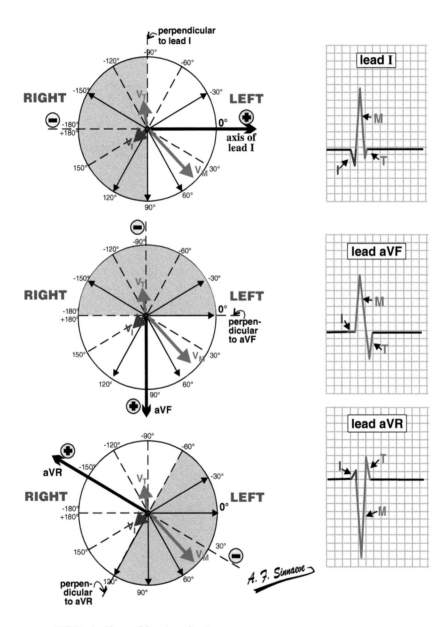

White half: positive hemisphere
Dark half: negative hemisphere

A. F. Sinnaeve

SUMMARY OF THE FRONTAL PLANE
FOR A NORMAL HEART

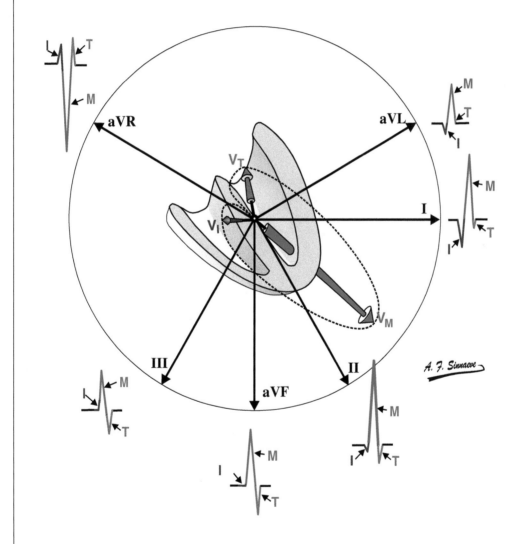

A. F. Sinnaeve

I = initial ; M = main ; T = terminal

SUMMARY OF THE PRECORDIAL PLANE FOR A NORMAL HEART

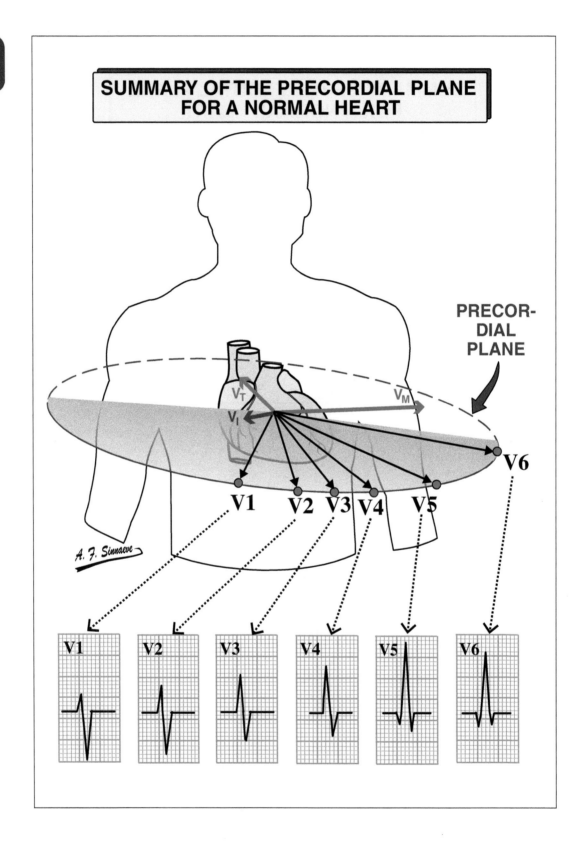

PRECOR-
DIAL
PLANE

A. F. Sinnaeve

In the normal ECG looking at the precordial leads, the r wave usually progresses from showing an rS complex in V1, with an increasing R and a decreasing S wave when moving towards the left side. There is usually a qR complex in V5 and V6 (the q wave reflecting septal activation) but the absence of q waves in V5 and V6 may be normal. The R wave amplitude is usually taller in V5 (and occasionally in V4) than in V6 because of the attenuating effect of the lungs. The transition zone is the lead with equal R and S wave voltage (i.e. R/S = 1) and occurs normally in V3 or V4. It may be normal to have the transition zone at V2 (called "early transition"), and at V5 (called "delayed transition"). It is normal to have a narrow QS or rSr' pattern in V1.

Normal progression in the precordial plane

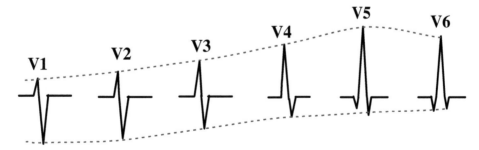

ROTATION OF THE HEART

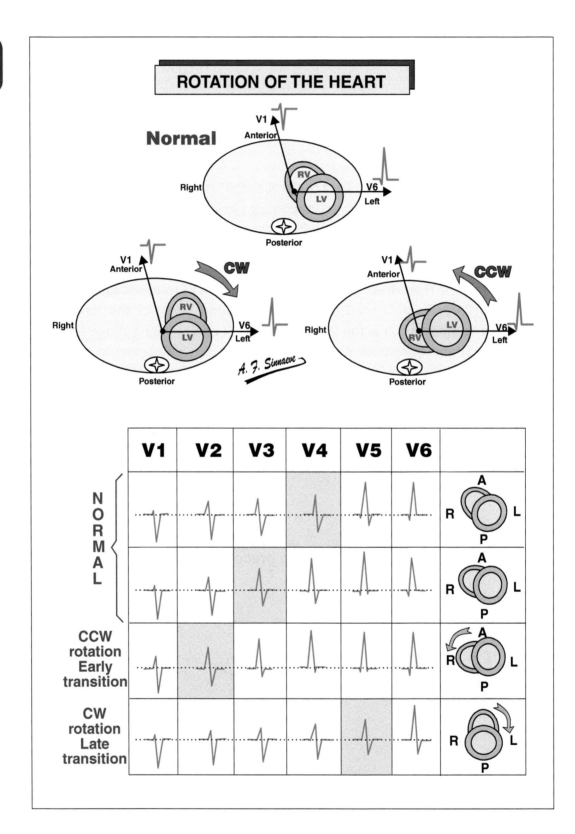

> **In cardiac rotation the heart is always visualized from under the diaphragm looking up. Hence, the anterior and posterior orientation of the body with its precordial leads is turned upside down.**

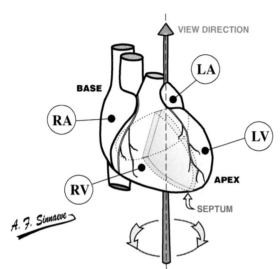

rotation possible in both directions

R WAVE PROGRESSION

In the normal ECG looking at the precordial leads, the r wave usually progresses from showing an rS complex in V1, with an increasing R and a decreasing S wave when moving towards the left side. There is usually an qR complex in V5 and V6 (the q wave reflecting septal activation) but the absence of q waves in V5 and V6 may be normal. The R wave amplitude is usually taller in V5 (and occasionally in V4) than in V6 because of the attenuating effect of the lungs. The transition zone is the lead with equal R and S wave voltage (R/S = 1) and occurs normally in V3 or V4. It may be normal to have the transition zone at V2 (called "early transition"), and at V5 (called "delayed transition"). It is normal to have a narrow QS or rSr' pattern in V1.

The definition of poor R wave progression in the literature varies considerably. A common definition relies on an R wave being less than 2-4 mm in leads V3 and V4. In addition it requires one or more of the following criteria: R in V4 < R in V3, R in V3 < R in V2, R in V2 < R in V1. If transition occurs at/or before V2 it is called CCW rotation. If it occurs after V4 it is called CW rotation. Poor R wave progression is also defined as a late transition seen in V5 or V6. In other words, poor R wave progression is present when the R wave height does not become progressively taller from leads V1 to V3 or V4, or even remains of low amplitude across the entire precordium. Poor R wave progression is abnormal but is not a diagnosis provided faulty ECG technique is ruled out, remembering that it can also be a normal variant.

MEAN FRONTAL PLANE ELECTRICAL QRS AXIS

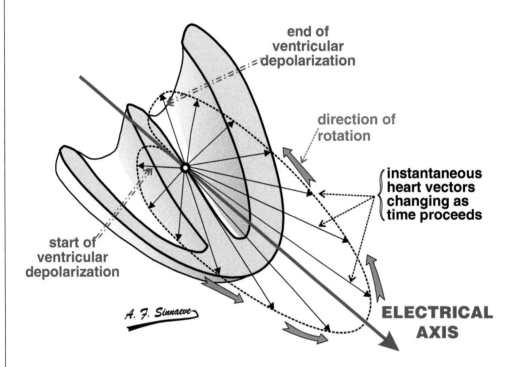

end of
ventricular
depolarization

direction of
rotation

instantaneous
heart vectors
changing as
time proceeds

start of
ventricular
depolarization

A. F. Sinnaeve

ELECTRICAL
AXIS

The **electrical QRS axis in the frontal plane** refers to the direction of a single vector representing the summation or mean of all the instantaneous frontal plane vectors generated by ventricular depolarization. It depicts the net overall direction of the electrical activity in the frontal plane. The mean frontal plane electrical QRS axis (abbreviated as "electrical axis") usually points to the left and inferiorly in the normal heart because of left ventricular dominance.

The mean QRS axis in the horizontal plane is rarely, if ever, used clinically. Determining the mean QRS axis in the horizontal plane may be useful for determining the origin of ventricular premature beats and ventricular tachycardias.

DETERMINATION OF THE MEAN QRS AXIS IN THE FRONTAL PLANE 1

 STEP 1 : LOOK AT LEADS I & aVF TO DETERMINE IN WHICH QUADRANT THE FRONTAL PLANE AXIS IS SITUATED

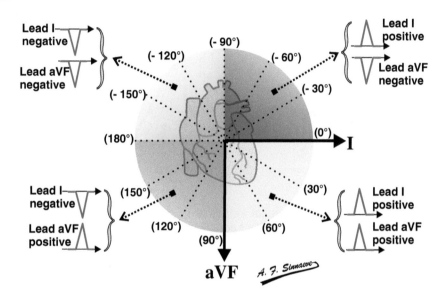

Leads I and aVF divide the thorax into 4 quadrants equal in size. Examine the direction of the QRS complex in leads I and aVF. The combination should place the electrical axis in one of the 4 quadrants of the hexaxial diagram.

1. If leads I and aVF are both upright, the axis is in the left inferior quadrant (yellow area). There is no point in going further to obtain the precise site of the mean axis as it is always normal in this quadrant.

2. If lead I is upright and lead aVF is downward, the axis is in the left superior quadrant (red area) where it may be normal or abnormal because the normal site extends from 90° to –30° moving in a counterclockwise fashion. The site of the axis can be more precisely determined by one step which involves looking at lead II (discussed later). The axis in this quadrant is called left superior axis deviation if it is more superior or more negative than –30°.

3. If lead I is downward and aVF is upright, the axis is in the right inferior quadrant (green area). It is simply called right axis deviation.

4. If both leads I and aVF are downwards, the axis is in the right superior quadrant (blue area). This quadrant has been described by a variety of names: no man's land, marked right axis deviation, marked left axis deviation, indeterminate axis, right shoulder axis and northwest quadrant. It is best called a right superior axis.

Another method related to the quadrant technique involves determining the frontal plane axis by seeking the QRS complex with the greatest amplitude. The axis is parallel to this lead (see step 2).

DETERMINATION OF THE MEAN QRS AXIS IN THE FRONTAL PLANE 2

 STEP 2 : LOOK IN THE APPROPRIATE QUADRANT FOR THE TALLEST R WAVE OR THE DEEPEST S WAVE

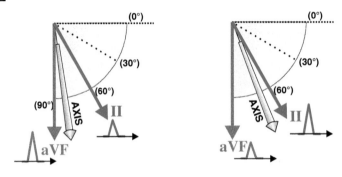

The lead nearest to (or parallel along) the QRS axis has the largest positive deflection. If two leads have equal positive deflections, the axis is exactly in the middle between these two leads.

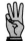 **STEP 3 : FIND THE LEAD WHICH IS PERPENDICULAR TO THE ELECTRICAL QRS AXIS**

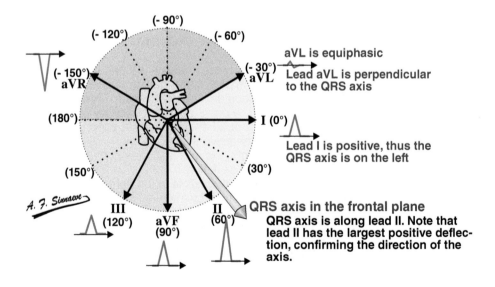

aVL is equiphasic
Lead aVL is perpendicular to the QRS axis

Lead I is positive, thus the QRS axis is on the left

QRS axis in the frontal plane
QRS axis is along lead II. Note that lead II has the largest positive deflection, confirming the direction of the axis.

A. F. Sinnaeve

The electrical QRS axis is perpendicular to the lead with an isoelectric (equiphasic) QRS complex or the lead with the smallest net amplitude (most equiphasic lead). Since there are two perpendicular directions to each isoelectric lead, choose the direction (positive or negative) that best fits to the adjacent leads.

This method can determine the axis within ± 10°–15°. If there is no isoelectric lead, there are usually *two* leads that are nearly isoelectric, and these are always 30° apart. Find the perpendiculars for each lead and choose an approximate QRS axis within the 30° range.

Occasionally each of the 6 frontal plane leads is small and/or isoelectric. The axis cannot be determined and is called indeterminate.

Normal & abnormal QRS axes of the heart

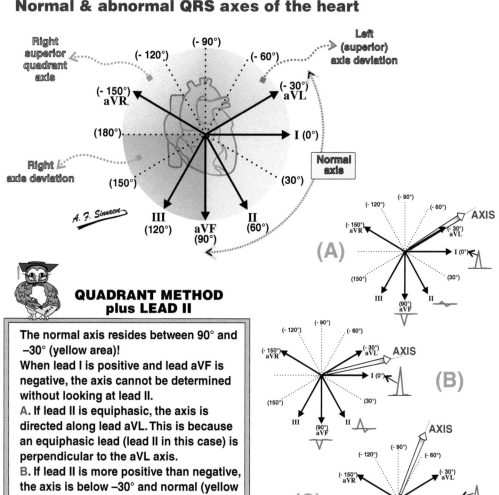

QUADRANT METHOD plus LEAD II

The normal axis resides between 90° and −30° (yellow area)!

When lead I is positive and lead aVF is negative, the axis cannot be determined without looking at lead II.

A. If lead II is equiphasic, the axis is directed along lead aVL. This is because an equiphasic lead (lead II in this case) is perpendicular to the aVL axis.

B. If lead II is more positive than negative, the axis is below −30° and normal (yellow area).

C. If lead II is more negative than positive, the axis is more negative than −30° and is in the left superior quadrant (red area).

MEAN QRS AXIS IN THE FRONTAL PLANE
EXAMPLES 1

lead I   lead II   lead III   lead aVR   lead aVL   lead aVF

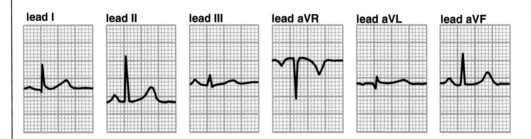

Normal electrogram
QRS axis at + 60°

I and aVF both positive: left inferior quadrant
tallest R wave in II: QRS axis is along II
most equiphasic in aVL: perpendicular to aVL

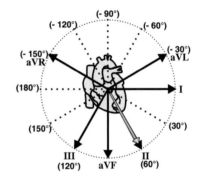

lead I   lead II   lead III   lead aVR   lead aVL   lead aVF

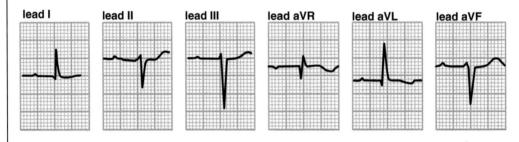

Left Axis Deviation (LAD)
QRS axis at − 60°

I positive; aVF negative: left superior quadrant
tallest S wave in III: QRS axis is along III
most equiphasic in aVR: perpendicular to aVR

A. F. Sinnaeve

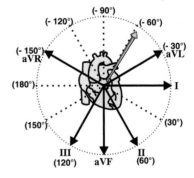

MEAN QRS AXIS IN THE FRONTAL PLANE
EXAMPLES 2

lead I	lead II	lead III	lead aVR	lead aVL	lead aVF

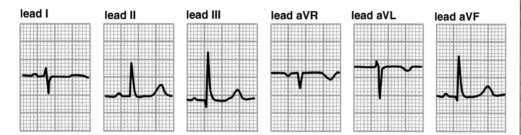

Right Axis Deviation (RAD)
QRS axis at about + 110°

aVF is + and lead I is –: QRS is in the right inferior quadrant
tallest R wave in III: QRS axis is close to III
lead III > aVF: axis near III

Note that the sum of R and S waves in lead I is negative which places the axis in the right inferior quadrant

A. F. Sinnaeve

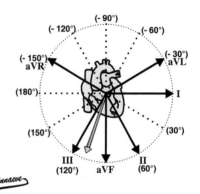

lead I	lead II	lead III	lead aVR	lead aVL	lead aVF

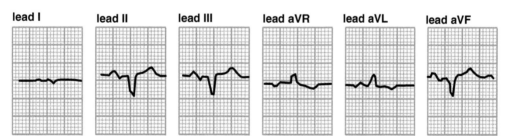

Right Superior Axis
QRS axis at about –100°

aVF is negative: QRS is oriented superiorly
most equiphasic in lead I: QRS axis is nearly perpendicular to lead I

Note that the largest QRS deflections are in leads II and aVF. Therefore the axis is diametrically opposite the line that bisects the angle between the lead II axis and the aVF axis.

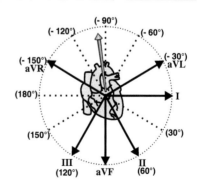

72 Further Reading

Burchell HB, Tuna N. The interpretation of gross left axis deviation in the electrocardiogram. Eur J Cardiol. 1979;10:259-77.

Pahlm US, O'Brien JE, Pettersson J, Pahlm O, White T, Maynard C, Wagner GS. Comparison of teaching the basic electrocardiographic concept of frontal plane QRS axis using the classical versus the orderly electrocardiogram limb lead displays. Am Heart J. 1997;134:1014-8.

Perloff JK, Roberts NK, Cabeen WR Jr. Left axis deviation: a reassessment. Circulation. 1979;60:12-21.

Prajapat L, Ariyarajah V, Spodick DH. Utility of the frontal plane QRS axis in identifying non-ST-elevation myocardial infarction in patients with poor R-wave progression. Am J Cardiol. 2009;104:190-3.

Spodick DH, Frisella M, Apiyassawat S. QRS axis validation in clinical electrocardiography. Am J Cardiol. 2008;101:268-9.

Stephen JM, Dhindsa H, Browne B, Barish R. Interpretation and clinical significance of the QRS axis of the electrocardiogram. J Emerg Med. 1990;18:757-63.

CHAPTER 4

THE COMPONENTS OF THE ECG WAVES AND INTERVALS

* What can be seen on the normal ECG – waves and complexes
* Intervals and segments
* The QT interval and the U wave
* T wave polarity and morphology
* The QRS complex – designation of special cases

ECG from Basics to Essentials: Step by Step. First Edition. Roland X. Stroobandt, S. Serge Barold and Alfons F. Sinnaeve.
Published 2016 © 2016 by John Wiley & Sons, Ltd. Companion Website: www.wiley.com/go/stroobandt/ecg

WHAT CAN BE SEEN ON THE NORMAL ECG

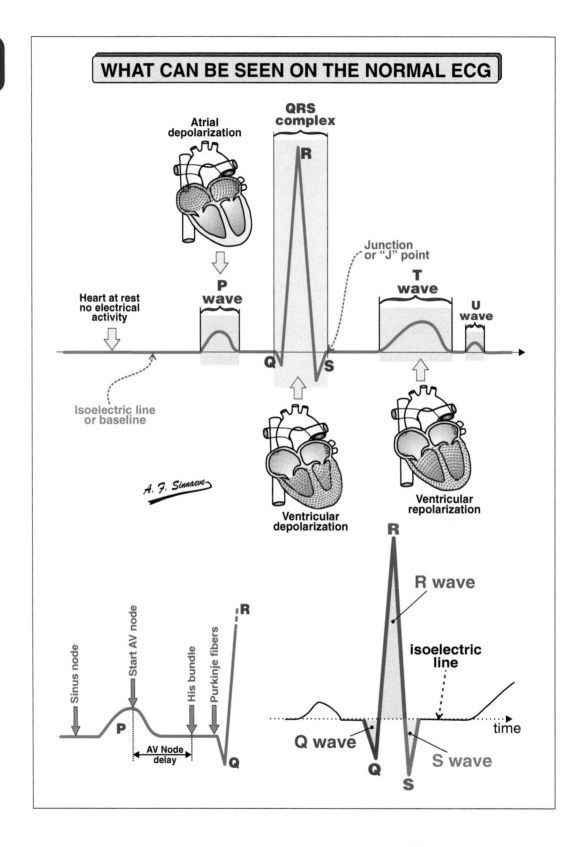

QRS complex

Atrial depolarization

R

Junction or "J" point

T wave

U wave

Heart at rest no electrical activity

P wave

Q S

Isoelectric line or baseline

A. F. Sinnaeve

Ventricular depolarization

Ventricular repolarization

Sinus node

Start AV node

His bundle

Purkinje fibers

R

P

Q

AV Node delay

R

R wave

isoelectric line

time

Q wave

Q

S wave

S

* Only electrical activity can be seen !
Mechanical action (contraction) is not registered by the ECG.

* Atrial repolarization is not seen in the ECG.

* The depolarization of sinus node, AV node, His bundle and bundle branches is not marked on the normal ECG because they do not contain sufficient cells to produce a voltage that can be measured on the skin of the body.

* An obvious U wave is seldom seen on a normal ECG.

> * The P wave represents the depolarization of both the right and left atria.

> * The QRS complex is the representation of ventricular depolarization.

> * The Q wave is the first downward deflection of the QRS complex and is followed by the upward R wave.

> * The R wave is the first upward deflection of the QRS complex and is followed by a downward S wave.

> * The S wave is the downward deflection preceded by an upward deflection.

> Note: differentiation between downward Q and S waves depends on whether the downward stroke occurs before or after the R wave.

> * The T wave represents the repolarization of both the right and left ventricles.

ABOUT INTERVALS AND SEGMENTS

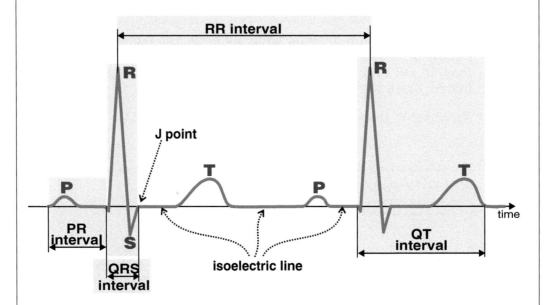

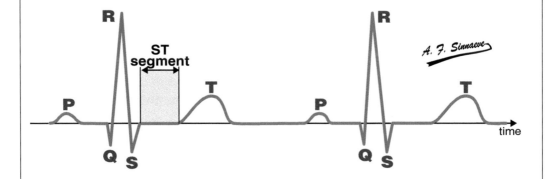

A. F. Sinnaeve

* **Intervals** are periods of time including waves and complexes. **Segments** are always measured between waves but never include them.

* The **baseline** or **isoelectric line** is a straight flat line seen when no electric activity of the heart is detected.

PR interval

The PR interval begins at the onset of the P wave and ends at the onset of the QRS complex. This interval represents the time taken by the cardiac impulse to reach the ventricles starting from the sinus node and high right atrium. It is called PR interval because the Q wave is frequently absent. Normal values are between 0.12 and 0.20 s ; prolongation defines 1st-degree atrioventricular block.

RR interval

The RR interval starts at the peak of one R wave to the peak of the next R wave and represents the time between two QRS complexes. This measure-ment is useful in calculating the heart rate.

QRS complex

The QRS complex represents the duration of ventricular depolarization. The short duration of the QRS complex indicates that ventricular depolarization normally occurs very rapidly (0.06 to 0.10 s). The QRS complex begins at the onset of the Q wave and ends at the endpoint of the S wave. The deflections are still termed QRS complexes even if one or more of the 3 waves (Q, R, S) are not visible. Hence the traditional use of the term RR interval to indicate the time between two QRS complexes regardless of their configurations.

The ventricles have a much larger muscle mass compared to the atria, causing the QRS complex to exhibit a much larger amplitude than the P wave. The amplitude of the QRS complex is increased secondary to a larger myo-cardial mass in left ventricular hypertrophy.

If the QRS complex is prolonged (> 0.1 s) conduction is impaired within the ventricles.

ST segment

The ST segment begins at the endpoint of the S wave and ends at the onset of the T wave, lasting 0.08 to 0.12 s. During the ST segment, the atria are relaxed and the ventricles are contracting but no electricity is noted. Electrical activity is not visible so that the ST segment is normally isoelectric but ST eleva-tion with a slight upward concavity may also be normal thereby complicating the diagnostic value of the ST segment.

The length of the ST segment shortens with increasing heart rate. A change from baseline producing ST segment depression or elevation occurs in pathological situations.

QT interval

The QT interval represents the duration from depolarization to repolarization of the ventricles. (See next page.)

THE QT INTERVAL

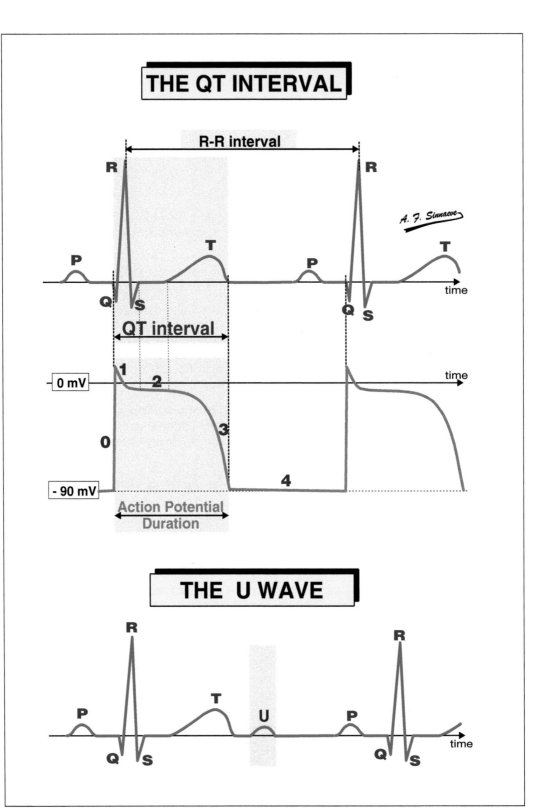

THE U WAVE

The QT interval represents the duration from depolarization to repolarization of the ventricles. It is measured from the beginning of the QRS complex to the end of the T wave. Therefore it roughly estimates the duration of an average ventricular action potential. Ventricular action potentials shorten in duration at faster rates which decrease the QT interval. The QT interval also varies according to gender (longer in females), and age (increases slightly with age). The QT interval can range from 0.2 to 0.4 s approximately depending upon the heart rate. Because prolonged QT intervals can indicate susceptibility to certain types of ventricular tachyarrhythmias and sudden death (see later), it is important to determine if a given QT interval is truly excessively long, especially in patients receiving drugs that lengthen the QT interval.

In practice, the QT interval is expressed as a "corrected QT interval" (QTc) by taking the QT interval (in s) and dividing it by the square root of the RR interval (in s). This is known as the Bazett formula:

$$\text{QTc (in s)} = \frac{\text{QT interval (in s)}}{\sqrt{\text{R-R interval (in s)}}}$$

The Bazett formula allows an assessment of the QT interval that is independent of heart rate. The normal corrected QTc is < 0.44 s in men and < 0.46 s in women. Easy to remember: at a heart rate of 60 bpm, the RR interval is 1 s and QTc = QT. The QT interval should be determined as the average value obtained from 3 to 5 cardiac cycles.

Modern ECG machines give the QTc. However, the machines are not always capable of making the correct determination of the end of the T wave. Therefore, it is important to check the QT time manually. The methodology of QT measure-ment has not been standardized!

The U wave is not always seen. It is typically low amplitude, and, by definition, follows the T wave. The U wave may be seen in some leads, especially the right precordial leads V2 to V4. U waves are associated with metabolic disturbances, typically hypokalemia. Additionally, it may be seen closely following the T wave and can make interpretation of the QT interval especially difficult.

T-WAVE POLARITY AND MORPHOLOGY

Depolarization
from endo- to epi-cardium

Purkinje fibers

direction of wavefront

R

equivalent dipole moving to epicardium

electrode

endocar-dium

epicar-dium

free wall

Repolarization
from epi- to endo-cardium

Purkinje fibers

direction of wavefront

T

equivalent dipole moving to endocardium

electrode

endocar-dium

epicar-dium

free wall

A. F. Sinnaeve

❀ ACTION POTENTIAL of myocardial cells

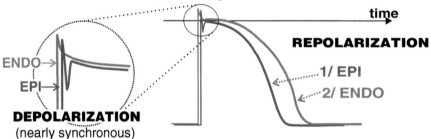

time

REPOLARIZATION

ENDO→

EPI→

1/ EPI

2/ ENDO

DEPOLARIZATION
(nearly synchronous)

(A notch is seen only in epicardial action potentials)

❀ SPREAD OF WAVEFRONTS in myocardial tissue

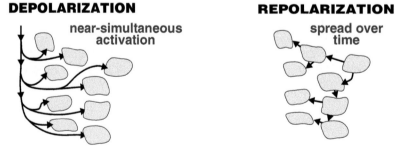

DEPOLARIZATION
near-simultaneous activation

REPOLARIZATION
spread over time

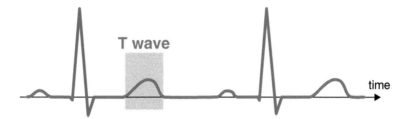

> * **The T wave represents the repolarization of the ventricles and roughly corresponds to phase 3 of the action potential of an average myocardial cell.**
> * **The T wave is broader and not as large as the R wave because ventricular repolarization is less synchronous than depolarization.**

The T wave is the most variable wave in the ECG. T wave changes including low-amplitude T waves and abnormally inverted T waves may be the result of many cardiac and non-cardiac conditions. The normal T wave is usually in the same direction as the QRS except in the right precordial leads. In the normal ECG the T wave is always upright in leads I, II, V3 to V6, and always inverted in lead aVR. The other leads are variable depending on the direction of the QRS and the age of the patient. The shape of the T wave is normally rounded and smooth. Also, the normal T wave is asymmetric with the first half moving more slowly than the second half.

The action potential duration in epicardial cells is shorter than in endocardial cells. Hence, the repolarization starts in the tissue that was depolarized last. Repolarization occurs from epicardum towards endocardium, i.e. opposite to the direction of depolarization. However, the voltage vector (the +/– dipole) is still pointing to the epicardium and towards the recording electrode and again causes a positive deflection (T wave) on the ECG. The heterogeneity of ventricular repolarization is in large part due to the presence of M cells constituting 30% to 40% of the mid-myocardium between the endocardial and epicardial layers of the heart. The hallmark of the M cells is their different electrophysiologic properties that pro-long their action potential duration even beyond those of epicardial and endocardial cells. Full repolarization of the epicardial cells coincides with the peak of the T wave and repolarization of the M cells corresponds to the end of the T wave.

Repolarization takes longer and is more diffuse than depolarization because the process spreads from cell to cell so that the T wave has a lower amplitude and a longer duration than the QRS complex.

THE QRS COMPLEX
Designation of special cases

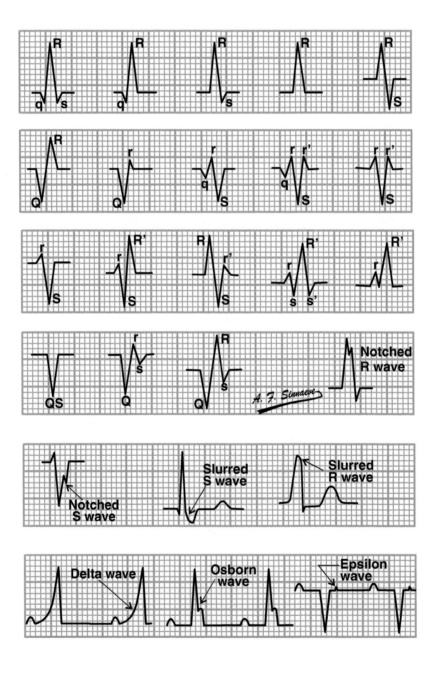

The waves composing the QRS complex are usually identified by upper or lower case letters depending on the relative size of the waves. The large waves that form the major deflections are identified by upper case letters (Q, R, S, QS). The smaller waves that are less than one-half the amplitude of the major deflections are identified by lower case letters (q, r, s). Thus, the ventricular depolarization complex can be accurately described by using combinations of upper and lower case letters (qrS, rS, Qrs, ...).

A QS wave is a QRS complex that consists entirely of a single large negative deflection.
A QS complex should not be called or equated to a Q or q wave especially when comparing the significance of a QS complex with one showing a qR, QR or Qr configuration.

More than one deflection in the same direction
Altough there may be only one Q wave, there can be more than one R wave and S wave in the QRS complex. A second upward or downward deflection is indicated by an accent (R' = R prime or S' = S prime). A rare subsequent deflection may be indicated by a double accent (e.g. R'' = R double prime).

Concordance
Positive or negative concordance indicates that the QRS complex in all 6 precordial leads has the same polarity. The 6 leads are either all positive or all negative.

Notches
A notch is a change in direction of the QRS complex and may involve the Q, R and S waves. A notch does not cross the baseline (causes and clinical significance will be discussed later).

Slurring
Slurring reflects a change in the rate of rise or fall of a wave within the QRS complex.

Delta wave
The slow and slurred upstroke of the QRS complex is called a "delta wave" because of its resemblance to the Greek capital letter delta (symbol Δ). Delta waves are due to premature ventricular excitation caused by an accessory pathway between atrium and ventricle (discussed later : WPW syndrome and preexcitation). The delta wave is a form of slurring of the initial portion of the QRS complex.

Osborn wave
When the J point is exaggerated and the downward deflection resembles the letter "h", the QRS complex displays an Osborn wave (named after Osborn who described the association of this wave with hypothermia). Osborn waves also occur in hypercalcemia (discussed later).

Epsilon wave
Epsilon waves are often seen in patients with right ventricular dysplasia. The waves are best seen as small wiggles in the ST segment of leads V1 and V2. They are caused by late excitation of myocytes in the right ventricle and constitute post-excitation.

Isbister GK, Page CB. Drug induced QT prolongation: the measurement and assessment of the QT interval in clinical practice. Br J Clin Pharmacol. 2013;76:48-57.

Johnson JN, Ackerman MJ. QTc: how long is too long? Br J Sports Med. 2009;43:657-62.

Malik M. Errors and misconceptions in ECG measurement used for the detection of drug induced QT interval prolongation. J Electrocardiol. 2004;37 Suppl:25-33.

Postema PG, Wilde AA. The measurement of the QT interval. Curr Cardiol Rev. 2014;10:287-94.

Surawicz B. U wave: facts, hypotheses, misconceptions, and misnomers. J Cardiovasc Electrophysiol. 1998;9:1117-28.

Surawicz B, Macfarlane PW. Inappropriate and confusing electrocardiographic terms: J-wave syndromes and early repolarization. J Am Coll Cardiol. 2011;57:1584-6.

Zareba W, Cygankiewicz I. Long QT syndrome and short QT syndrome. Prog Cardiovasc Dis. 2008;51:264-78.

CHAPTER 5

P WAVES AND ATRIAL ABNORMALITIES

* Topographical anatomy of the heart
* The normal P wave in the frontal plane
* The normal P wave in the horizontal plane
* Left atrial abnormality
* Right atrial abnormalitiy
* Biatrial abnormality

ECG from Basics to Essentials: Step by Step. First Edition. Roland X. Stroobandt, S. Serge Barold and Alfons F. Sinnaeve.
Published 2016 © 2016 by John Wiley & Sons, Ltd. Companion Website: www.wiley.com/go/stroobandt/ecg

TOPOGRAPHICAL ANATOMY OF THE HEART

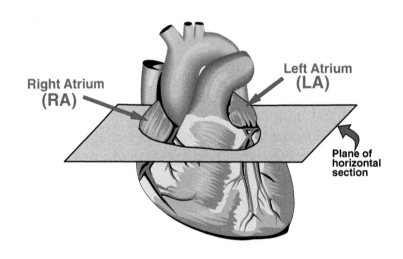

Right Atrium
(RA)

Left Atrium
(LA)

Plane of
horizontal
section

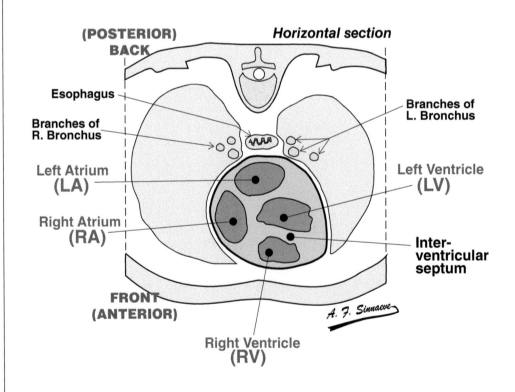

Horizontal section

(POSTERIOR)
BACK

Esophagus

Branches of
R. Bronchus

Branches of
L. Bronchus

Left Atrium
(LA)

Left Ventricle
(LV)

Right Atrium
(RA)

Inter-
ventricular
septum

FRONT
(ANTERIOR)

A. F. Sinnaeve

Right Ventricle
(RV)

Due to rotation of the heart along its long axis the right heart is located anteriorly with regard to the left heart. The right atrium (RA) is located to the right, while the right ventricle (RV) is the most anteriorly located structure. The left ventricle (LV) lies behind the RV and points towards the left. The LV is situated mostly in the anterior part of the chest. The left atrium (LA) is the most posteriorly (dorsally) located heart chamber. The wall thickness of a cardiac chamber reflects the amount of muscle tissue needed to produce its level of pressure. Therefore a cross-section of the chambers shows that the atrial walls and the interatrial septum (wall) are relatively thin. The right ventricular wall is much thicker. The left ventricular wall is again several times thicker than that of the right. The increased thickness of the left ventricle enables it to generate the high pressure required for the systemic circulation. In contrast, the right ventricle is a low pressure system sustaining the pulmonary arterial circulation. The ventricular septum separates the two ventricles. It is mostly muscular but partly membranous in its superior portion. The septum is directed obliquely backward and to the right, and is curved with the convexity toward the right ventricle.
Note: The anatomic heart axis differs from the electrical axis.

THE NORMAL P WVE 1

THE FRONTAL PLANE

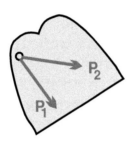

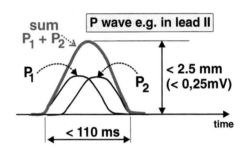

P wave e.g. in lead II

sum
$P_1 + P_2$

P_1

P_2

< 2.5 mm
(< 0,25mV)

< 110 ms

time

What is the sum $P_1 + P_2$?

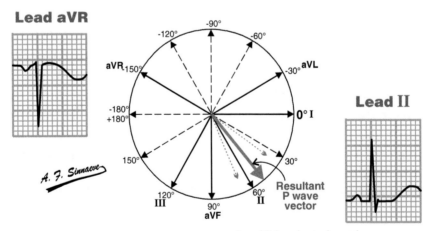

$P_1 + P_2$ P_1 P_2 $P_1 + P_2$ P_1 P_2

Lead aVR

Lead II

-90°
-120°   -60°
aVR -150°   -30° aVL
-180°
+180°   0° I
150°   30°
120°   60°
III   II
90°
aVF

Resultant
P wave
vector

A. F. Sinnaeve

Lead II is oriented nearly
parallel to atrial activation

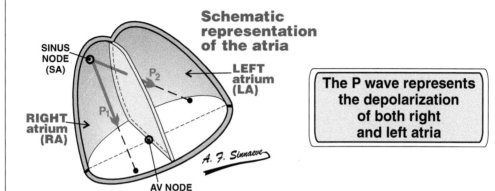

Schematic representation of the atria

SINUS NODE (SA)

LEFT atrium (LA)

RIGHT atrium (RA)

P₂

P₁

AV NODE

A. F. Sinnaeve

> **The P wave represents the depolarization of both right and left atria**

☆ The sinoatrial node is situated near the top of the right atrium near the inlet of the superior vena cava.

☆ Atrial depolarization starts at the sinus node and progresses from right to left.

✳ The right atrium depolarizes first and the wave front (P1) travels from the top (superior) to the bottom (inferior).

✳ Electrical activation is transmitted from the sinoatrial node to the high left atrium via Bachmann's bundle which serves as the only atrial specialized conduction system or tract conducting electrical activity to the high left atrium. This arrangement causes a slight delay in left atrial compared to right atrial depolarization as the activation then travels to the left and posteriorly (P2). This delay causes continuing left atrial depolarization after right atrial depolarization has finished.

Since activation starts at the sinus node, the P wave is always negative in lead aVR during normal sinus rhythm. The P wave vector is directed towards lead II and hence the P wave is always positive in lead II during sinus rhythm.

The mean frontal plane axis of the P wave is between 0° and 75°. It is usually between 45° and 60°. The axis of the P wave is usually the first measurement in ECG interpretation to determine whether normal sinus rhythm is present. An abnormal P wave axis may suggest the presence of a non-sinus rhythm, dextrocardia or reversal of the ECG limb leads. The normal P wave has a smooth contour and is never peaked or pointed.

THE NORMAL P WAVE 2

THE HORIZONTAL PLANE

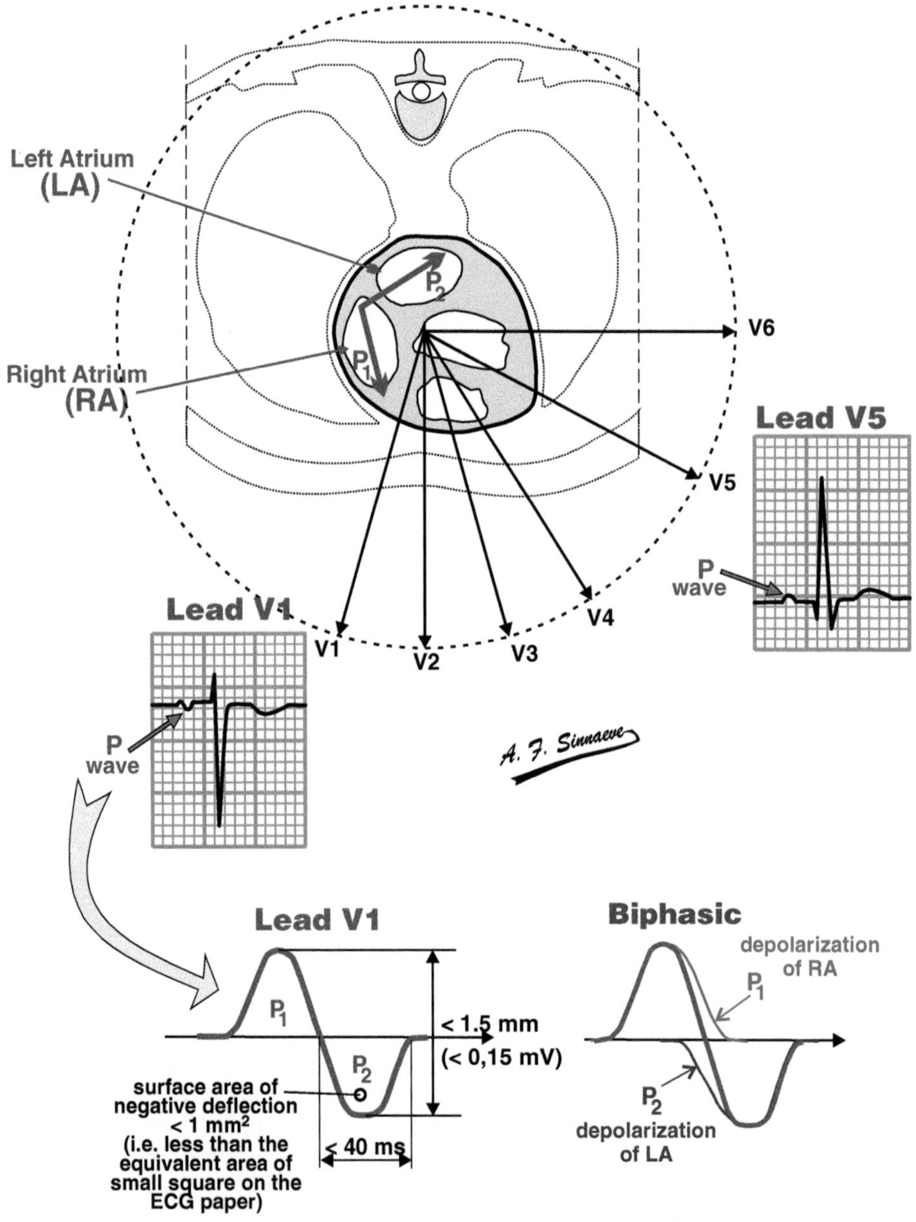

Left Atrium (LA)

Right Atrium (RA)

P_2

P_1

V6

V5

V4

V3

V2

V1

Lead V5

P wave

Lead V1

P wave

A. F. Sinnaeve

Lead V1

P_1

P_2

< 1.5 mm
(< 0,15 mV)

surface area of negative deflection
< 1 mm² (i.e. less than the equivalent area of small square on the ECG paper)

≤ 40 ms

Biphasic

depolarization of RA

P_1

P_2

depolarization of LA

The best two leads to examine the P wave are leads II and V1 as they look at the atria in opposite directions (lead II looks along the axis of the atria, while V1 looks across the atria).

Lead V1 allows the easy separation of the two components of atrial depolarization.

The P wave consists of two components: the depolarization of the right atrium (P1) and the depolarization of the left atrium (P2). The first part of the P wave is positive in lead V1 as the depolarization vector of the RA is directed towards lead V1 which is oriented to the right and anteriorly. The terminal part of the P wave is negative in V1 as the depolarization vector of the left atrium (P2) is directed towards the left and posteriorly (i.e. in the opposite direction of lead V1). Thus, the P wave in lead V1 is often biphasic as the mean P wave vector travels perpendicular to the axis of lead V1.

Atrial depolarization generates a positive deflection in the leads that look at the heart from below (frontal plane). The chest leads (apart from V1) do not detect atrial depolarization well because atrial depolarization is downwards (i.e. inferiorly). As five of the six (excluding V1) chest leads are mostly on the left side of the body and approximately at the same level in the horizontal plane, the P wave will not exhibit the P wave variations typical of the frontal plane leads. There will generally not be much difference in the P wave in these leads with small positive deflections seen in each. Lead V1 with its different view on the heart looks at the atrial depolarization passing across its axis.

LEFT ATRIAL ABNORMALITY

> **Look at leads where the P wave is most prominent: usually lead II, but also leads III and aVF, and V1.**

The P wave becomes broadened (P wave duration ≥ 0.11 s) because of prolonged total atrial activation time. P wave amplitude generally remains unchanged. The P wave may be notched, or double-peaked (M shape pattern) with an interpeak interval ≥ 0.04 s due to the delay in left atrial activity which also causes wider separation of right and left atrial depolarization. These features are best seen in lead II. The left atrial vector may increase toward the left and become more pronounced, resulting in a negative terminal deflection of the P wave in leads III and aVF. Leads V1 and V2 may show a deeply inverted or negative portion of the P wave reflecting left atrial activation directed posteriorly. The terminal inverted P wave in V1 should be ≥ 1 mm in depth and ≥ 1 mm (0.04 s) in duration. The product of amplitude and duration should have an area greater than that of the initial upright portion of the P wave (reflecting right atrial activation which is directed anteriorly) or greater than the area of a small square on the ECG paper.

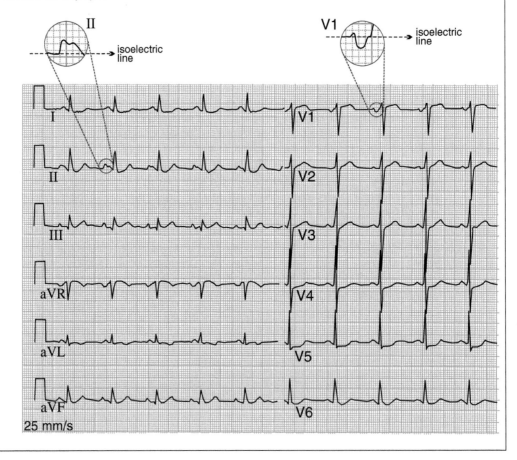

LEFT ATRIAL ABNORMALITY

"Atrial abnormality" (or delay of left atrial activation) is a term being used increasingly in place of "atrial enlargement", "atrial dilatation", "atrial distention", "atrial hypertrophy", "atrial overload", and "P mitrale" or even in the presence of atrial conduction delay.

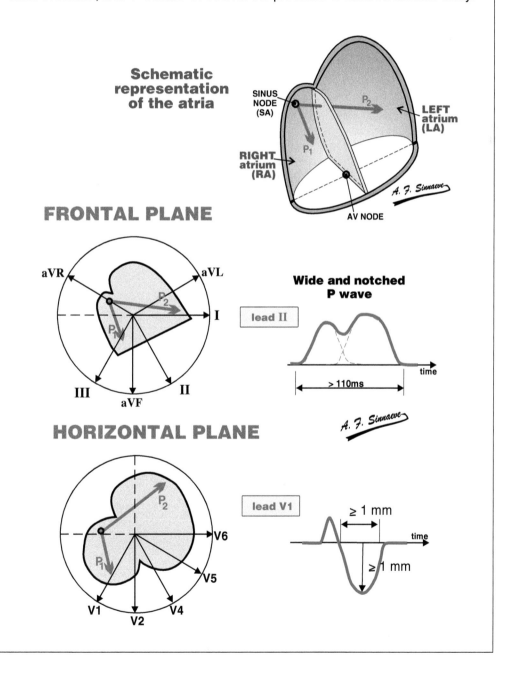

Schematic representation of the atria

SINUS NODE (SA)

P₂

LEFT atrium (LA)

P₁

RIGHT atrium (RA)

AV NODE

A. F. Sinnaeve

FRONTAL PLANE

aVR   aVL

P₂

I

P₁

III   aVF   II

Wide and notched P wave

lead II

> 110ms

time

A. F. Sinnaeve

HORIZONTAL PLANE

P₂

V6

P₁

V5

V1   V2   V4

lead V1

≥ 1 mm

time

≥ 1 mm

RIGHT ATRIAL ABNORMALITY

> **Left atrial abnormality causes wider P waves with no significant change in amplitude.**
> **RA abnormality does not cause a significant change in P wave duration (though the P waves appear somewhat more narrow) but it increases the P wave amplitude.**

Right atrial (RA) abnormality refers to delayed activation of the right atrium as a result of dilatation, hypertrophy, scarring or a conduction abnormality. RA abnormality is also known as P pulmonale because it is often the result of severe lung disease. An RA abnormality is reflected in the early portion of the P wave.

RA abnormality leads to simultaneous activation of the two atria resulting in relatively narrow tall pointed and peaked P waves which are increased in amplitude (> 2.5 mm in leads II, III and aVF). This reflects the summation of the enhanced RA component with the left atrial component.

In leads V1 and V2 the positive part of a biphasic P wave may display prominent positivity and be > 1.5 mm which is larger than the negative component.

The P wave axis in the frontal plane is deviated to 75° or greater. Therefore the tallest P wave may be seen in lead III rather than lead II.

> **The criteria for the diagnosis of RA abnormality are not specific nor sensitive**

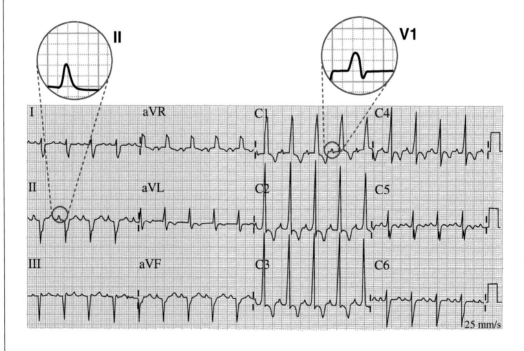

RIGHT ATRIAL ABNORMALITY

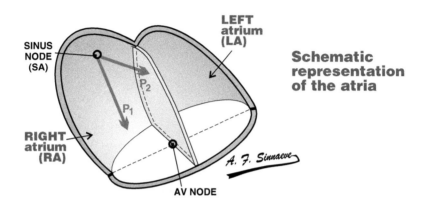

SINUS NODE (SA)

LEFT atrium (LA)

RIGHT atrium (RA)

P₂

P₁

AV NODE

Schematic representation of the atria

A. F. Sinnaeve

FRONTAL PLANE

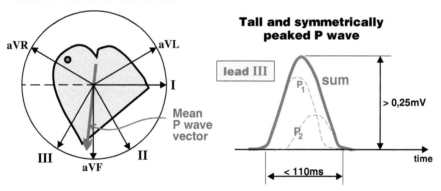

aVR

aVL

I

III

aVF

II

Mean P wave vector

Tall and symmetrically peaked P wave

lead III

P₁

sum

P₂

> 0,25mV

< 110ms

time

HORIZONTAL PLANE

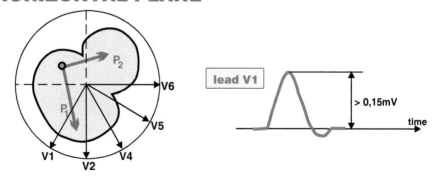

P₂

V6

V5

V4

V2

V1

P₁

lead V1

> 0,15mV

time

BIATRIAL ABNORMALITY

Biatrial or combined atrial abnormality demonstrates essentially some of the features of both RA and LA abnormalities. The P wave in lead II is > 2.5 mm and > 0.12 s in duration. The initial positive component of the P wave in lead V1 is > 1.5 mm tall and the terminal portion of the P wave is prominent with a negative amplitude > 1 mm. Little evidence is available regarding the accuracy of the ECG in combined atrial abnormality.

INTERATRIAL CONDUCTION DELAY

The Bachmann Bundle (interatrial bundle) plays a fundamental role in interatrial conduction as the preferential interatrial connection which ensures rapid inter-atrial conduction leading to physiologic near-simultaneous right and left atrial contraction. Delay in this pathway causes an interatrial conduction delay (IACD) manifested by the typical ECG pattern of left atrial abnormality but not all the features may be present. Typically there is widening of the P wave with one or two notches. The ECG configuration is not surprising because the general features of left atrial abnormality from a variety of causes are more dependent on IACD than on actual atrial dilatation.

Isolated IACD due to atrial fibrosis or scarring is a diagnosis of exclusion and should be suspected when there is no clinical suspicion or evidence of left atrial enlargement. The situation is compounded by the fact that primary IACD may be associated with left atrial enlargement as a result of the conduction disorder itself. Furthermore, an ECG pattern of left atrial abnormality may be produced by primary left atrial enlargement. IACD is not uncommun in patients with sick sinus syndrome and is a precursor to atrial fibrillation. For patients undergoing dual chamber pacemaker implantation, measurement of the electrocardiographic P wave duration is essential. IACD may cause significant left atrial electromechanical dysfunction which may necessitate placement of an atrial pace-maker lead at a site other than the traditional right atrial appendage.

BIATRIAL ABNORMALITY

Leads II, III or aVF

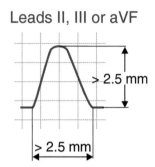

> 2.5 mm

> 2.5 mm

Lead V1

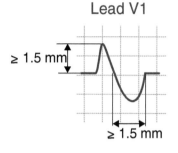

≥ 1.5 mm

≥ 1.5 mm

INTERATRIAL CONDUCTION DELAY

Diagrammatic representation of interatrial conduction delay due to a lesion in Bachmann's bundle

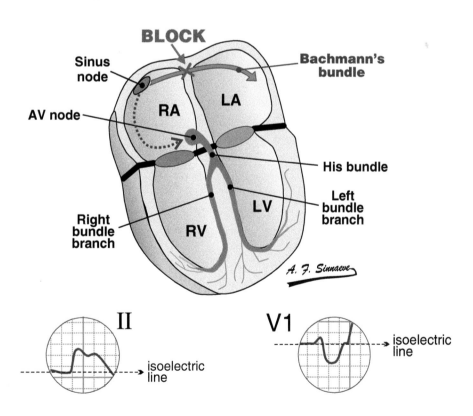

BLOCK

Sinus node

Bachmann's bundle

AV node

RA

LA

His bundle

Right bundle branch

RV

LV

Left bundle branch

A. F. Sinnaeve

II

isoelectric line

V1

isoelectric line

Further Reading

Heikkilä J, Hugenholtz PG, Tabakin BS. Prediction of left heart filling pressure and its sequential change in acute myocardial infarction from the terminal force of the P wave. Br Heart J. 1973;35:142–51.

Kitkungvan D, Spodick DH. Interatrial block: is it time for more attention? J Electrocardiol. 2009;42:687-92.

Michelucci A, Bagliani G, Colella A, Pieragnoli P, Porciani MC, Gensini G, Padeletti L. P wave assessment: state of the art update. Card Electrophysiol Rev. 2002;6:215-20.

Platonov PG. Atrial conduction and atrial fibrillation: what can we learn from surface ECG? Cardiol J. 2008;15:402-7.

Platonov PG. P-wave morphology: underlying mechanisms and clinical implications. Ann Noninvasive Electrocardiol. 2012;17:161-9.

Tereshchenko LG, Shah AJ, Li Y, Soliman EZ. Electrocardiographic deep terminal negativity of the P wave in V1 and Risk of Mortality: The National Health and Nutrition Examination Survey III. J Cardiovasc Electrophysiol. 2014;25:1242-8.

CHAPTER 6

CHAMBER ENLARGEMENT AND HYPERTROPHY

* Left ventricular hypertrophy
* Right ventricular hypertrophy

ECG from Basics to Essentials: Step by Step. First Edition. Roland X. Stroobandt, S. Serge Barold and Alfons F. Sinnaeve.
Published 2016 © 2016 by John Wiley & Sons, Ltd. Companion Website: www.wiley.com/go/stroobandt/ecg

LEFT VENTRICULAR HYPERTROPHY

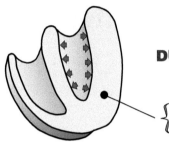

LEFT VENTRICULAR HYPERTROPHY DUE TO SYSTOLIC OVERLOAD

{ The left ventricular wall is much thicker than normal

SOME CRITERIA TO DIAGNOSE LEFT VENTRICULAR HYPERTROPHY

① In the horizontal plane
(Sokolow index)
S + R ⩾ 35 mm

V1 or V2   **V5 or V6**

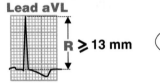 +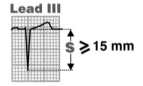

② In the frontal plane
(for a horizontal heart axis)

Lead aVL

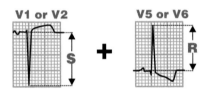

R ⩾ 11 mm

In the frontal plane (if left axis deviation)

Lead aVL   **Lead III**

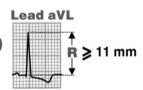 **R ⩾ 13 mm**   (AND)   **S ⩾ 15 mm**

③ In the frontal plane   **(R in I) + (S in III) > 25 mm**

Lead I   **Lead III**

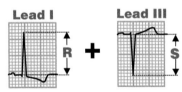 +

R   **S**

Lead V6

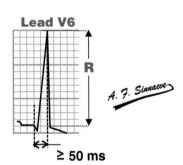

R

A. F. Sinnaeve

④ Delayed intrinsicoid deflection
(Time from QRS onset to peak R is ⩾ 50 ms)

⩾ 50 ms

> **Left ventricular hypertrophy (LVH) refers to an increase in the size of myocardial fibers. Such hypertrophy is usually the response to a chronic volume or pressure overload.**
> *** The two most important pressure overload states are systemic hypertension and aortic stenosis.**
> *** The major conditions associated with LV volume overload are aortic or mitral valve regurgitation and dilated cardiomyopathy.**

Hypertrophic cardiomyopathy is an example of an inherited condition in which LVH (usually with asymmetric septal hypertrophy) occurs in the absence of any apparent hemodynamic pressure or volume overload unless there is LV outflow tract obstruction.

A physiologic type of hypertrophy with increase in wall thickness and diastolic volume overload may occur in trained athletes. The "athletic heart" is often associated with ECG voltage criteria for LVH.

The electrocardiogram is a useful but imperfect tool for detecting LVH. The utility of the ECG relates to its being relatively inexpensive and widely available. The limitations of the ECG relate to its poor sensitivity depending upon which of the many proposed sets of criteria are applied. The ECG is often used as a screening test to determine who should undergo further testing with an echocardiogram.

> **Commonly used ECG criteria for diagnosis of LVH :**
> *** S in V1 + R in V5 or V6 (whichever is larger) ≥ 35 mm (or 3.5 mV)**
> *** R in aVL ≥ 11 mm**
> ** or if left axis deviation R in aVL ≥ 13 mm plus S in III ≥ 15 mm**
> *** R in I + S in III > 25 mm**
> *** Delayed intrinsicoid deflection in V6 ≥ 50 ms**

The ECG criteria for diagnosing LVH are very insensitive (about 20–50%) meaning that many patients with LVH cannot be recognized by ECG (false negatives!). However, the criteria are very specific (about 90%) which means it is very likely that LVH is present if the criteria are met.

> **The power of some of the more commonly used ECG criteria to rule out the diagnosis of LVH in patients with hypertension is poor.**

RIGHT VENTRICULAR HYPERTROPHY

The causes of RVH involve mostly congenital disease and lung disease. Because the electrical activity of the RV is overshadowed by that of the LV, RVH has to be significant to cause ECG abnormalities.

The diagnosis requires a QRS duration < 0.12 s and a right axis deviation of approximately 100° or larger. There are a number of criteria but the diagnosis is usually made on the basis of a constellation of supportive findings.

R wave in lead V1.
As expected RVH increases the height of the R waves in the RV leads (V1 to V3).
1. Lead V1 shows > 7 mm in height (with an s wave < 2 mm) and the R/S ratio is > 1.
2. Lead V1 may show a qR pattern.
3. If there is an rSR' complex the R' > 10 mm
   In the normal ECG the S wave is dominant in lead V1. A dominant R wave can occasionally be a normal variant. A posterior myocardial infarction (MI) may cause a dominant R wave in lead V1 but the T waves are often upright in the right precordial leads. Such a posterior MI is commonly associated with an inferior MI which is easily recognizable on the ECG.

Deep S waves in the left ventricular leads. The S wave > R wave.

ST - T wave changes in leads V1 to V3. There is T wave inversion in lead V1 and often in V2 and V3. The ST segment is depressed secondary to RVH. The changes are opposite in polarity to the QRS complex. This pattern used to be called RV strain.

R wave in lead aVR. The R wave in lead aVR is > q wave in the same lead. The R > 5 mm.

Right axis deviation. At least 100°.

Right atrial enlargement provides indirect proof of RVH.

Delayed intrinsicoid deflection in lead V1. This is similar to the corresponding changes in the left ventricular leads in left ventricular hypertrophy.

The specificity varies according to the underlying pathology. The diagnosis of RVH can be made with an ECG in only 50% of patients with chronic obstructive pulmonary disease who have definite RVH documented echocardiographically. However the specificity is higher.

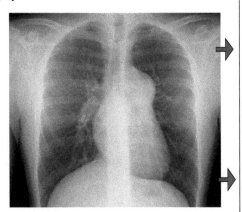

Chest X-ray in a patient with primary pulmonary hypertension showing marked prominence of the main pulmonary artery.

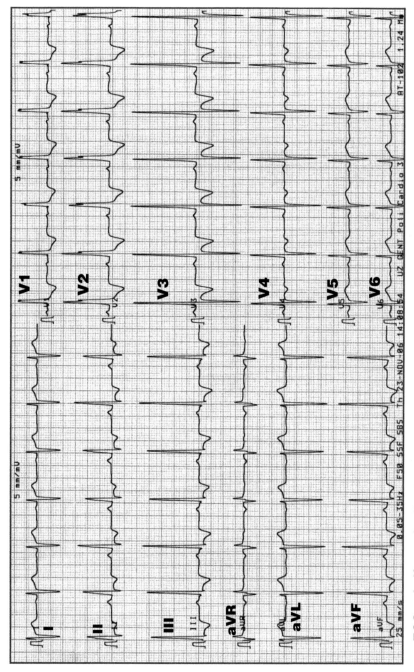

ECG at half standardization (1 mV = 5 mm) of a patient with primary pulmonary hypertension showing right ventricular hypertrophy. Note the tall 22 mm R wave in lead V1. The initial and remaining QRS vectors are directed rightward and anteriorly. There is right axis deviation of +110° and ST segment depression and inverted T waves in leads V1 to V4.

Devereux RB, Koren MJ, de Simone G, Okin PM, Kligfield P. Methods for detection of left ventricular hypertrophy: application to hypertensive heart disease. Eur Heart J. 1993;14 Suppl D:8-15.

Griep AH. Pitfalls in the electrocardiographic diagnosis of left ventricular hypertrophy: a correlative study of 200 autopsied patients. Circulation. 1959;20:30-4.

Hancock EW, Deal BJ, Mirvis DM, Okin P, Kligfield P, Gettes LS, Bailey JJ, Childers R, Gorgels A, Josephson M, Kors JA, Macfarlane P, Mason JW, Pahlm O, Rautaharju PM, Surawicz B, van Herpen G, Wagner GS, Wellens H; American Heart Association Electrocardiography and Arrhythmias Committee, Council on Clinical Cardiology; American College of Cardiology Foundation; Heart Rhythm Society. AHA/ACCF/HRS recommendations for the standardization and interpretation of the electrocardiogram: part V: electrocardiogram changes associated with cardiac chamber hypertrophy: a scientific statement from the American Heart Association Electrocardiography and Arrhythmias Committee, Council on Clinical Cardiology; the American College of Cardiology Foundation; and the Heart Rhythm Society: endorsed by the International Society for Computerized Electrocardiology. Circulation. 2009;119:e251-61.

Levy D, Labib SB, Anderson KM, Christiansen JC, Kannel WB, Castelli WP. Determinants of sensitivity and specificity of electrocardiographic criteria for left ventricular hypertrophy. Circulation. 1990;81:815-20.

Roberts WC, Filardo G, Ko JM, Siegel RJ, Dollar AL, Ross EM, Shirani J. Comparison of Total 12-Lead QRS Voltage in a Variety of Cardiac Conditions and Its Usefulness in Predicting Increased Cardiac Mass. Am J Cardiol. 2013;112:904-9.

Sokolow M, Lyon TP. The ventricular complex in left ventricular hypertrophy as obtained by unipolar precordial and limb leads. Am Heart J. 1949;17:161-86.

Surawicz B. Electrocardiographic diagnosis of chamber enlargement. J Am Coll Cardiol. 1986;8:711-24.

CHAPTER 7

INTRAVENTRICULAR CONDUCTION DEFECTS

* Right bundle branch block
* Left bundle branch block
* LBBB versus RBBB
* Left anterior hemiblock
* Left posterior hemiblock
* LAH versus LPH
* Incomplete right bundle branch block
* Left hemiblock and right bundle branch block
* Rate-dependent bundle branch block
* Phase 3 and phase 4 blocks

ECG from Basics to Essentials: Step by Step. First Edition. Roland X. Stroobandt, S. Serge Barold and Alfons F. Sinnaeve.
Published 2016 © 2016 by John Wiley & Sons, Ltd. Companion Website: www.wiley.com/go/stroobandt/ecg

RIGHT BUNDLE BRANCH BLOCK

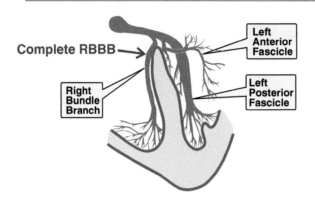

Complete RBBB

Left Anterior Fascicle

Right Bundle Branch

Left Posterior Fascicle

Sequence of Ventricular Depolarization

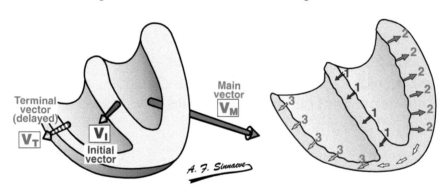

Terminal vector (delayed)

V_T

V_I
Initial vector

Main vector V_M

A. F. Sinnaeve

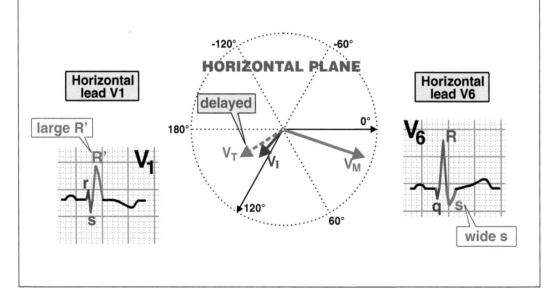

HORIZONTAL PLANE

Horizontal lead V1

large R'

V_1

B'

r

s

-120°   -60°

delayed

180°   0°

V_T V_I

V_M

120°   60°

Horizontal lead V6

V_6

R

q   s

wide s

Complete RBBB – Criteria

➡ **1.** QRS duration ≥ 120 ms in adults, > 100 ms in children 4 to 16 years of age, and > 90 ms in children less than 4 years of age.

➡ **2.** rsr', rsR', rSr', or rSR' in leads V1 or V2. The R' or r' deflection is usually wider than the initial R wave. In a minority of patients, a wide and often notched R wave pattern may be seen in lead V1 and/or V2.

➡ **3.** S wave of greater duration than R wave or > 40 ms in leads I and V6 in adults.

➡ **4.** Normal R peak time in leads V5 and V6 but > 50 ms in lead V1.

Incomplete RBBB

➡ Incomplete RBBB is defined by QRS duration between 110 and 120 ms in adults, between 90 and 100 ms in children between 8 and 16 years of age, and between 86 and 90 in children less than 8 years of age.

➡ Other criteria are the same as for complete RBBB. The ECG pattern of incomplete RBBB may be present in the absence of heart disease, particularly when the V1 lead is recorded higher than or to the right of normal position and r' is less than 20 ms.

The terms rsr' and normal rsr' are not recommended to describe such patterns, because their meaning can be variously interpreted. In children an rsr' pattern in V1 and V2 with a normal QRS duration is a normal variant.

Functional RBBB

A transient form of RBBB may be observed in patients with premature atrial contractions (Ashman phenomenon) or supraventricular tachycardia (rate dependent functional right bundle branch block). This occurs when an early impulse is conducted from the atrioventricular node to the His bundle while the right bundle branch but not the left bundle branch is still refractory. Conduction down the right bundle branch is therefore delayed or blocked, resulting in a **transient** RBBB.

The right bundle branch is a superficial and fragile structure on the right side of the septum. Thus, the right bundle branch may be traumatized and transiently blocked during any form of right heart catheterization.

RBBB is a conduction disorder seen in the mid- or late portion of the QRS complex. Thus, initial septal q waves (not more than 0.02 s) are seen in the left lateral leads. Only the first 60–80 ms of the QRS complex corresponds to LV activation. Therefore, analysis of the frontal plane axis should be done by using only the initial portion of the QRS.

The frontal plane axis is usually normal. A frontal plane axis of −30° or more superior almost always indicates associated left anterior hemiblock. Right axis deviation may be caused by a variety of conditions which have to be ruled out before making a diagnosis of associated left posterior hemiblock.

LEFT BUNDLE BRANCH BLOCK

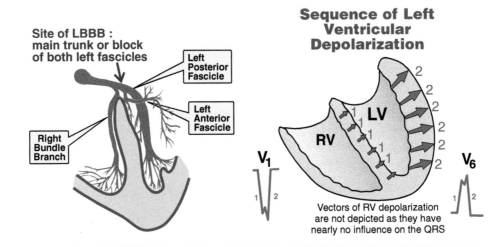

**Site of LBBB :
main trunk or block
of both left fascicles**

Left Posterior Fascicle

Left Anterior Fascicle

Right Bundle Branch

Sequence of Left Ventricular Depolarization

LV

RV

V$_1$

V$_6$

Vectors of RV depolarization
are not depicted as they have
nearly no influence on the QRS

LBBB is a conduction disorder that alters the initial forces of the QRS complex. Consequently LBBB may mask the electrocardiographic manifestations of conditions affecting the initial part of the QRS complex such as the Q waves of myocardial infarction.

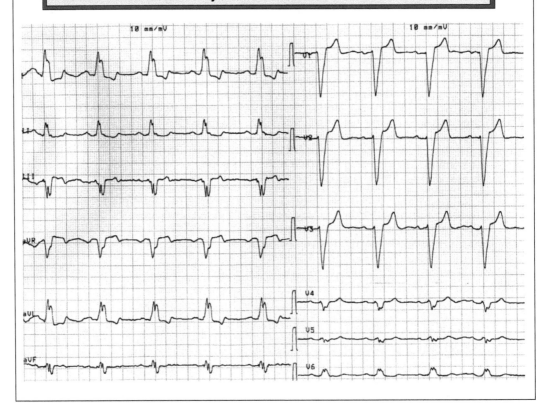

Complete LBBB – Criteria

➡ **1.** QRS duration ≥ 120 ms in adults, > 100 ms in children 4 to 16 years of age, and > 90 ms in children less than 4 years of age.

➡ **2.** Broad notched or slurred R wave in leads I, aVL, V5, and V6 and an occasional RS pattern in V5 and V6 attributed to displaced transition of QRS complex (or incorrect lead placement).

➡ **3.** Absent q waves in leads I, V5, and V6, but in lead aVL, a narrow q wave may be present in the absence of myocardial pathology.

➡ **4.** R peak time > 60 ms in leads V5 and V6 but normal in leads V1, V2, and V3. The latter exhibit either a small initial r wave or a QS complex.

➡ **5.** ST and T waves usually opposite in direction to QRS.

➡ **6.** Positive T wave in leads with upright QRS may be normal (positive concordance).

➡ **7.** Depressed ST segment and/or negative T wave in leads with negative QRS (negative concordance) are abnormal.

➡ **8.** The appearance of LBBB may change the mean QRS axis in the frontal plane to the right, to the left, or to a superior site, and in some cases in a rate-dependent manner.

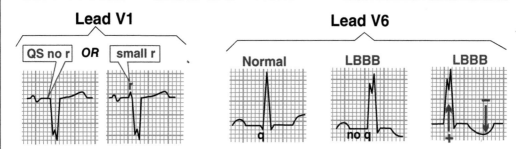

Lead V1 — QS no r OR small r

Lead V6 — Normal | LBBB (no q) | LBBB

Is complete LBBB overdiagnosed? This issue is important in the selection of heart failure patients for cardiac resynchronization implantable devices.
Stricter criteria have been proposed for complete LBBB that include a QRS duration ≥ 140 ms for men and ≥ 130 ms for women, QS or rS in leads V1 and V2, and mid-QRS notching or slurring in 2 leads of V1, V2, V5, V6, I, and aVL.

Incomplete LBBB

➡ **1.** QRS duration between 110 and 119 ms in adults (between 90 and 100 ms in children 8 to 16 years of age, and between 80 and 90 ms in children less than 8 years of age).

➡ **2.** Presence of left ventricular hypertrophy pattern.

➡ **3.** R peak time greater than 60 ms in leads V4, V5, and V6.

➡ **4.** Absence of q wave in leads I, V5, and V6.

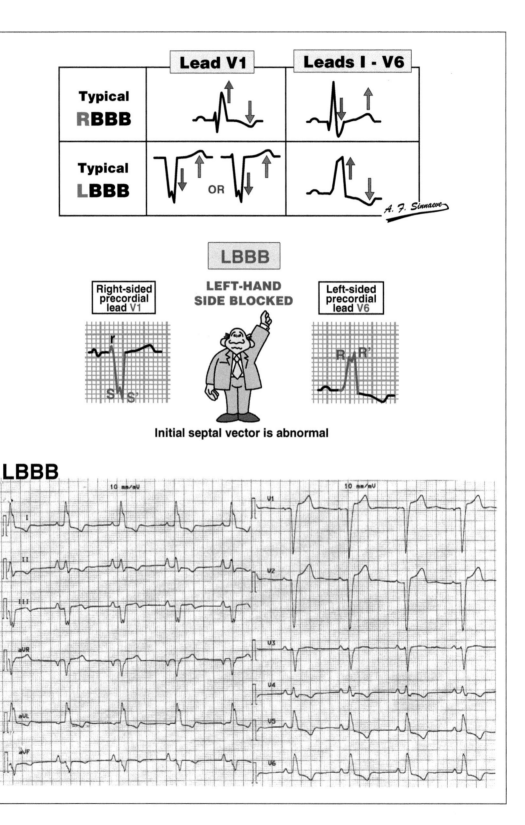

	Lead V1	**Leads I - V6**
Typical **R**BBB		
Typical **L**BBB	OR	

A. F. Sinnaeve

LBBB

Right-sided precordial lead V1	**LEFT-HAND SIDE BLOCKED**	Left-sided precordial lead V6

Initial septal vector is abnormal

LBBB

LBBB versus RBBB

An upright (positive) wide QRS complex in V1 clinches the diagnosis of RBBB. Occasionally RBBB does not produce a dominant R wave in V1. RBBB may then be recognized in V1 by an rSr' pattern, where the r' deflection is typical of a right-sided conduction delay or block.

If V1 is negative (and without an rSr' complex), the disorder is either LBBB or a nonspecific intraventricular conduction disorder. The next step is to look for the typical LBBB configuration in the left-sided leads.

RBBB

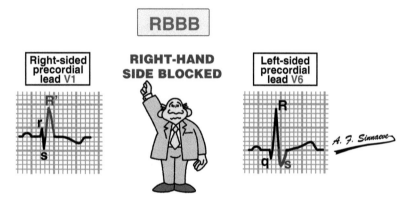

RIGHT-HAND SIDE BLOCKED

Right-sided precordial lead V1

Left-sided precordial lead V6

A. F. Sinnaeve

Initial septal vector is normal

RBBB

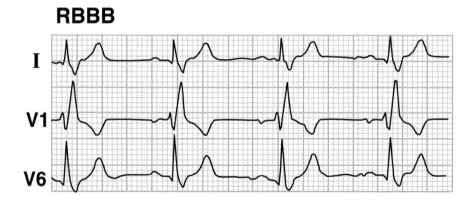

I

V1

V6

Lead V1 shows the typical pattern of RBBB.
Note the wide but shallow terminal S wave in leads I and V6.

LEFT ANTERIOR HEMIBLOCK

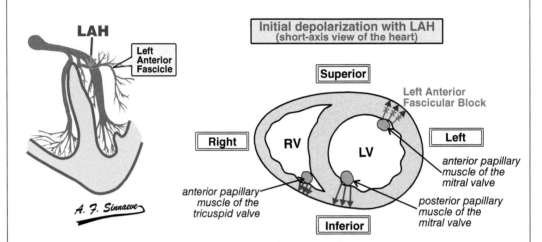

LAH

Left Anterior Fascicle

A. F. Sinnaeve

Initial depolarization with LAH
(short-axis view of the heart)

Superior

Left Anterior Fascicular Block

Right

RV

LV

Left

anterior papillary muscle of the mitral valve

anterior papillary muscle of the tricuspid valve

posterior papillary muscle of the mitral valve

Inferior

The left anterior fascicle crosses the LV outflow tract and terminates in the Purkinje system of the anterolateral wall of the LV. In "Left Anterior Hemiblock" (LAH), which is also known as "Left Anterior Fascicular Block" (LAFB), the impulse spreads first through the left posterior fascicle, causing a delay in activation of the anterior and lateral walls of the LV which are normally activated via the left anterior fascicle. The main vector moves superiorly and anticlockwise. Thus, the peak of the terminal R wave in aVR occurs later than the peak of the R wave in aVL.

LEFT ANTERIOR HEMIBLOCK
1. Frontal plane axis between −45° and −90°.
2. qR pattern in lead aVL.
3. R peak time in lead aVL of 45 ms or more.
4. QRS duration < 120 ms.

In LAH the inferior LV is activated first, giving rise to septal q waves in leads I and aVL and small initial r waves in leads II, III, and aVF. The R wave in I and aVL may be tall. The delayed and unopposed activation of the rest of the LV produces a shift in the QRS axis leftward and superiorly, causing a marked left axis deviation. This process takes about 20 ms longer than simultaneous activation by the 2 fascicles on the left side. This results in a QRS duration which is either normal or slightly prolonged but < 0.12 s.

WARNING !
1. **Low r waves in V1 to V3 (delayed transitional zone) may cause the erroneous diagnosis of anteroseptal myocardial infarction.**
2. **Because the initial vector points inferiorly and to the right, V2 and V3 may exhibit micro q waves simulating an anteroseptal myocardial infarction. These q waves occur in a small portion of patients and disappear with recording V2 and V3 one intercostal space lower.**
3. **The small inferior r waves differentiate LAH from an inferior myocardial infarction (although the two may coexist).**

LEFT ANTERIOR HEMIBLOCK

Quick diagnosis of LAH: lead I is predominantly positive, but leads II and III are predominantly negative and QRS < 0.12 s.

Projections of the main vector V$_M$

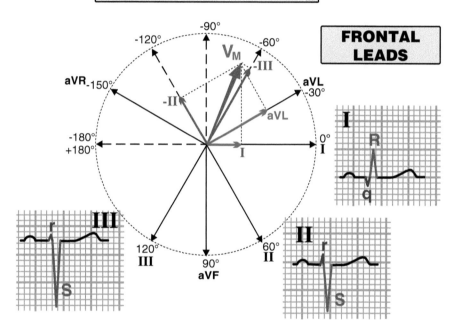

FRONTAL LEADS

FRONTAL PLANE VECTORS

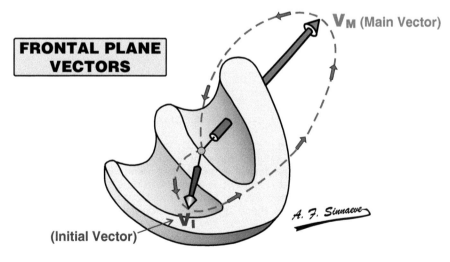

V$_M$ (Main Vector)

(Initial Vector)

A. F. Sinnaeve

LEFT POSTERIOR HEMIBLOCK

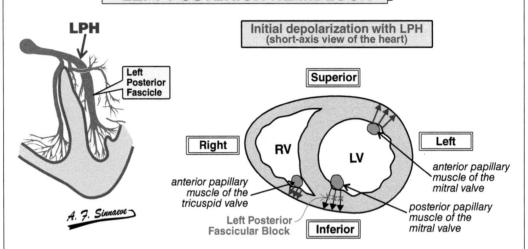

LPH

Left Posterior Fascicle

A. F. Sinnaeve

Initial depolarization with LPH
(short-axis view of the heart)

Superior

Right

RV

LV

Left

anterior papillary muscle of the tricuspid valve

anterior papillary muscle of the mitral valve

posterior papillary muscle of the mitral valve

Left Posterior Fascicular Block

Inferior

The left posterior fascicle courses along the inflow tract of the LV a site less turbulent than the site of the left anterior fascicle. "Left Posterior Hemiblock" (LPH) is rare as an isolated abnormality and it usually occurs together with right bundle branch block. The ECG manifestations of LPH are opposite to those of LAH. The cardiac impulse emerges from the unblocked left anterior fascicle and spreads superiorly and leftward. This causes small q waves in leads II, aVF and III, and small r waves in I and aVL. The major wave of depolarization then spreads in an inferior and rightward direction (in areas normally activated by the left posterior fascicle) generating tall R waves in the inferior leads and large negative voltages (deep S waves) in the lateral leads I and aVL. This leads to the characteristic rightward axis of +90° to +180°. As with LAH the QRS complex may be normal in duration or increased by < 20 ms. The precordial leads do not contain any diagnostic data.

LEFT POSTERIOR HEMIBLOCK

1. **Frontal plane axis between 90° and 180° in adults. Owing to the more rightward axis in children up to 16 years of age, this criterion should only be applied to them when a distinct rightward change in axis is documented.**
2. **rS pattern in leads I and aVL.**
3. **qR pattern in leads III and aVF**
4. **QRS duration < 120 ms.**

WARNING !

There are a number of settings which may produce ECG findings similar to LPH which is a diagnosis of exclusion.
1. The diagnostic criteria apply only in the absence of other causes for right axis deviation such as right ventricular hypertrophy or lung disease with cor pulmonale.
2. A high lateral or anterolateral myocardial infarction can mimic LPH. With an infarct, however, the initial r wave in leads I and aVL is absent and only a Q wave is seen.
3. The deep terminal S wave in leads I, aVL, V5 and V6 in RBBB should not be mistaken for right axis deviation because these S waves reflect delayed right ventricular activation, not left ventricular forces.
4. The small q waves in the inferior leads in LPH may cause confusion with an inferior wall myocardial infarction.

LEFT POSTERIOR HEMIBLOCK

Projections of the main vector V$_M$

R in lead III > R in lead aVF > R in lead II
S in lead aVL > S in lead I

FRONTAL LEADS

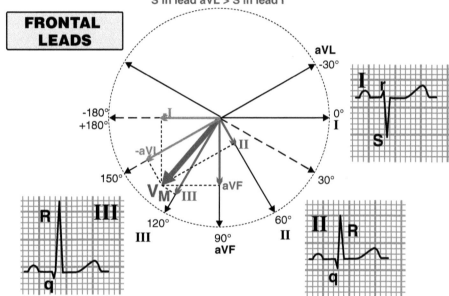

FRONTAL PLANE VECTORS

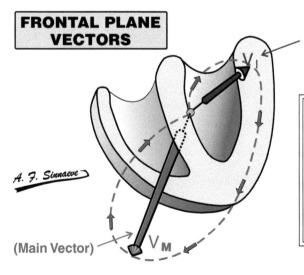

A. F. Sinnaeve

(Initial Vector)
(or Septal Vector)

(Main Vector)

V$_M$

The initial forces oriented superiorly and to the left are caused by early activation of the anterolateral wall of the left ventricle. These forces are responsible for the small r waves in leads I and aVL and the small q waves of leads II, III, and aVF.

LAH versus LPH

For both LAH & LPH: QRS duration < 120 ms
LAH and LPH are mirror images of each other

LAH

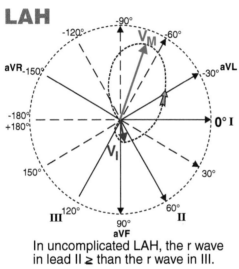

In uncomplicated LAH, the r wave
in lead II ≥ than the r wave in III.

LPH

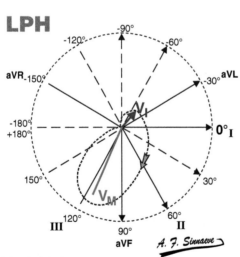

Vᵢ : initial vector
V_M : main vector

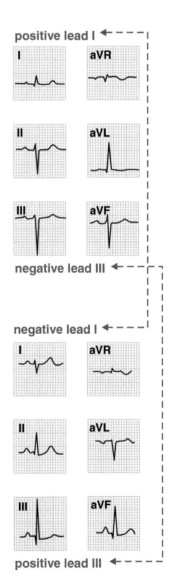

positive lead I

negative lead III

negative lead I

positive lead III

LAH versus LPH

LAH

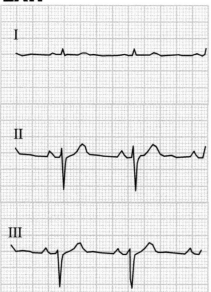

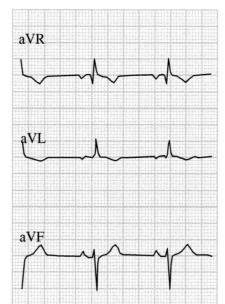

LPH

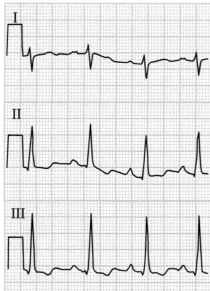

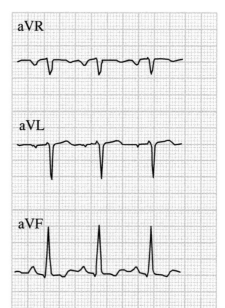

INCOMPLETE
RIGHT BUNDLE BRANCH BLOCK

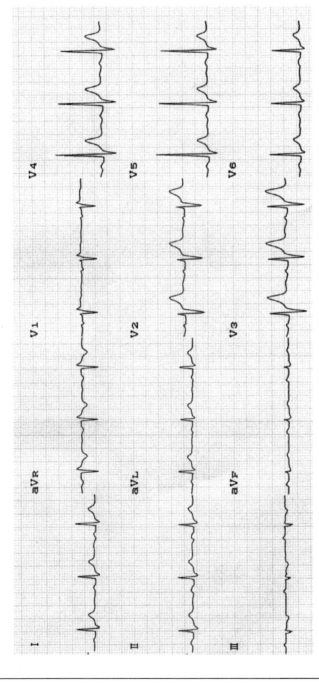

Incomplete RBBB with an rSr' complex in V1. QRS duration of 0.10 – 0.11 s. Such an ECG may indicate a problem which may eventually progress to complete RBBB or a normal variant. An rSr' pattern may occur in normal subjects when V1 is recorded higher than the 4th right intercostal space. As a rule a normal variant consists of a normal QRS duration with a very low r' in V1 and typically occurs in young patients or patients with a flat chest.

LEFT HEMIBLOCK AND RIGHT BUNDLE BRANCH BLOCK

RBBB & LAH

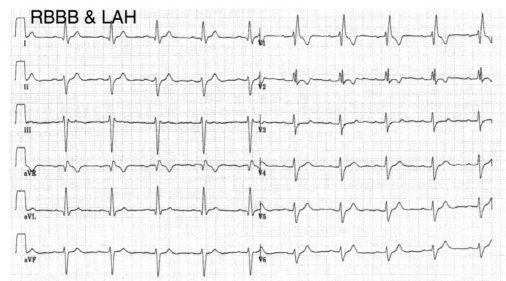

The tracing shows the typical pattern of RBBB. Looking at an upright QRS complex in lead I and a downward QRS complex in lead III raises the possibility of left axis deviation. Then, by looking at lead II with an rS and a deeply negative QRS complex, the frontal plane axis must be more negative than −45°, a finding consistent with LAH. This ECG therefore shows bifascicular block.

RBBB & LPH

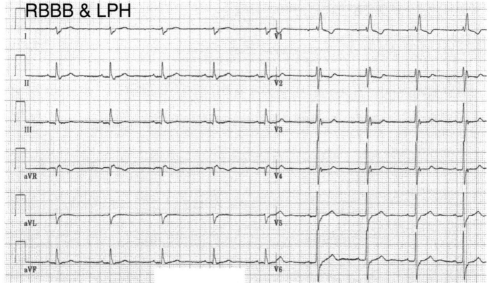

The tracing shows the typical pattern of RBBB. Looking at an upright QRS complex in lead II and III and a downward QRS complex in lead I immediately indicates the presence of right axis deviation compatible with the diagnosis of additional LPH (and thus bifascicular block), provided all other causes of right axis deviation are ruled out.

RATE-DEPENDENT
LEFT BUNDLE BRANCH BLOCK

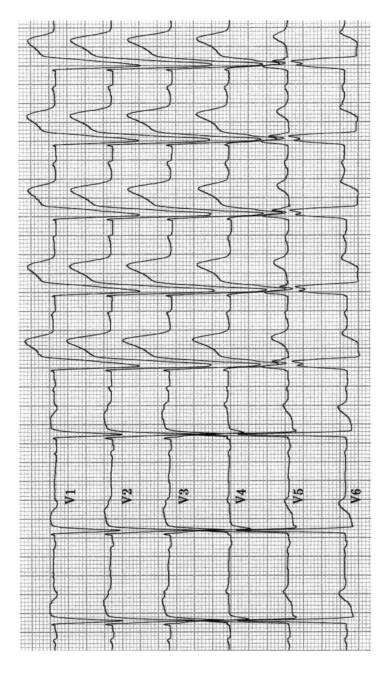

V1

V2

V3

V4

V5

V6

On the left, there is sinus rhythm with a slightly prolonged PR interval and the pattern of incomplete left bundle branch block (LBBB) prolonging the QRS duration to 0.10 - 0.11 s. Note the characteristic absence of a q wave in lead V6. Tachycardia-dependent (phase 3) complete LBBB (QRS = 0.16 s) supervenes when the third RR interval shortens to 0.72 s (720 ms). Complete LBBB will continue until the sinus rate drops below a critical value to restore the baseline intraventricular conduction.

PHASE 3 AND PHASE 4 BLOCKS

In the normal heart, a very premature impulse arriving in the ventricles may exhibit aberrant conduction or functional bundle branch block (BBB). An early atrial premature beat may traverse the AV node and then encounter a still refractory bundle branch. The beat is then conducted with functional BBB (usually right BBB because the right bundle branch has a longer refractory period than the left bundle branch). Such aberrant conduction may also occur with fast supraventricular tachycardias. The combination of a long RR interval and then a following short interval may lead to aberrant ventricular conduction as seen in atrial fibrillation (Ashman phenomenon).

Tachycardia dependent BBB is abnormal and occurs at relatively slower rates than those associated with functional aberrancy. This form of His-Purkinje block is called phase 3 block because it occurs during phase 3 of the action potential. The abnormal bundle branch has a prolonged refractory period that allows a critical cycle length to encroach on it. The critical rate at which BBB occurs may be relatively slow or fast if BBB occurs as a result of exercise. Normal conduction returns at a slower rate. In some cases normalization of intraventricular conduction occurs at an RR interval significantly longer than the RR interval which initiated BBB. This rate discrepancy is usually due to reset of the refractory periods from retrograde invasion of the blocked bundle branch coming from the activation of the unaffected bundle branch.

Bradycardia dependent BBB or phase 4 block is rare and due to disease in the His-Purkinje system. Abnormal His-Purkinje cells may acquire the property of spontaneous phase 4 depolarization. During a long pause, the site of the diseased His-Purkinje abnormality continues to depolarize and becomes less responsive to subsequent impulses which are then blocked.

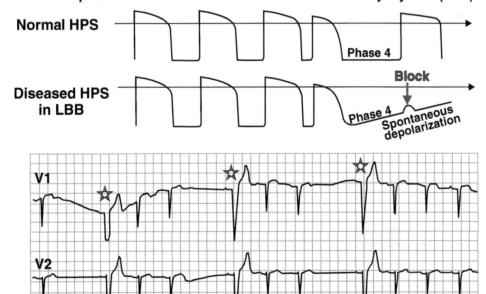

Simultaneous recording of leads V1 and V2. There is intermittent sinus arrest. The pause is terminated by a sinus beat conducted to the ventricle with left bundle branch block (LBBB). This is known as phase 4 block because it is believed that the block is due to spontaneous depolarization. This form of conduction block is not due to excessive vagal tone.

Elizari MV, Acunzo RS, Ferreiro M. Hemiblocks revisited. Circulation. 2007;115:1154-63.

Garcia D, Mattu A, Holstege CP, Brady WJ. Intraventricular conduction abnormality–an electrocardiographic algorithm for rapid detection and diagnosis. Am J Emerg Med. 2009;27:492-502.

Gettes LS, Kligfield P. Should electrocardiogram criteria for the diagnosis of left bundle-branch block be revised? J Electrocardiol. 2012;45:500-4.

Rosenbaum MB, Elizari MV, Lazzari J, Nau GJ, Levi RJ, Halpern MS. Intraventricular trifascicular blocks. Review of the literature and classification. Am Heart J. 1969;78:450-9.

Rosenbaum MB, Elizari MV, Lazzari JO, Nau GJ, Levi RJ, Halpern MS. Intraventricular trifascicular blocks. The syndrome of right bundle branch block with intermittent left anterior and posterior hemiblock. Am Heart J. 1969;78:306-17.

Strauss DG, Selvester RH, Wagner GS. Defining left bundle branch block in the era of cardiac resynchronization therapy. Am J Cardiol. 2011;15;107:927-34.

Surawicz B, Childers R, Deal BJ, Gettes LS, Bailey JJ, Gorgels A, Hancock EW, Josephson M, Kligfield P, Kors JA, Macfarlane P, Mason JW, Mirvis DM, Okin P, Pahlm O, Rautaharju PM, van Herpen G, Wagner GS, Wellens H; American Heart Association Electrocardiography and Arrhythmias Committee, Council on Clinical Cardiology; American College of Cardiology Foundation; Heart Rhythm Society. AHA/ACCF/HRS recommendations for the standardization and interpretation of the electrocardiogram: part III: intraventricular conduction disturbances: a scientific statement from the American Heart Association Electrocardiography and Arrhythmias Committee, Council on Clinical Cardiology; the American College of Cardiology Foundation; and the Heart Rhythm Society. Endorsed by the International Society for Computerized Electrocardiology. J Am Coll Cardiol. 2009 17;53:976-81.

CHAPTER 8

CORONARY ARTERY DISEASE AND ACUTE CORONARY SYNDROMES

* Electrophysiologic concepts of ischemia
* ST segment and T wave changes during ischemia
* Coronary artery disease and acute coronary syndromes
* Pathophysiology of acute coronary syndromes
* Common causes of myocardial infarction
* Manifestations of acute ST elevation MI
* Reciprocal changes in ST elevation MI
* ST elevation MI vs early repolarization
* Q waves in ST elevation MI
* Conditions that mimic MI
* T waves in ST elevation MI
* Right-sided leads and right ventricular infarction
* Non-STEMI and unstable angina
* ST segment depression
* Other features – poor R wave progression; persistent ST elevation
* Reperfusion
* Takotsubo cardiomyopathy
* Localization of STEMI
* Myocardial infarction and bundle branch block
* Diagnosis of MI during pacing
* Arrhythmias in acute myocardial infarction
* Diagnosis of coronary artery disease – exercise testing

ECG from Basics to Essentials: Step by Step. First Edition. Roland X. Stroobandt, S. Serge Barold and Alfons F. Sinnaeve.
Published 2016 © 2016 by John Wiley & Sons, Ltd. Companion Website: www.wiley.com/go/stroobandt/ecg

ELECTROPHYSIOLOGIC CONCEPTS OF ISCHEMIA 1

ORIGIN OF ISCHEMIC VECTORS

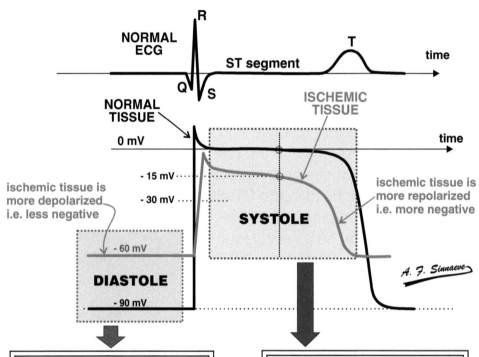

NORMAL ECG

R

ST segment

T

time

Q S

NORMAL TISSUE

ISCHEMIC TISSUE

0 mV

time

- 15 mV

- 30 mV

ischemic tissue is more depolarized i.e. less negative

ischemic tissue is more repolarized i.e. more negative

SYSTOLE

- 60 mV

DIASTOLE

A. F. Sinnaeve

- 90 mV

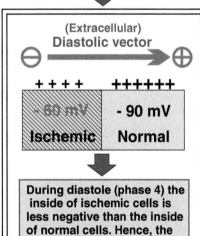

(Extracellular)
Diastolic vector

⊖ ⟶ ⊕

+ + + +   + + + + +

− 60 mV	− 90 mV
Ischemic	Normal

During diastole (phase 4) the inside of ischemic cells is less negative than the inside of normal cells. Hence, the outside of the ischemic cells is less positive in relation to normal cells.

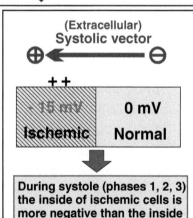

(Extracellular)
Systolic vector

⊕ ⟵ ⊖

+ +

− 15 mV	0 mV
Ischemic	Normal

During systole (phases 1, 2, 3) the inside of ischemic cells is more negative than the inside of normal cells. Hence, the outside of the ischemic cells is more positive in relation to normal cells.

ISCHEMIA DURING DIASTOLE

When a region of the heart becomes ischemic it loses its ability to maintain ionic pumps and the cells become depolarized. During diastole the transmembrane potential of ischemic cells becomes less negative than that of the surrounding normal tissue. As a consequence, during diastole, their outside surface is less positive relative to nonischemic cells. Hence, during phase 4 of the action potential (corresponding to the segment between the T wave and the next Q wave) an *"ischemic voltage vector during diastole"* is created directed from the less positive ischemic area towards the relatively more positive normal myocardium. A surface electrode placed over the ischemic zone will record a shift of the segment between T wave and next Q wave in the direction of the diastolic ischemic vector (i.e. positive if this vector points toward the electrode).

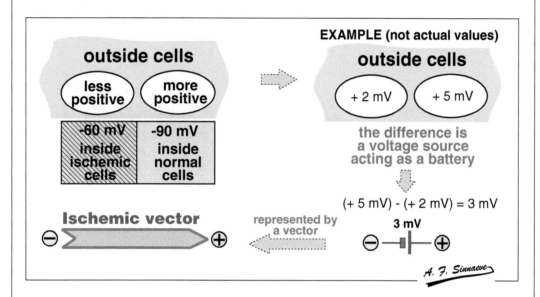

EXAMPLE (not actual values)

A. F. Sinnaeve

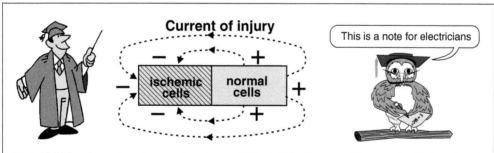

Current of injury

This is a note for electricians

Many books describe the mechanism of ST shift in terms of "current of injury" pointing to the ischemic region (during diastole) or pointing away from the ischemic zone (during systole). This is not correct because the ECG leads only record voltages (or potentials). Conventional electrical current flows from positive to negative zones and cannot be determined clinically by ECG.
The ST shift should be described in terms of ischemic voltage vectors!

ELECTROPHYSIOLOGIC CONCEPTS OF ISCHEMIA 2

ISCHEMIA DURING SYSTOLE

Ischemia also decreases the rate of rise and the amplitude of phase 0 of the action potential and shortens its duration resulting in a faster and earlier repolarization of ischemic cells. Therefore, during systole the interior of ischemic cells becomes more negative causing their outside to become more positive relative to nonischemic cells. Again, a voltage difference is created between the surroundings of ischemic cells and those of healthy cells. This voltage difference can be symbolized by an *"ischemic voltage vector during systole"* pointed from normal towards ischemic myocardium. Since this situation occurs as well during the ST segment as during the T wave (i.e. during repolarization of the cells) both will be affected by the systolic voltage vector. A surface electrode will record an ST shift in the direction of the systolic vector and sometimes tall (or hyperacute) T waves may be reigstered.

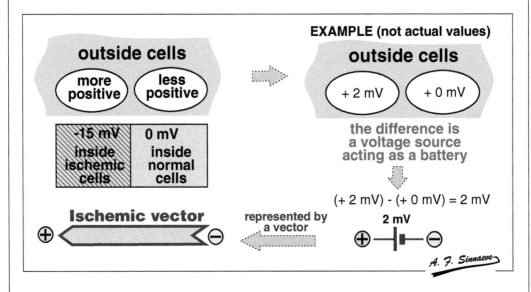

The line through the flat segments of the ECG is called the "baseline" and is used as a reference for measuring amplitudes.

For a normal healthy heart the baseline is also the "zero-voltage line"

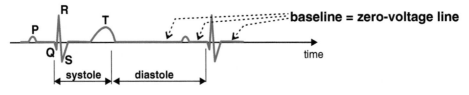

Note: the real zero-voltage line is not seen on real ECGs ! An accepted zero level can be established on the ECG machine.

INFLUENCE OF ISCHEMIA ON THE ECG – EXAMPLES

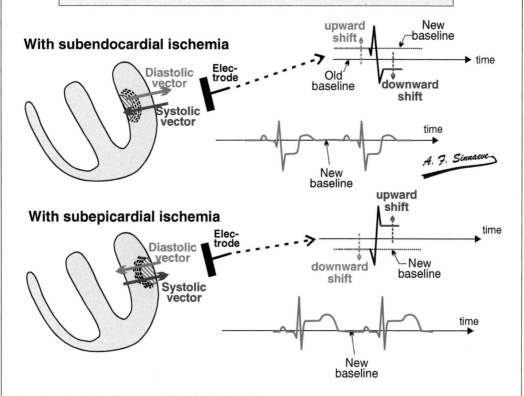

With subendocardial ischemia

With subepicardial ischemia

TOTAL SHIFT OF THE ST SEGMENT

Since the systolic vector and the diastolic vector work in opposite directions, their effect is cummulative and the apparent shift of the ST segment consists of the sum of both diastolic and systolic shifts.

However, as the assumed new baseline coincides with the position of the diastolic shift of the TQ segment, only the resulting global or apparent shift of the ST segment is seen on the ECG. This apparent shift is always in the direction of the systolic vector, i.e. from normal healthy tissue towards ischemic tissue (or from less ischemic towards more ischemic tissue).

* Note: for clarity the T-P, P-Q and Q-T are depicted as flat (isoelectric) although they are often curved (convex or concave).

Rules to remember

1. The shift of the ST segment, due to the combined action of both the systolic and the diastolic vectors, is always directed from normal towards ischemic tissue.
2. The ST elevation or ST depression depends upon the position of the electrode (or lead) with respect to the ischemic zone.

T WAVE CHANGES DURING ISCHEMIA 1

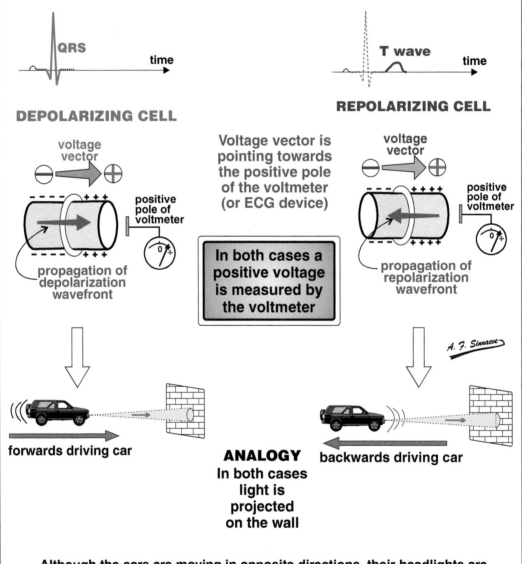

DEPOLARIZING CELL

voltage vector

positive pole of voltmeter

propagation of depolarization wavefront

Voltage vector is pointing towards the positive pole of the voltmeter (or ECG device)

In both cases a positive voltage is measured by the voltmeter

REPOLARIZING CELL

voltage vector

positive pole of voltmeter

propagation of repolarization wavefront

A. F. Sinnaeve

forwards driving car

ANALOGY
In both cases light is projected on the wall

backwards driving car

Although the cars are moving in opposite directions, their headlights are pointing in the same direction. In a normal healthy cell depolarization and repolarization are also propagating in opposite directions, but their voltage vectors are both pointing towards the positive pole of the voltmeter (or ECG recorder) resulting in the same deflection.

A. NORMAL T WAVE

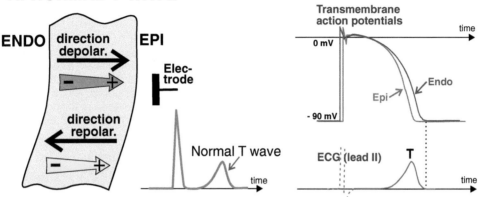

Depolarization in normal healthy myocardium starts at the endocardium. However, as the action potential duration (APD) is shorter in the epicardial cells, repolarization starts in the epicardium and the direction of repolarization goes from epicardium to endocardium. Although the directions of depolarization and repolarization are each opposite, the voltage vector (from negative tail to positive head) is oriented towards the epicardium. Therefore, an electrode located at the epicardium will record a positive QRS complex as well as a positive T wave.

In a normal heart the T wave and the QRS complex are *concordant*.

B. SUBENDOCARDIAL ISCHEMIA

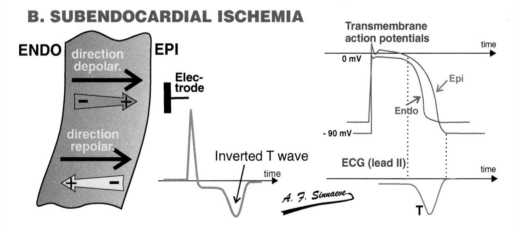

During subendocardial ischemia the duration of the endocardial action potential becomes shorter than the epicardial action potential. Depolarization starts in the endocardium as normal but as the endocardium repolarizes first, repolarization will occur earlier than in the epicardium. Both depolarization and repolarization directions are oriented from endo- to epicardium. The voltage vector, however, is oriented away from the epicardium and therefore an electrode positioned over the epicardium will record a negative T wave.

T WAVE CHANGES DURING ISCHEMIA 2

C. TRANSMURAL ISCHEMIA

During transmural ischemia the action potential duration (APD) of both the endocardial and the epicardial cells of the wall shortens. However, the electrophysiologic changes are most prominent in the subepicardium. Subepicardial cells have the highest ATP(*) sensitive potassium channels. Due to the high ATP concentration inside the cells of normal myocardium, these potassium channels are closed. However, they open when the intracellular ATP decreases during ischemia. This leads to an outward movement of potassium ions resulting in an increase of extracellular potassium. (*) ATP: adenosine triphosphate

Hyperacute T wave

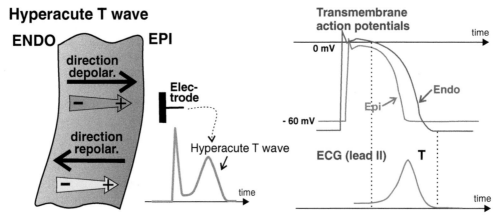

During the hyperacute phase of ischemia – that is seldom recorded on ECG – the subepicardial action potential duration (APD) becomes shorter than in normal myocardium. Therefore repolarization starts earlier in the epicardium resulting in an earlier inscription of the T wave. The ascending limb of the T wave will come closer to the QRS complex. The increased speed of repolarization of phase 3 causes a tall T wave while the larger difference between the endo- and epicardial APD is responsible for the broadening of the T wave. The T wave is positive as the voltage vector is oriented towards the epicardium.

Transmural Ischemia (later stage)

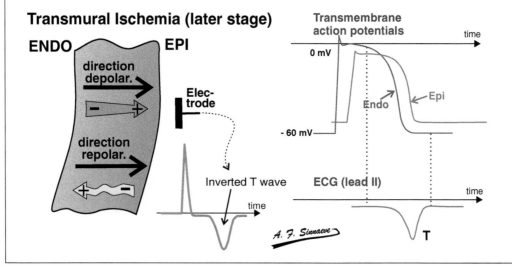

Very soon after the hyperacute phase – but still during the acute phase – the speed of depolarization of phase 0 decreases and transmural conduction slows. Depolarization starts in the subendocardial cells but due to the slow conduction from endo- to epicardium, the subepicardium having an even shorter APD depolarizes and repolarizes later than the endocardium. The direction of both depolarization and repolarization is the same from endo- to epicardium. However, the voltage vector is directed away from the epicardium during repolarization causing a negative T wave. QRS complex and T wave become ***discordant***.

⭐ **The heart is a complex organ with a multitude of cells with different properties. Moreover a lot of cells are involved in an ischemic zone. It follows that the explanation of the T wave by two cells (endocardial and epicardial action potentials) is only a good approximation to understand ischemia and myocardial infarction.**

⭐ **The conduction speed of the repolarization depends on several factors. Therefore, the shift of epicardial transmembrane action potentials with respect to the endocardial action potentials is patient dependent as well as time dependent and so is the T wave.**

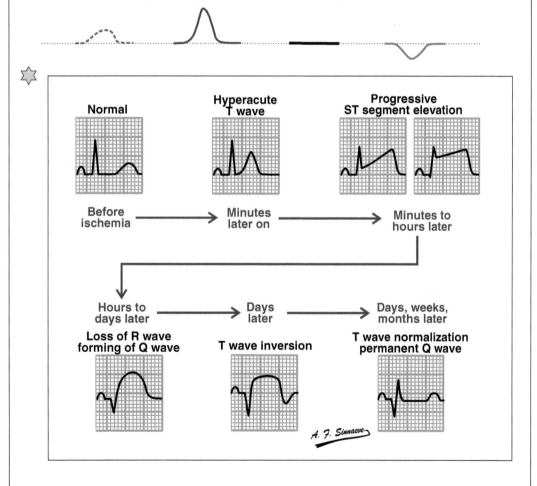

CORONARYARTERY DISEASE AND ACUTE CORONARY SYNDROMES 1

CORONARY ARTERY DISEASE

It is well known that the sensitivity of current 12-lead ECG criteria is poor for detecting acute myocardial infarction (MI). There are three reasons for this. 1. The infarct may be too small. 2. The location of the MI might not be seen by a 12-lead ECG due to its limited coverage of the precordium. 3. The location of ischemia in acute infarction might be "seen" by the 12-lead ECG as ST depression when it should in fact be considered "ST elevation equivalent" exemplified by lead –aVR. Lead aVR may show ST depression but lead –aVR (– aVR or *minus* aVR is an inferolateral lead) may show ST elevation usually in association with ST elevation in leads II, III, and aVF in an inferior wall MI.

The number of leads used and the electrode placement in a standard ECG have remained the same for over half a century though the technology of ECG recording has made great progress. Many alternative lead systems have been proposed to enhance the diagnostic ability of the ECG, but these additional leads have not become popular because the standard 12-lead ECG is so well established.

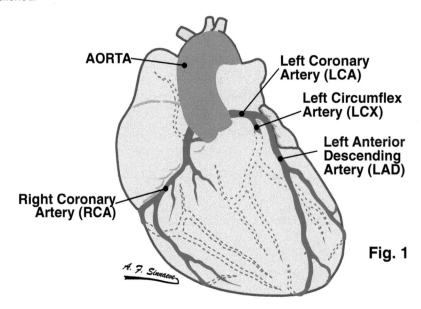

Fig. 1

Acute coronary syndrome is a term used for any condition brought on by sudden, reduced blood flow to the heart (Fig. 2). The term includes acute myocardial infarction (MI) which refers to two subtypes of acute coronary syndromes, namely non-ST-elevated MI and ST-elevated MI, which are most frequently (but not always) a manifestation of coronary artery disease. The absence of MI defines unstable angina as the third component of acute coronary syndromes. The acute coronary syndromes account for over 1.5 million hospital admissions in the US (Fig. 3).

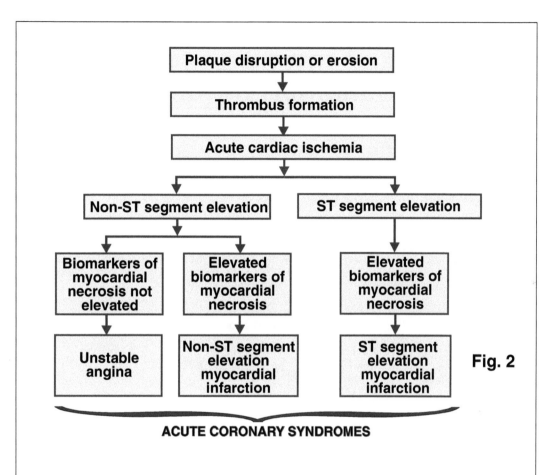

Fig. 2

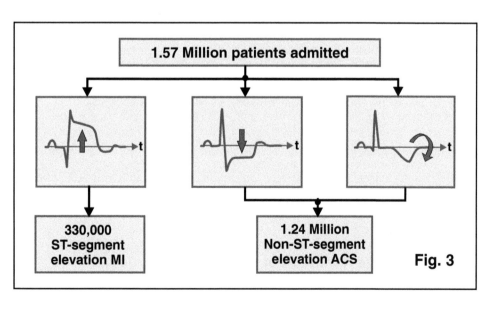

Fig. 3

CORONARY ARTERY DISEASE AND ACUTE CORONARY SYNDROMES 2

PATHOPHYSIOLOGY of ACUTE CORONARY SYNDROMES

Plaques in atherosclerosis consist of gradual buildup of cholesterol and fibrous tissue in the wall of arteries. Slowly developing, high-grade coronary artery stenoses usually do not precipitate acute myocardial infarction (MI) because of the development of a rich collateral network over time. Instead, acute coronary syndromes occur when a coronary artery thrombus develops rapidly at a site of vascular injury. Histologic studies indicate that the coronary plaques prone to rupture are those with a rich lipid core and a thin fibrous cap.

The 3 components of acute coronary syndrome share the same mechanism based on rupture of an unstable plaque (with erosion of the fibrous cap) in a large epicardial coronary artery. Thrombus formation either partially or completely occludes the coronary artery (Fig. 4).

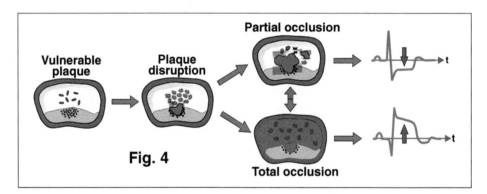

Fig. 4

The degree of thrombotic occlusion of an unstable and disrupted plaque defines which of the 3 acute coronary syndromes will occur clinically. With a major or complete thrombotic obstruction some of the heart muscle cells begin to die if the blood clot persists for more than just a few minutes. The death of heart muscle is what defines an MI. The diagnosis of MI is made by the presence of cardiac biomarkers in the blood such as troponin. When a patient presents with a potential acute coronary syndrome, the ECG findings are immediately used to classify the patient into one of the three groups selected to determine the most appropriate diagnostic and management strategies (Fig. 5).

After the onset of myocardial ischemia, cell death is not immediate but takes a finite period to develop. Necrosis starts after about 20 minutes. Complete necrosis of myocardium at risk requires at least 2-4 hours or longer depending on the collateral circulation, the sensitivity of the myocytes to ischemia and preconditioning. The latter refers to a greater resistance to ischemia acquired from repeated episodes of reversible ischemia that occurred before MI.

> **Most cases of acute myocardial infarction (AMI) are due to the formation of an occluding thrombus on the surface of an atheromatous plaque.**

> **The ECG in acute MI is quite variable. It is related to size, location and rapidity of reperfusion (if any).**

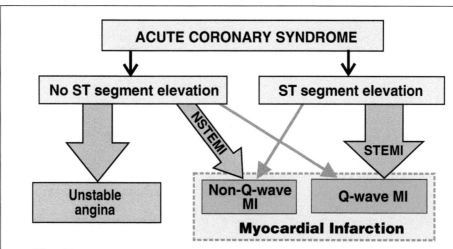

Fig. 5 Nomenclature of acute coronary syndromes

Patients with ischemic discomfort may present with or without ST-segment elevation on the ECG. The majority of patients with ST-segment elevation (large arrow) ultimately develop a Q-wave MI, whereas a minority (small arrow) develop a non-Q-wave MI. Patients who present without ST-segment elevation are experiencing either unstable angina or an non-ST-segment elevation myocardial infarction (NSTEMI). The distinction between these 2 diagnoses is ultimately made by the presence or absence of a cardiac biomarker detected in the blood. Most patients with NSTEMI do not develop a Q wave on the 12-lead ECG and are subsequently referred to as having sustained a non-Q-wave MI; only a minority of NSTEMI patients develop a Q wave and are later diagnosed as having Q-wave MI. Not shown is Prinzmetal's angina considered to be due to coronary artery spasm. It presents with transient chest pain and ST-segment elevation but rarely MI. The spectrum of clinical conditions that range from unstable angina to non-Q-wave AMI is referred to as acute cardiac syndromes.

COMMON CAUSES OF MYOCARDIAL INFARCTION

* Rupture of an atheromatous plaque.
* Vasospasm (including cocaine).
* In-stent thrombosis (early).
* In-stent fibrosis (late).
* Coronary artery surgery (poor surgical technique).

OLD TERMINOLOGY OF MI

The terms transmural and nontransmural (subendocardial) MI are no longer used because ECG findings in patients are not closely correlated with pathologic myocardial changes. Therefore, a transmural MI may occur in the absence of Q waves in the ECG, and many Q-wave MIs may be subendocardial, as noted pathologically. It should be noted that the term "subendocardial" can be rightfully used to describe subendocardial ischemia which occurs in non-STEMI or unstable angina (Fig. 6).

CORONARY ARTERY DISEASE AND ACUTE CORONARY SYNDROMES 3

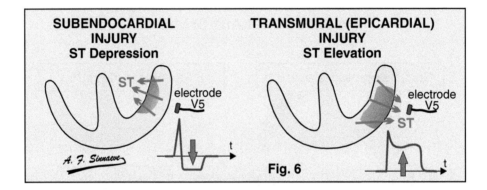

SUBENDOCARDIAL INJURY
ST Depression

TRANSMURAL (EPICARDIAL) INJURY
ST Elevation

Fig. 6

MANIFESTATIONS OF ACUTE ST ELEVATION MI

ST elevation MI (STEMI) occurs when a coronary artery is completely blocked, so that a large proportion of the heart muscle being supplied by that artery becomes damaged or necrotic. The patient with STEMI has (1) cardiac chest pain; (2) serologic evidence of myonecrosis (i.e. elevation of serum troponin or creatine kinase MB isoenzyme concentration); and (3) persistent (> 20 mins) ST segment elevation. In a patient without chest pain, ST-segment elevation incidentally noted, suggests the presence of a nonischemic cardiac condition. When the ECG identifies a STEMI, the diagnosis dictates the need for immediate reperfusion therapy for an optimal outcome. The potential size of an STEMI and the amount of myocardium at risk can be estimated by the larger number of ECG leads with ST-segment elevation. If ST elevation involves many leads, extensive ST elevation (if a large proximal coronary artery is involved) correlates with a higher mortality.

> **The prognosis of STEMI depends on the size of the MI, the site and timely medical therapy**

Hyperacute T wave changes

The earliest manifestation of acute MI is the hyperacute T wave, which is treated in the same way as ST-segment elevation. It only exists for 20–30 minutes after the onset of MI and represents transmural ischemia before the beginning of necrosis. Hyperacute T waves must be differentiated from the peaked T waves seen with hyperkalemia. Such T waves are often asymmetric with a broad base. Because of the rapid progression from the hyperacute T wave to frank ST elevation, most ECGs fail to show this pattern and patients usually present with significant ST-segment elevation.

Current of injury: ST-segment elevation

Under normal conditions, the ST segment is usually isoelectric (flat along the baseline) because normal myocardial cells attain the same potential during repolarization. Ischemia causes complex time-dependent effects on the electrophysiology of myocardial cells. Severe acute ischemia lowers the resting membrane potential and shortens the duration of the action potential in the ischemic area, and also decreases the rate of rise and amplitude of phase 0. These changes generate a **voltage gradient** between normal and ischemic zones, causing a current-flow of injury between these regions. This voltage difference is represented on the surface ECG by elevation of the ST segment.

> ## ECG manifestations of acute myocardial ischemia (in absence of left ventricular hypertrophy and left bundle branch block) (Current guidelines as accepted by ESC/ACCF/AHA/WHF, 2012)
>
> **New ST elevation at the J-point in two contiguous leads with the cut-points: ≥ 0.1 mV in all leads other than leads V2 and V3 where the following cut-points apply: ≥ 0.2 mV in men ≥ 40 years; ≥ 0.25 mV in men < 40 years; or ≥ 0.15 mV in women.**

ECG diagnosis of STEMI

The ST-segment elevation must be present in anatomically contiguous leads (I, aVL, V5, V6 correspond to the lateral wall; V1 to V4 correspond to the anterior wall; II, III, aVF correspond to the inferior wall). The ECG from the acute phase contains important information about the site and the size of the area at risk. Like STEMI, new onset left bundle branch block is also considered an indication for urgent revascularization.

> **Acute MI is not the most common cause of ST-segment elevation in chest pain patients. So-called ECG mimics of acute MI include left ventricular hypertrophy, left bundle branch block, paced rhythm, early repolarization, pericarditis, hyperkalemia, and left ventricular aneurysm.**

The evolution of a STEMI may take different pathways. In most cases without reperfusion therapy, the ST elevation resolves in 7–12 hours and the T wave becomes inverted, usually with the development of pathologic Q waves depending on the resulting amount of necrosis (Fig. 7). Even normalization of the ECG is possible after a short episode of vessel occlusion (with spontaneous recanalization) as is the case in aborted thrombotic MI or vasospastic (Prinzmetal) angina.

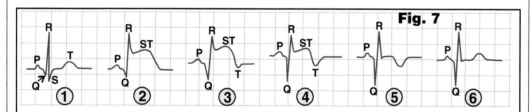

Fig. 7

Evolution of STEMI: (1) Normal ECG. The q wave originates from septal depolarization and is normal in this particular lead. (2) STEMI with ST elevation. No distinct T wave is seen. There is no increase in the amplitude of the q wave. (3) A deep Q wave has developed and T wave inversion appears with persistence of the elevated ST-segment. (4) Inverted T wave is more prominent but ST elevation is less prominent. (5) ST elevation has disappeared and there is now obvious T wave inversion. (6) Pattern of old myocardial infarction after more than 1–2 weeks. Note that a q wave appears relatively early in 2 and increases in amplitude thereafter. The Q wave remains indefinitely in most patients.

CORONARYARTERY DISEASE AND ACUTE CORONARY SYNDROMES 4

ECG diagnosis of ST elevation MI : "concave" versus "convex" ST elevation

It is commonly taught that the elevated ST-segment configuration which is convex (looking from above the ECG) or straight is more specific for an STEMI than one with ST elevation displaying a concave morphology. It is also believed that STEMI is less likely if the upward-directed ST-segment changes are concave rather than convex. However, concave morphology of ST elevation in the anterior leads does not exclude STEMI. A concave morphology in STEMI may evolve into a convex pattern. A convex morphology is 97% specific for STEMI.

ECG diagnosis of STEMI : "tombstoning"

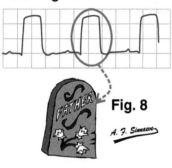

Fig. 8

A. F. Sinnaeve

Tombstoning ST elevation MI is a STEMI with a special form of ST elevation. This MI is associated with extensive myocardial damage, reduced left ventricular function, serious hospital complications and poor prognosis. The peak of the ST segment attains the level of the R wave or may even be higher than the R wave. The ST segment merges with the T wave. Thus, ST segment elevation surpassing the R wave exhibits a morphological appearance that reminds of a tombstone (Fig. 8). The QRS, ST-segment and T wave all blend together to form a large monophasic complex similar to that of an action potential. Tombstoning is not rare and more common in anterior MI.

It appears that tombstoning ST elevation is caused by sudden occlusion of a coronary artery supplying a large area of unprepared myocardium, i.e. myocardium not protected by collaterals or ischemic preconditioning. This results in complete transmural injury rapidly progressing to complete MI with the characteristic tombstone ECG pattern.

RECIPROCAL CHANGES IN ST ELEVATION MI

Patients with ST elevation in in one territory often have ST depression in other territories. The additional ST deviation may represent ischemia in a myocardial region other than the area of infarction or may represent pure reciprocal changes. Reciprocal change refers to ST-segment depression in leads that are 180 degrees (or nearly 180°) opposite to those that are exhibiting ST elevation. Also, reciprocal change does not describe ST-segment depression related to altered depolarization as seen in patients with left bundle branch block (LBBB) or left ventricular hypertrophy (LVH). Therefore, the definition includes the absence of confounding ECG patterns (LVH, LBBB, or ventricular paced rhythm).

Most of the common patterns of remote ST depression probably represent reciprocal changes and not "ischemia at a distance". In patients with inferior STEMI, ST depression in lead aVL is a pure reciprocal change and is found in almost all patients, a minor ST depression may even be seen in lead I (Fig. 10). ST depression in leads V1 to V3 in inferior MI probably does not represent "ischemia at a distance", but rather reciprocal changes due to more posterior, inferoseptal, apical, or lateral left ventricular involvement. Reciprocal ST-segment depression can therefore occur in the setting of a large amount of myocardium at risk with extensive ST elevation. In contrast, among patients with inferior STEMI, ST depression in leads V4 to V6 is associated with concomitant left anterior descending coronary artery stenosis or three vessel disease. Thus, presence of an atypical pattern of ST depression, and especially ST depression in leads V4 to V6 in inferior STEMI may signify "ischemia at a distance".

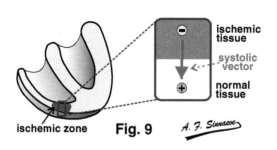

ischemic tissue
systolic vector
normal tissue
ischemic zone **Fig. 9** *A. F. Sinnaeve*

As pointed out in the previous chapter about "Electrophysiologic Concepts" the amplitude and the duration of action potentials in ischemic tissue are smaller than those in normal healthy tissue. Ischemic tissue is partially depolarized and therefore it is negative in relation to surrounding normal tissue during the repolarization of myocardial tissue. Consequently, a potential difference is created represented by the ischemic vector during systole. This is seen on the ECG as an elevation of the ST segment.

In patients with an inferior STEMI the ischemic vector during systole is directed downwards and a ST elevation may be expected in the inferior leads (III; aVF; II). A complete reciprocal ST depression can be observed in a true opposite position (Fig. 10A). However, no posterior electrodes are provided with the standard 12-lead ECG and only incomplete reciprocal ST depression may be observed in the left lateral leads (aVL and eventual lead I) (Fig. 10B).

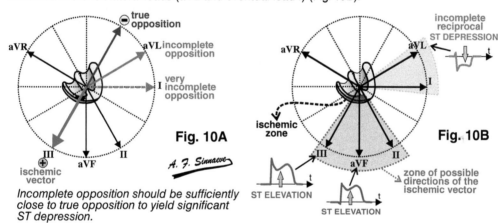

Fig. 10A *A. F. Sinnaeve*

Incomplete opposition should be sufficiently close to true opposition to yield significant ST depression.

Fig. 10B

Occasionally the magnitude of ST-segment elevation is small, whereas the reciprocal ST-segment depression is more prominent. In fact, in the absence of LVH or LBBB, reciprocal ST-segment depression may gain great importance. It is of great utility in patients with acute symptoms and mild elevation of ST segments of 1 to 1.5 mm in two contiguous leads, because it strongly suggests the diagnosis of STEMI rather than other causes of mild ST-segment elevation (1–1.5 mm). This avoids overlooking the less pronounced ST-segment elevation and having the patient erroneously diagnosed with non-ST-segment elevation acute coronary syndrome rather than STEMI.

Since there are no posterior electrodes in a standard 12-lead ECG, the diagnosis of posterior MI is dependent upon ST depression in anterior leads.

ST ELEVATION MI VS EARLY REPOLARIZATION

The typical pattern of early repolarization nonischemic ST elevation shows an elevation of 1–4 mm in the lateral leads (mainly V5 and V6). It may also involve the inferior leads. There is a characteristic notch at the J-point . The ST-segment is usually concave and tall while peaked T waves may be present. Early repolarization nonischemic ST elevation is commonly seen in young males. In many cases, ST elevation is transient and ameliorates or even disappears with tachycardia and with hyperventilation. Thus, dynamic changes in the degree of ST elevation are not always indicative of ischemia.

CORONARYARTERY DISEASE AND ACUTE CORONARY SYNDROMES 5

The ECG alone cannot reliably be used to diagnose acute MI as many conditions result in deviation of ST segments and may be misinterpreted as acute MI. Serial ECGs are essential because acute coronary syndrome is an evolving process.

Q WAVES IN ST ELEVATION MI

Small septal Q waves in the left ventricular leads result from depolarization of the septum from left to right. A Q wave in lead III alone may be positional and represents a normal finding. Q waves in lead III are not pathologic as long as abnormal Q waves are absent in leads II and aVF (the contiguous leads).

Q waves may be a marker of electrical silence which, when pathologic, implies myocardial necrosis in the past. Most STEMI develop Q waves and a few non-STEMI also develop Q waves (see Fig. 7). A Q wave reflects normal endocardial to epicardial depolarization of the ventricular wall on the opposite side of the heart, moving away from the positive electrode of the recording lead. Therefore Q waves are negative because they are effectively windows through which the opposite side of the heart can be seen. Regardless of the underlying mechanism, presence of abnormal Q waves in the leads with ST elevation on the admission ECG is associated with larger final infarct size and increased in-hospital mortality.

Q waves may occur as early as 2 hours with a STEMI. Q waves typically appear within the first 9 hours with a range of only a few minutes to 24 hours. Q waves should not be considered a marker of late MI presentation thereby denying a patient potentially beneficial reperfusion therapy. The time it takes for the development of Q waves depends on the collateral circulation that connects with the occluded coronary artery. The collateral network supplies circulation retrogradely to the distal part of the occluded artery responsible for the MI. A rich collateral network may delay or may actually prevent the appearance of Q waves.

Transient Q waves

Transient Q waves occur uncommonly during ischemia in the absence of MI and reflect transient loss of electrophysiologic function without irreversible cellular damage ("myocardial concussion"). Q waves of MI may sometimes disappear after early successful revascularization.

EXAMINATION of a Q WAVE
* Width.
* Depth (not as important as width).
* Lead or leads where Q wave(s) are recorded.
   Look for grouping or contiguous leads.
* Age of the individual.
* Relevant clinical findings.

Q waves of old MI

The ECG changes associated with prior MI as accepted by the ESC / ACCF /AHA / WHF criteria (2012) may be too nonspecific resulting in an inappropriately high number of false positive results.

ECG changes associated with prior myocardial infarction

* Any Q wave in leads V2 and V3 ≥ 0.02 s or QS complex in leads V2 and V3
* Q wave ≥ 0.03 s and ≥ 0.1 mV deep or QS complex in leads I, II, aVL, aVF or V4 to V6 in any two leads of a contiguous lead grouping (I, aVL; V1 to V6; II, III, aVF). [a]
* R wave ≥ 0.04 s in V1 and V2 and R/S ≥ 1 with a concordant positive T wave in the absence of a conduction defect.

[a] *The same criteria are used for supplemental leads V7 to V9*

> **Misplacement of chest lead electrodes is an important cause of anterior pseudo-infarction patterns. Poor R wave progression in the precordial leads sometimes with actual QS waves may be due to improper placement of chest electrodes above their usual position or on, rather than under the left breast.**

Normal Q or q waves

> **Despite differences in some of the guidelines and the definitions, the following is a useful rule of thumb. Normal septal q waves (seen in leads I, aVL, V5 and V6) are < 25% of the depth of the succeeding R wave and last for < 0.03 s. A Q wave may not be pathologic in lead III as long as there are no accompanying Q waves in aVF and II – these Q waves often disappear on deep inspiration. Lead aVR is usually a predominantly negative QRS complex with frequent Q waves. Lead V1 may occasionally show a QS pattern in the absence of heart disease.**

A complete transmural MI represents a zone without any electrical activity. An electrode placed in front of such zone is looking as it were through a window and only sees the activity in the ventricular septum and the right free wall (Fig. 12).

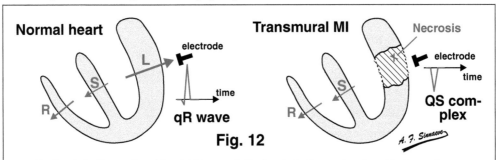

Fig. 12

R : depolarization vector of the right free wall; S : depolarization vector of ventricular septum; L : depolarization vector of the left free wall

CORONARY ARTERY DISEASE AND ACUTE CORONARY SYNDROMES 6

Conditions that mimic MI either by simulating pathologic Q waves or QS complexes or mimicking the typical ST-T changes of acute MI

* Normal variant "septal" Q wave in leads I, aVL, V5, V6
* Normal variant Q waves as in lead III
* Early repolarization
* Transient short-lived severe myocardial ischemia. Transient Q waves without MI.
* Preexcitation (Wolff-Parkinson-White syndrome): negative delta wave may mimic a pathologic Q waves.
* Left ventricular aneurysm with persistent ST elevation after acute MI
* Hypertrophic cardiomyopathy (septal hypertrophy may make normal septal Q waves "fatter" thereby mimicking pathologic Q waves).
* Hypertrophic cardiomyopathy: ST elevation in V3 to V5 (sometimes V6)
* Cardiomyopathy (dilated, infiltrative - such as sarcoid, amyloid).
* Left ventricular hypertrophy (may have QS pattern or poor R wave progression in leads V1 to V3).
* Right ventricular hypertrophy (tall R waves in V1 or V2 may mimic true posterior MI).
* Acute myocarditis
* Complete or incomplete LBBB (QS waves or poor R wave progression in leads V1 to V3).
* Left anterior fascicular block (may see small q waves in anterior chest leads).
* Pneumothorax (loss of right precordial R waves).
* Acute pericarditis (ST elevation in all leads except aVR; the ST segment elevation may mimic acute transmural injury)
* Pulmonary emphysema and cor pulmonale (loss of R waves in V1 to V3 and/or inferior Q waves with right axis deviation).
* Pulmonary embolism: ST elevation in V1 and aVR
* Artificial cardiac pacemaker.
* Central nervous system disease and raised intracranial pressure (acute neurologic events may mimic non-Q-wave MI causing diffuse ST-T abnormalities primarily in V1 to V6.)
* Idioventricular rhythm
* Hyperkalemia: ST elevation in V1 and V2
* Brugada syndrome: leads V1 and V2
* Hypothermia: ST elevation in V3 to V6, II, III, and aVF
* Cardiac contusion
* Following electrical cardioversion (transient ST elevation)

T waves in ST elevation MI

An evolving MI usually causes T wave inversion within hours or days. These T waves are symmetrical and affect the same leads that demonstrate ST elevation. Reperfusion therapy promotes the earlier development of T wave inversion. The significance of negative T waves in leads with ST elevation before reperfusion therapy is currently unclear.

Right-sided leads and right ventricular infarction

Right ventricular myocardial infarctions (RVMI) rarely occur alone or in isolation, but usually in conjunction with inferior MI. RVMI occurs in association with about 30–40% of inferior MI. The diagnosis of associated RVMI is important because its presence requires therapy different from that of an inferior MI without RVMI. Patients with RVMI have a poorer prognosis and a high risk of developing high-degree AV block. Usually, there are only inconclusive signs of RVMI in the standard 12-lead ECG. Right-sided leads usually V4R are now widely used for the diagnosis of RVMI (leads V3R and V4R are located on the right side of the chest in the same location as the left-sided V3 and V4). The V3R or V4R leads are the mirror image to their placement on the left side. Many studies have found a high but variable sensitivity and specificity of V4R for detecting RVMI.

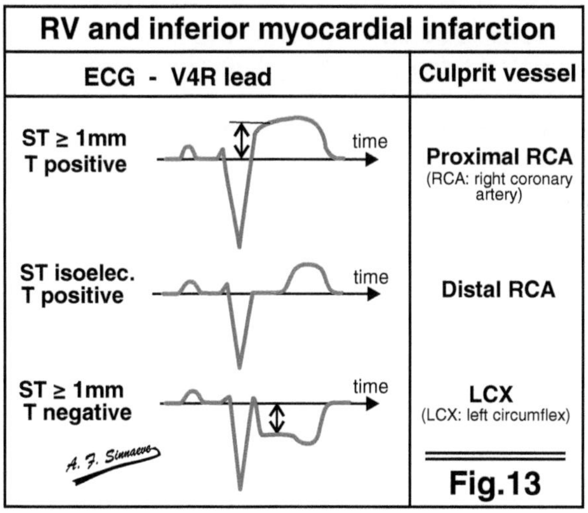

RV and inferior myocardial infarction

ECG - V4R lead	Culprit vessel
ST ≥ 1mm T positive	**Proximal RCA** (RCA: right coronary artery)
ST isoelec. T positive	**Distal RCA**
ST ≥ 1mm T negative	**LCX** (LCX: left circumflex)

A. J. Sinnaeve

Fig.13

Lead V4R is used most commonly and a 1 mm elevation of the ST-segment in lead V4R (with positive T wave) is highly specific for RVMI. The ST-segment elevation in V4R is transient, disappearing in less than 10 hours following its onset in half of patients. A dominant right coronary artery is always the culprit vessel in RVMI where a proximal occlusion compromises flow to one or more of the major RV branches. Distal right coronary artery occlusions or circumflex occlusions spare the RV branch and therefore do not show the ST elevation in lead V4R of RVMI. When the right coronary occlusion is distal to the RV branch, V4R will show a positive T wave but no ST elevation. ST depression with negative T wave in lead V4R is suggestive of an LCX occlusion (Fig. 13).

Pulmonary embolism and pericarditis also cause elevation of the ST-segment in the right-sided precordial leads. Uncommonly, lead V1 may show ST elevation in a RVMI in association with an inferior myocardial infarction.

Isolated RVMI is rare and may develop from occlusion of a nondominant right coronary artery or following balloon angioplasty complicated by acute occlusion of a large right ventricular branch of the right coronary artery. The ECG changes of isolated acute RVMI are not obscured by the coexisting dominant electrical forces of the inferior wall of the left ventricle as occurs in inferior MI. Therefore, when isolated RVMI occurs, the ECG may show an acute anterior ST segment elevation pattern (leads V1 to V3 which can be misinterpreted as signs of an anteroseptal infarction) and right ST segment elevation (lead V4R).

In patients with anterior left ventricular infarction, ST segment elevation is the lowest in lead V1, increasing in amplitude as precordial leads move to the left. On the other hand, patients with an isolated RV infarction display the greatest amplitude of ST segment elevation in lead V1, which progressively decreases as the precordial leads move to the left.

CORONARY ARTERY DISEASE AND ACUTE CORONARY SYNDROMES 7

Limitations of the ECG in the diagnosis of myocardial infarction

1 It provides a snapshot view of a highly dynamic process.

2 Lack of perfect detection in areas of myocardium supplied by a coronary artery.

3 Small areas of ischemia or infarction may not be detected.

4 Conventional leads do not directly examine right ventricle, posterobasal or lateral walls very well.

5 Baseline changes like hemiblocks (fascicular blocks) and left bundle branch block, early repolarization, left ventricular hypertrophy and arrhythmias make interpretation difficult.

6 Acute myocardial infarctions in the left circumflex territory are likely to have non-diagnostic ECG.

7 ECG is not a very sensitive test and should always be considered a supplement to, rather than a substitute for, physician judgment.

A normal ECG during symptoms suggests a low likelihood of acute coronary syndrome.
A normal ECG does not rule out acute myocardial infarction.

NON-STEMI AND UNSTABLE ANGINA

Non-ST-elevation myocardial infarction (NSTEMI) occurs when the occlusion in the coronary artery is not complete, so that a relatively small proportion of heart muscle becomes damaged or necrotic. Up to 25% of patients with NSTEMI and elevated CPK-MB or troponin enzymes go on to develop a Q-wave MI during their hospital stay, whereas the remaining 75% have a non-Q-wave MI. Although electrocardiography is necessary, it cannot distinguish acute ischemia (unstable angina) from NSTEMI. Cardiac biomarkers are required for the diagnosis of MI. Sometimes there is no myocardial damage either because the resultant blockage is not sufficiently extensive, or because the clot does not persist long enough, to produce cell death. The body's protective mechanisms try to dissolve blood clots that form within the affected coronary artery.

ST SEGMENT DEPRESSION

When ischemia is confined primarily to the subendocardium, the combination of the ischemic QT vector and the ischemic TQ vector results in depression of the ST segment on the ECG (see "Electrophysiologic Concepts - 8"). This subendocardial ischemic pattern is a frequent finding during spontaneous episodes of angina at rest and represents the typical ECG finding during exercise tests for cardiac ischemia.

ST segment depression associated with unstable angina/NSTEMI is transient and dynamic. It is important to obtain serial ECGs especially during symptoms because ischemia is an evolving process. Serial ECGs are essential if the first ECG is obtained during a pain-free episode.

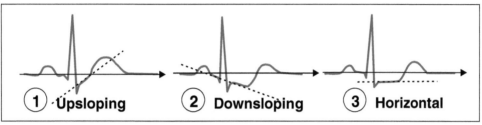

| ① Upsloping | ② Downsloping | ③ Horizontal |

Fig. 14 *Various forms of ST segment depression*

ECG manifestations of acute myocardial ischemia
(in absence of left ventricle hypertrophy and left bundle branch block)

ST elevation

New ST elevation at the J-point in two contiguous leads with the cut-points: ≥ 0.1 mV in all leads other than leads V2 and V3 where the following cut-points apply: ≥ 0.2 mV in men ≥ 40 years; ≥ 0.25 mV in men < 40 years; or ≥ 0.15 mV in women.

ST depression and T wave changes

New horizontal or downsloping ST depression ≥ 0.05 mV in two contiguous leads and/or T inversion ≥ 0.1 mV in two contiguous leads with prominent R wave or R/S ratio > 1.

According to the guidelines of the "Joint ESC/ACCF/AHA/WHF Task Force for the Universal Definition of Myocardial Infarction" European Heart Journal, 2012

Note that the criteria for cardiac ischemia are the same as for STEMI. In ischemia the duration of ST elevation is shorter and reversible.

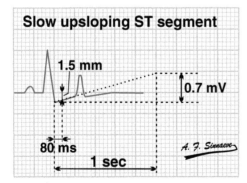

Slow upsloping ST segment

1.5 mm

0.7 mV

80 ms

1 sec

A. J. Sinnaeve

Fig. 15A *Slow upsloping (0.7 mV/s) with 1.5 mm ST depression at 80 ms after J point*

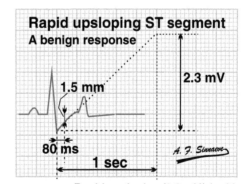

Rapid upsloping ST segment
A benign response

1.5 mm

2.3 mV

80 ms

1 sec

A. J. Sinnaeve

Fig. 15B *Rapid upsloping (2.3 mV/s) with 1.5 mm ST depression at 80 ms after J point*

CORONARY ARTERY DISEASE AND ACUTE CORONARY SYNDROMES 8

Upsloping ST depression is far less specific for myocardial ischemia than horizontal or down-sloping ST depression. The presence of slow upsloping ST depression (0.15 mV, 80 ms after the J point) should be considered as being ischemic in the setting of suspected coronary syndrome until proven otherwise.

Because a single 12-lead ECG recording provides only a snapshot view of a dynamic process, the usefulness of obtaining serial ECG tracings or performing continuous ST segment monitoring is obvious. Concurrent T wave inversion may or may not be present. A recording made during an episode of the presenting symptoms is particularly valuable. Importantly, transient ST segment changes (greater than or equal to 0.05 mV (i.e. 0.5 mm) that develop during a symptomatic episode at rest and that resolve when the patient becomes asymptomatic strongly suggest acute ischemia. Minor (0.5 mm) ST depression may be difficult to measure in clinical practice. Comparison with a previous ECG, if available, is valuable, particularly in patients with coexisting cardiac disorders such as left ventricular hypertrophy or a previous MI. ECG recordings should be repeated at least at 6 and 24 h, and in case of recurrence of chest pain/symptoms.

> **In the absence of ST elevation, additional recordings should be obtained when the patient is symptomatic and compared with recordings obtained in an asymptomatic state.**

More relevant for diagnosis and prognosis is ST depression of $\geq$ 1 mm (0.1 mV) or ST depression of $\geq$ 2 mm both of which carry a poor long-term prognosis. Patients with ST depression have a higher risk for subsequent cardiac events compared with those with isolated T wave inversion (> 1 mm) in leads with predominant R waves, who in turn have a higher risk than those with a normal ECG.

> **It is not possible to immediately distinguish between unstable angina and NSTEMI before the results of the cardiac biomarkers.**

The ST segment in unstable angina (UA)

In unstable angina (in the absence of left ventricular hypertrophy and left bundle branch block) the ECG may show the following abnormalities :
* **Transient ST segment elevations.** This is like a STEMI but is transient. It is sometimes called variant or Prinzmetal's angina and may be due to coronary artery spasm.
* **Dynamic T wave changes.** Inversions, normalizations, or hyperacute changes or transient ST segment elevations.
* **ST depressions.** May be downsloping, horizontal or slow upsloping.

Upsloping ST depression

Although ST segment depression – especially an upsloping ST segment depression – may be considered the baseline (and stable), ST segment depression associated with UA/NSTEMI is transient and dynamic. Its appearance is usually flat or downsloping. Concurrent T wave inversion may or may not be present.

Normal T wave inversion

The normal T wave is usually in the same direction as the QRS complex. The T wave is always upright in leads I, II, V3 to V6. It is normally inverted in lead aVR and may be normally inverted in leads III and V1. In lead aVL, the T wave should be in the same direction as the QRS complex. The T wave can be inverted in the right precordial leads in normal persons. T waves are commonly inverted in all precordial leads at birth but usually become upright as time passes. T wave inversions in V1 to V3 are relatively common in athletes < 16 years and probably represent the juvenile electrocardiogram pattern. In adolescent athletes, T wave inversions may occur beyond V2 if > 16 years. A persistent juvenile pattern with inverted T waves in V1 to V3 occurs in 1–3% of adults (19 to 45 years of age) and is more common in women than in men and is more common in black people. T wave inversions in the inferior/lateral leads and deep T wave inversions in any lead are unusual, warranting further investigations for underlying cardiomyopathy.

> **Marked (i.e. ≥ 2 mm or 0.2 mV) deep symmetrical T wave inversion in the precordial leads (V1 to V4) strongly suggests severe acute ischemia and a critical lesion in the proximal left anterior descending artery requiring emergency reperfusion therapy. These abnormalities may appear some time after an episode of chest pain.**

OTHER FEATURES OF MYOCARDIAL INFARCTION

Poor R wave Progression

Poor R wave progression is a vague term used to describe the transition in voltage in the precordial leads of an ECG. It is not a diagnosis but simply describes a pattern frequently noted. This finding is often inconclusively interpreted as suggestive, but not diagnostic, of anterior MI. The ECG report often states that "cannot rule out anterior myocardial infarction". Normal R wave progression in the precordial leads shows an rS-type complex in lead V1 with a steady increase in the relative size of the R wave toward the left chest and a decrease in the S wave amplitude (Fig. 16A). If the height of the r wave in leads V1 to V4 remains extremely small, we say there is "poor R wave progression" (Fig. 16B). In the literature, definitions of poor R wave progression have been variable.

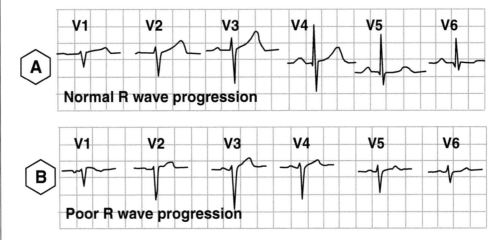

Fig. 16 *Normal versus poor R wave progression*

CORONARY ARTERY DISEASE AND ACUTE CORONARY SYNDROMES 9

Poor R wave progression may be secondary to previous anterior MI that produced Q waves in the right and midprecordial leads (V1 to V4). When the Q waves do not persist small r waves take their place. It is also conceivable that an MI may initially produce poor R wave progression when full transmural necrosis has not occurred.

The placement of the precordial leads is of paramount importance to obtain reliable ECG patterns. Frequently the precordial leads are placed in the wrong position in haste to obtain the ECG. Verification of proper lead placement should be the first response followed by echocardiography if there remains concern that there has been prior myocardial injury.

Poor R wave progression in the precordial leads

The differential diagnosis of these QRS abnormalities depends on other ECG findings as well as clinical evaluation. Note that the list resembles that of conditions that interfere with the diagnosis of STEMI.

* Normal variant (if the rest of the ECG is normal).
* Misplaced ECG leads.
* Dextrocardia.
* Left ventricular hypertrophy (look for voltage criteria and ST-T changes of LV "strain").
* Complete or incomplete left bundle branch block (increased QRS duration).
* Left anterior fascicular block (should see left axis deviation in frontal plane).
* Anterior or anteroseptal MI.
* Emphysema and COPD (look for R/S ratio in V5 and V6 < 1)
* Diffuse infiltrative or dilated cardiomyopathy.
* WPW preexcitation (look for delta waves, short PR).
* Right ventricular hypertrophy (should see RAD in frontal plane and or P pulmonale).

COPD = chronic obstructive pulmonary disease ; WPW = Wolff-Parkinson-White ; MI = myocardial infarction ; RAD = right axis deviation ; LV = left ventricle

Persistent ST elevation

Persistent ST elevation (convex or concave upwards) after an MI suggests the presence of a LV aneurysm manifested by a thinned dyskinetic LV wall with a broad neck and bulging during systole and diastole. About 3-15% of STEMI develop a left ventricular aneurysm after several weeks. Most LV aneurysms occur after a large anterior or apical MI and ECG changes occur in V1 to V6, I and aVL. Q waves occur in the leads showing ST elevation. The T wave is usually inverted. The ST elevation may be convex upwards or concave. Persistence of ST segment elevation for at least 2 weeks is suggestive of a left ventricular aneurysm. The mechanism of the ST elevation is not well known. Sometimes the ECG is indistinguishable from that of an acute MI in patients with an old MI. This may lead to errors in therapy. Comparison of the ECGs with old tracings is crucial.

Reperfusion

Without reperfusion ST elevation recedes in 12–24 hours. Reperfusion may be achieved with the administration of thrombolytic drugs or emergency angioplasty. Sometimes reperfusion is spontaneous. A resolution of more than 50% of ST segment elevation at 60 to 90 minutes after the initiation of therapy is a good indicator of improved myocardial perfusion and is associated with relief of chest pain, enhanced recovery of LV function, and improved prognosis. A 70% reduction of ST elevation is associated with the most favorable outcome. Q waves may even disappear with early therapeutic reperfusion suggesting that the Q waves may have been the result of a small STEMI or severe ischemia rather than myocardial necrosis. Q waves may also disappear with spontaneous reperfusion. On the other hand, successful reperfusion may cause more rapid evolution of the ECG with the early appearance of Q waves. The appearance of Q waves within < 6 hours of MI onset does not signify irreversible damage and does not preclude myocardial salvage with appropriate reperfusion therapy.

In contrast, persistence of unrelenting ischemic chest pain, absence of resolution of the ST segment elevation, and hemodynamic or electrical instability are generally indicators of failed reperfusion. T wave inversion is a highly specific sign of reperfusion that occurs during the first few hours of successful reperfusion therapy in the leads with the highest ST elevation.

An accelerated idioventricular rhythm occurs in about 50% of reperfused patients (defined as a heart rate of 60 to 120 bpm). It is a highly specific marker of reperfusion but insensitive for the diagnosis of reperfusion. This rhythm is benign and should not be suppressed with medication.

Isolated ventricular premature depolarizations may also be seen with reperfusion. Polymorphic ventricular tachycardia and ventricular fibrillation may be seen with reperfusion but are rare and should arouse suspicion of ongoing arterial occlusion.

Normalization of the ECG in acute coronary syndromes

It is a well-known electrocardiographic principle that electrical forces in a zone that creates QRS changes in a lead, can create reciprocal changes in an opposite lead. An old inferior Q wave MI can be masked by acute anterior MI (countercoup effect). The unmasking of an inferior MI can also be observed after the surgical revascularization of an anterior MI. When an ECG shows persistent T wave inversion accompanying the changes of a previous acute MI, superimposed ischemia in the same territory may cause "normalization" of the T wave (return to an upright position). Alternatively, further ischemia makes the T wave inversion more pronounced.

Takotsubo cardiomyopathy

Takotsubo cardiomyopathy (TCM) mimics acute coronary syndrome. It is accompanied by reversible LV ballooning in the absence of angiographically significant coronary artery stenosis. In Japanese, "takotsubo" means "fishing pot for trapping octopus" (Fig. 17). The LV of a patient diagnosed with this condition resembles that shape during systole, hence the name. It is a transient entity typically precipitated by acute emotional stress. It is called "takotsubo cardiomyopathy", "stress cardiomyopathy", "broken-heart syndrome", or apical ballooning syndrome.

Enhanced sympathetic activity appears to play a very important role in the pathophysiology of takotsubo cardiomyopathy. Triggering factors, such as intense emotional stress, are frequently seen in patients with this syndrome. Catecholamine surge due to intense physical or emotional stress is believed to be the major pathogenic factor in TCM. Plasma catecholamine levels are 2 or 3 times higher in patients as compared with those with MI. The ECG resembles acute

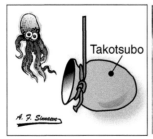
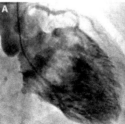
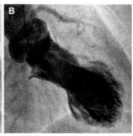

Fig. 17 *The Japanese pot and the left ventricle. (A) Diastole (B) Systole*

CORONARY ARTERY DISEASE AND ACUTE CORONARY SYNDROMES 10

coronary syndrome. The ST elevation evolves into deep T wave inversion but Q waves rarely appear. 95% of ST elevations have been found to involve precordial leads and to be maximal in V2 and V3. When compared with patients with STEMI from left anterior descending coronary artery (LAD) occlusion, the amplitude of ST elevation in patients with TCM is significantly less.

LOCALIZATION OF STEMI

Determination of regions of infarction may be done by analysis of the ECG. Therefore, it should be kept in mind that different leads are looking at different parts of the heart (Fig. 18 – and also chapter 2). To be certain that changes of ST segments or T waves are truly due to ischemia or MI, changes have to be seen in a regional distribution of leads.

I High Lateral	aVR	V1 Anteroseptal	V4 Anterior
II Inferior	aVL High Lateral	V2 Anteroseptal	V5 Low Lateral
III Inferior	aVF Inferior	V3 Anterior	V6 Low Lateral

Fig. 18 *Regions of the heart seen by the leads in the frontal and the precordial plane*

Anterior STEMI

Anterior wall ischemia/infarction is invariably due to occlusion of the left anterior descending artery (LAD) expressed as ST elevation in some or all of leads V1 to V6 and changes in the high lateral leads I and aVL. The location of the occlusion within the LAD whether proximal or distal, is suggested by the precordial leads in which the ST segment elevation occurs and the presence of ST elevation or depression in other leads (extremity and lateral leads) (Fig., p.128). Reciprocal ST depression occurs in the inferior leads (mainly III and aVF) and is determined by the magnitude of the ST elevation in I and aVL (as these high lateral leads are electrically opposite to III and aVF. Reciprocal changes may be minimal or absent in anterior STEMIs that do not involve the high lateral leads.

Sites of anterior STEMI in the precordial leads
* Septal = V1 and V2
* Anterior = V2 to V5
* Anteroseptal = V1 to V4
* Anterolateral = V3 to V6; I + aVL
* Extensive anterior/anterolateral = V1 to V6; I + aVL

Three other important ECG patterns to be aware of:
* Anterior-inferior STEMI due to occlusion of a "wrap around" LAD: simultaneous ST elevation in the precordial and inferior leads due to occlusion of a variant LAD that wraps around the cardiac apex to supply both the anterior and inferior walls of the left ventricle.
* Left main coronary artery occlusion: widespread ST depression with ST elevation in aVR ≥ V1.
* Deep precordial T wave inversions or biphasic T waves in V2 and V3, indicate critical proximal LAD stenosis (a warning sign of imminent anterior infarction).

Sites of occlusion in the LAD

The site of occlusion in the LAD can be inferred from the pattern of ST changes in leads corresponding to the two most proximal branches of the LAD: the first septal branch (S1) and the first diagonal branch (D1).
* S1 supplies the basal part of the interventricular septum, including the bundle branches
  (corresponding to leads aVR and V1)
* D1 supplies the high lateral region of the heart
  (corresponding to leads I and aVL)

> ### Occlusion proximal to S1: Signs of basal septal involvement
> * ST elevation in V1 > 2.5 mm
> * ST elevation in aVR
> * Complete right bundle branch block
>
> ### Occlusion proximal to D1: Signs of high lateral involvement
> * ST elevation / Q wave formation in aVL
> * Reciprocal ST depression ≥ 1 mm in II, III or aVF (reciprocal to
>   ST elevation in aVL)

> **The early diagnosis of STEMI depends on deviation of the ST segment rather than the development of Q waves. The leads with ST segment deviation reflect the site and the size of the ischemic process. Analysis of the ST segment permits identification of the culprit artery.**

Occlusion of the proximal LAD above the first septal and first diagonal branches

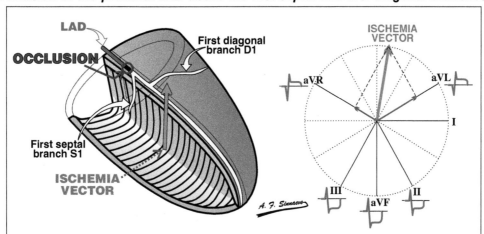

Fig. 19 *LAD occlusion proximal to both S1 and D1 and resulting ischemia vector*

This results in involvement of the basal portion of of the left ventricle, as well as the anterior and lateral walls and the interventricular septum (Fig. 19). This will result in ST segment elevation in leads V1 to V4 (lead V1 ST elevation > 2 mm) and also in lead I /aVL and often in aVR. It will also be associated with reciprocal ST segment depression in the inferior leads II, III, aVF, and often V5. Typically, ST elevation in aVL > aVR and more ST segment depression in lead III than in lead II. Acquired right bundle branch block may occur.

CORONARY ARTERY DISEASE AND ACUTE CORONARY SYNDROMES 11

Occlusion of the LAD between the first septal and first diagonal branches

The basal interventricular septum will be spared, and the ST segment in lead V1 will not be elevated. In that situation, the QT vector will be directed toward I and aVL and the ST segment will be elevated in these leads. On the contrary, the QT vector is directed away from lead III which will show a depression of the ST segment. ST depression in lead III > lead II. (Fig. 20)

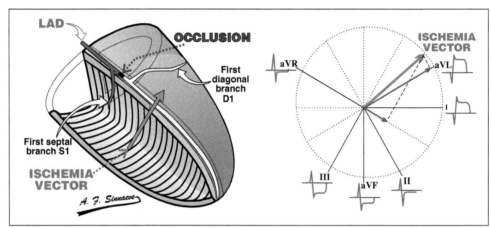

Fig. 20 *LAD occlusion between S1 and D1*

Occlusion of the LAD distal to the first diagonal branch but proximal to the first septal branch

Leads I and aVL will not show ST elevation. ST elevation in lead III > lead II. ST elevation in V1.

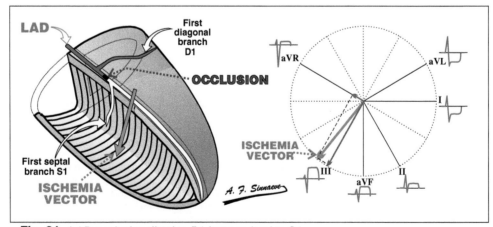

Fig. 21 *LAD occlusion distal to D1 but proximal to S1*

Occlusion of the distal LAD below both the first septal and first diagonal branches

The basal portion of the left ventricle will not be involved, and the QT vector will be oriented more inferiorly. Thus, the ST segment will not be elevated in leads V1, aVR, or aVL, and the ST segment will not be depressed in leads II, III, or aVF. Indeed, because of the inferior orientation of the QT vector, elevation of the ST segment in leads II, III, and aVF may occur (but these leads may be isoelectric). In addition, ST segment elevation may be more prominent in leads V3 to V6 and less prominent in V2 than in the more proximal occlusions.

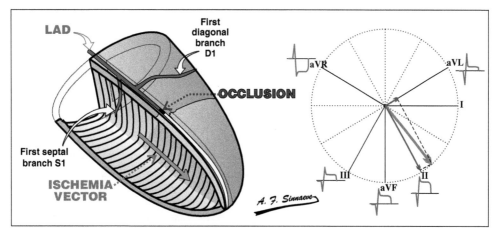

Fig. 22 *LAD occlusion distal to both D1 and S1*

Occlusion of the left main coronary artery

The ECG shows signs of coronary occlusion proximal to the first septal branch and marked ST depression in the inferior leads consistent with severe posterobasal ischemia. Typically lead aVR shows ST elevation ≥ 1 mm. The ST elevation in aVR is greater than the ST elevation in lead V1. The aVR/V1 relationship is enough to warrant a rapid trip to the cardiac catheterization laboratory for angioplasty. The ST segment may be depressed or elevated according to the timing of the pathologic changes. Right bundle branch block is common.

> **ST elevation in aVR is a reliable sign of ischemia in the posterobasal part of the heart (causing marked depression in II, III, and aVF), and the proximal interventricular septum which are supplied by the left main coronary artery.**

CORONARY ARTERY DOMINANCE

The artery that supplies the posterior descending artery (PDA) determines the coronary dominance. If the PDA is supplied by the right coronary artery (RCA) the circulation is "right-dominant." When the PDA is supplied by the left circumflex coronary artery (LCx), the coronary circulation is classified as "left-dominant." If the PDA is supplied by both RCA and LCx, the coronary circulation is classified as "co-dominant" (or balanced). Approximately 70–80% of the general population have a right-dominant system, 10–20% are co-dominant and 10% or less are left-dominant.

Occlusion of a dominant LCx may result in a very large MI involving the posterolateral and inferior wall. An RV MI (in lead V4R) rules out a dominant LCx occlusion. A non-dominant RCA is rarely occluded. Total occlusion of a tiny non-dominant RCA results in a small MI with changes confined to the right precordial leads but no Q waves are generated in the inferior leads.

CORONARY ARTERY DISEASE AND ACUTE CORONARY SYNDROMES 12

Inferior STEMI

The vast majority (80–90%) of inferior STEMIs (ST elevation in leads II, III and aVF) are due to occlusion of the dominant right coronary artery (RCA). Less commonly, the culprit vessel is a dominant left circumflex artery (LCx) depending on which provides the posterior descending branch, that is, which is the dominant vessel. Occasionally, inferior STEMI may result from occlusion of a "wraparound" LAD. Both RCA and LCx perfuse the inferior part of the left ventricle. While an occlusion in RCA or one in LCx may both cause infarction of the inferior wall, the precise area of infarction in each case is somewhat different.

> The RCA territory covers the medial part of the inferior wall, including the inferior septum. The LCx territory covers the lateral part of the inferior wall and the left posterobasal and lateral areas.

Occlusion of the right coronary artery

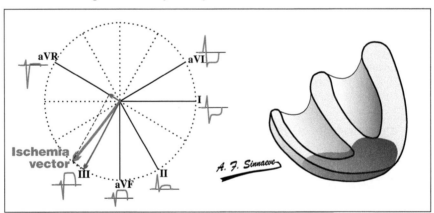

Fig. 23 *Inferior wall STEMI due to occlusion of the RCA*

The rightward and inferiorly directed ischemia vector results in ST segment elevation in lead III > lead II and will often be associated with reciprocal ST segment depression in the leads oriented to the left and superiorly, thus in lead I and in aVL (Fig. 23). ST segment depression in lead I and especially in aVL is highly predictive of RCA occlusion. When the RCA is occluded in its proximal portion, ischemia/infarction of the RV may occur and may be confirmed by recording lead V4R. This finding is important in the distinction between RCA and LCx occlusion and between proximal and distal RCA occlusion. LCx occlusion is suggested by ST elevation in lead II > lead III, absence of reciprocal ST depression in lead I and signs of lateral infarction: ST elevation in the lateral leads I and aVL or V5 and V6.

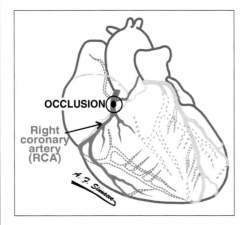

Right ventricular STEMI occurs only with proximal RCA occlusion

In inferior STEMI, ST segment depression in leads I and aVL is highly suggestive of RCA occlusion

Fig. 24 *Occlusion of the proximal part of a dominant RCA. Note that the RV branches are distal to the occlusion so that a RV MI may occur.*

Occlusion of the left circumflex artery

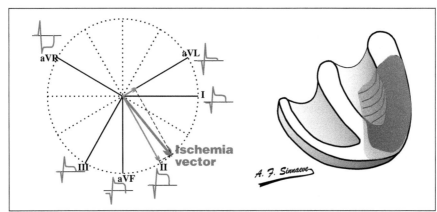

Fig. 25 *Inferior wall STEMI due to occlusion of the LCx*

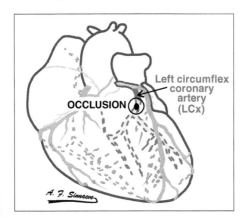

Fig. 26 *Occlusion of a nondominant LCx. The posterior distribution of the vessel is responsible for most cases of posterior MI.*

ST segment depression in leads V1, V2, and V3 that occurs in association with an inferior wall MI may be caused by occlusion of either the RCA or the LCx. This ECG pattern has been termed posterior or posterolateral ischemia. LCx-related STEMI less frequently shows reciprocal ST depression in lead aVL and more often shows an isoelectric or a raised ST segment in leads I and aVL compared to patients with RCA-related inferior MI.

In patients with inferior STEMI, ST depression in leads V1 to V3 has been shown to indicate a larger infarction with extension of the injury to the posterolateral and/or inferoseptal wall.

(continuation on next page)

CORONARY ARTERY DISEASE AND ACUTE CORONARY SYNDROMES 13

ST segment depression in the anterior leads V1 to V3 during STEMI is a reciprocal change and does not indicate concomitant left anterior descending (LAD) coronary artery disease. The changes in V1 to V3 may be seen in both RCA and LCx inferior infarctions. However, in inferior STEMI due to proximal RCA occlusion with concomitant RV infarction, posterior wall injury may be masked because the two opposed electrical vectors may cancel each other (i.e. ST elevation in leads V1 to V3 with RV MI and reciprocal ST depression in these same leads with concurrent posterior infarction). On this basis the absence of ST depression in leads V2 and V3 is strongly suggestive of RCA involvement.

Posterior STEMI

Posterior MI occurs when either the LCx or a branch of the right coronary artery (RCA) – supplying blood to the posterior wall of the left ventricle – is occluded. Posterior MI is the most common manifestation of LCx occlusion. Posterior infarction may accompany an inferior or lateral MI. Posterior extension of an inferior or lateral infarct indicates a much larger area of myocardial damage. Isolated posterior MI is less common.

Look for evidence of posterior MI in any patient with an inferior or lateral STEMI

For all other infarctions the ECG is an essential tool for identifying patients with STEMI who might benefit from reperfusion therapy. The standard 12-lead ECG is relatively poor at examining the posterobasal and lateral walls of the left ventricle so that LCx occlusions are often not recognized.

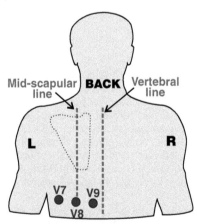

Patients with LCx acute coronary syndromes often present without ST segment elevation even when there is a total occlusion causing a full-thickness posterior or inferobasal MI. Recent registries and trials show over-representation of circumflex occlusions in non-STEMI and underrepresentation in ST elevation MI populations. This is because usually only the 12-lead ECG has been recorded.

The use of posterior leads (V7, V8, and V9) may help in the diagnosis of occlusion of the LCx artery (Fig. 27). Posterior leads V7 (left posterior axillary line), V8 (left midscapular line), and V9 (left border of the spine) are all located in the same horizontal plane as lead V6. ST segment elevation in posterior leads (V7 to V9) is significantly more common during occlusion of the LCx than during RCA occlusion.

Fig. 27 *Posterior leads*

Leads V7 to V9 should be recorded if there is a clinical suspicion of LCx territory involvement. This is important when posterior MI has to be differentiated from acute anterior ischemia by finding ST elevation in leads V7 to V9. The ECG pattern of ST segment elevation in posterior leads V7 to V9 without ST segment depression in lead aVL is highly sensitive and specific for occlusion of the LCx.

Diagnosis of MI according to the QRS complex
No conventional lead is oriented directly to the posterior wall of the heart

Any Q wave in leads V2 and V3 ≥ 0.02 s or QS complex in leads V2 and V3.

Q wave ≥ 0.03 s and ≥ 0.1 mV deep or QS complex in leads I, II, aVL, aVF or V4 to V6 in any two leads of a contiguous lead grouping (I, aVL; V1 to V6; II, III, aVF). The same criteria are used for supplemental leads V7 to V9.

R wave ≥ 0.04 s in V1 and V2 and R/S ≥ 1 with a concordant positive T wave in the absence of a conduction defect.

(Current guidelines (2012) as accepted by ESC/ACCF/AHA/WHF)

A posterior MI may be considered to produce in the right precordial leads the inverse or mirror-image of the opposite ECG leads V7 to V9. Because posterior electrical activity is recorded from the anterior side of the heart, the typical injury pattern of ST elevation and Q waves becomes inverted in the right precordial leads compared to leads V7 to V9.

* ST elevation becomes ST depression.
* Q waves become tall R waves (the equivalent of a Q wave associated with traditional STEMI). The diagnosis of posterior MI should not be ruled out by the absence of a tall R wave in V1 and V2.
* Terminal T wave inversion becomes upright and widened T wave or relatively tall T wave (opposite of T wave inversion).

Causes of a tall R wave in lead V1:
* True posterior infarct: ST↓, T↑ in V1 and V2; Q waves and ST↑ in V7 to V9.
* Right ventricular hypertrophy: right axis deviation, right atrial enlargement, secondary ST-T wave changes; V7 to V9 normal.
* Hypertrophic cardiomyopathy: Q waves; left ventricular hypertrophy; V7 to V9 normal or deep narrow Q waves.
* Right bundle branch block: wide QRS; typical rSR' pattern in V1; V7 to V9 normal or broad S waves
* Wolff-Parkinson-White syndrome with left-sided accessory pathway: short PR; delta wave.
* Left ventricular pacing.
* Normal variant: healthy children and healthy people with prominent forward QRS vectors.

Lateral wall infarction - RCA or LCx occlusion?

In patients with inferior STEMI, ST elevation in leads V5 and V6 is considered to indicate extension of the infarct to the lateral aspect of the cardiac apex. ST segment elevation in leads V5 and V6 is slightly more common in occlusions of the LCx than in occlusion of the RCA. The cause of such an extension may be occlusion of either the LCx or RCA with a posterior descending or posterolateral branch that extends to the lateral apical zone. ST elevation in lead V5 is more frequently associated with involvement of the apical portion of the inferior wall.

It is not unusual for occlusions of the LCx or its branches to show little on the ECG even though they represent a large amount of ischemic myocardium at risk for complete infarction. The circumflex territory is known as being "electrocardiographically" silent.

CORONARY ARTERY DISEASE AND ACUTE CORONARY SYNDROMES 14

Myocardial infarction and right bundle branch block

Right bundle branch block (RBBB) does not usually interfere with the diagnosis of a Q wave MI. RBBB primarily affects the terminal phase of ventricular depolarization, producing a wide R' wave in the right chest leads. These changes are due to delayed depolarization of the right ventricle, while depolarization of the left ventricle is not affected. The criteria for the diagnosis of a Q wave MI in a patient with RBBB are the same as in patients with normal intraventricular conduction. Complete RBBB may mask a posterior infarct.

The appearance of RBBB during an anterior MI strongly suggests an LAD occlusion proximal to the first septal and first diagonal branches and therefore carries a high mortality. The development of RBBB during an acute inferior MI also carries a high mortality but it is less pronounced than with an anterior MI. Transient RBBB is usually not associated with a higher mortality.

Myocardial infarction during left bundle branch block

The diagnosis of MI in the presence of left bundle branch block (LBBB) has long been considered problematic or even almost impossible. Many proposed ECG markers in the old literature have now been discarded. However, the advent of reperfusion therapy has generated greater interest in the ECG diagnosis of acute MI (based on ST segment abnormalities) though criteria for old MI (based on QRS changes) have not been reevaluated for almost 25 years. Electrocardiographic signs involving the QRS complex are not diagnostically useful in the acute setting.

Acute myocardial infarction

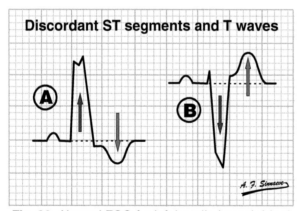

Discordant ST segments and T waves

A. J. Sinnaeve

Fig. 28 *Normal ECG for left bundle branch block*

ST segment deviation is the only useful electrocardiographic sign for the diagnosis of acute MI in the presence of LBBB. In uncomplicated LBBB, ECG leads with a predominantly negative QRS complex show ST segment elevation with positive T waves (Fig. 28).

The diagnosis of acute MI is based on three criteria with relatively poor sensitivity but high specificity (Fig. 29). (1) At least one lead exhibiting ST segment elevation ≥ 1 mm concordant with (i.e. in the same direction as) a predominantly positive QRS complex. (2) Discordant ST segment elevation ≥ 5 mm with (in the opposite direction from) a predominantly negative QRS complex. (3) ST segment depression ≥ 1 mm in V1, V2, or V3. With regard to the weakest criterion (ST segment elevation ≥ 5 mm discordant with the QRS), this sign may occur in clinically stable patients with LBBB without an acute MI in the presence of unusually large QRS complexes in V1 to V3 in which leads the ST segment elevations are also large. Such patients frequently have severe left ventricular hypertrophy or markedly dilated hearts. So-called primary T wave changes (T waves in the same direction as the QRS complex) carry no important diagnostic value. The above markers should be utilized together with the clinical findings because the ECG markers alone miss acute MI in many patients who would benefit from aggressive treatment. The published studies showing poor sensitivity of the ECG markers support the recommendations of the American College of Cardiology and the American Heart Association that all patients with new LBBB, irrespective of ECG features and with symptoms of acute MI, should receive reperfusion therapy.

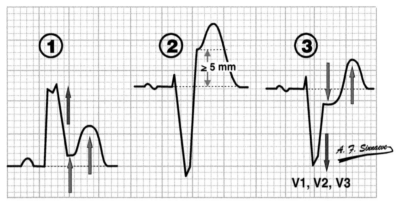

Fig. 29 *Acute myocardial infarction during left bundle branch block*

Old myocardial infarction

The diagnosis of MI in the presence of LBBB is considerably more complicated and confusing than that of RBBB. The reason is that LBBB alters both the early and the late phases of ventricular depolarization. In uncomplicated LBBB septal activation occurs from right to left because the left septal mass cannot be activated via the left bundle branch. Consequently LBBB does not generate a septal q wave in the lateral leads (I and V6). Lead V1 may show an initial r wave because of the anterior component of right-to-left septal activation but leads V1 to V3 may also show QS complexes in the absence of MI. After crossing the ventricular septum, the activation reaches the left ventricle which is depolarized via ordinary myocardium. Secondary ST segment and T wave abnormalities are oriented in the opposite direction to the QRS complex (Fig. 30).

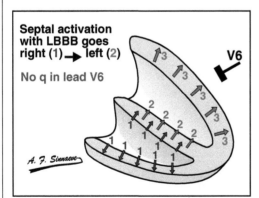

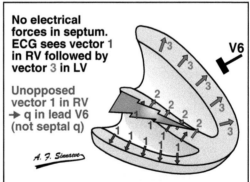

Fig. 30 *Uncomplicated left bundle branch block. The septal vector is oriented from left to right in the normal situation. In LBBB the septal vector is oriented from right to left.*

Fig. 31 *LBBB with extensive anteroseptal MI. In a large septal MI the septal forces are so attenuated that lead V6 records as first deflection the predominance of the RV forces (1). This generates a q wave in V6 but it should not be labeled a restoration of septal forces.*

CORONARY ARTERY DISEASE AND ACUTE CORONARY SYNDROMES 15

During LBBB, an extensive anteroseptal MI will alter the initial QRS vector, with forces pointing to the right because of unopposed activation of the right ventricle. This causes (initial) q waves in leads I, aVL, V5, and V6 producing a Qr or qR pattern (Fig. 31).

A Q or q wave in leads I, aVL or V6 (regardless of size or duration) is highly specific and a relatively insensitive sign for the diagnosis of old anteroseptal MI in the presence of complete LBBB. Late notching of the upstroke of the S wave (Cabrera's sign) in at least 2 leads V3 to V5 is helpful for the diagnosis of anterior MI. Again the sensitivity is low but the specificity is high.

Diagnosis of MI during right ventricular pacing

The ECG diagnosis of MI and ischemia in pacemaker patients can be challenging. The criteria are moderately insensitive for the diagnosis of acute MI and exhibit even lower sensitivity for the diagnosis of old MI. The diagnosis can be made in a limited number of cases because of the high specificity of some criteria. ST-T wave abnormalities are useful only for the diagnosis of acute MI and QRS abnormalities are useful only for the diagnosis of old MI.

Acute myocardial infarction

Three ST segment abnormalities are useful in the diagnosis of acute MI during right ventricular pacing. Their specificity is high but their sensitivity is low or moderate. (1) ST elevation ≥ 5 mm in predominantly negative QRS complexes (inappropriate discordance in ST deviation). (2) ST depression ≥ 1 mm in V1, V2, and V3. (3) ST elevation ≥ 1 mm in leads with a concordant QRS polarity (concordance in ST deviation). ST depression concordant with the QRS complex may occur in leads V3 to V6 during uncomplicated RV pacing. Leads V1 to V3 sometimes show marked ST elevation during right ventricular pacing in the absence of myocardial ischemia or infarction.

> **The diagnosis of MI during RV pacing and that of MI during LBBB are quite similar. The difference of the ECG between both cases might be found in the presence of spikes during pacing.**

Old myocardial infarction

Because the QRS complex during RV pacing resembles (except for the initial forces) that of spontaneous LBBB, many of the criteria for the diagnosis of MI in LBBB also apply to MI during RV pacing. RV pacing almost invariably masks a relatively small anteroseptal MI. During RV pacing, as in LBBB, an extensive anteroseptal MI will alter the initial QRS vector, with forces pointing to the right because of unopposed activation of the RV. This causes (initial) q waves in leads I, aVL, V5, and V6, producing a stimulus-qR (St-qR) pattern. The abnormal q wave is usually 0.03 s or more but a narrower one is also diagnostic. The sensitivity of the St-qR pattern varies from 10 to 50% but the specificity is close to 100%. An extensive anterior MI may produce notching of the ascending limb of the S wave in the precordial leads usually V3 and V4 (Cabrera's sign) > 0.03 s and present in 2 leads. The sensitivity varies from 25 to 50% according to the size of MI but again the specificity is close to 100% if notching is properly defined.

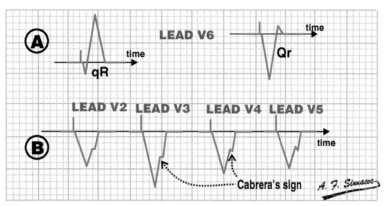

Fig. 32 *Diagnosis of old myocardial infarct (MI)*
(A) A qR or Qr pattern in leads V5 and V6 often indicates an old anteroseptal MI. This pattern may also occur in leads I and aVL.
(B) A shelf-like notch (0.03–0.04 s) on the ascending limb of the S wave, called Cabrera's sign, in leads V2 to V5 often indicates an old anterior MI.

> **In the case of Cabrera's sign, rule out ventricular fusion beats and retrograde P waves.**

Diagnosis of coronary artery disease: Exercise testing

The conventional 12-lead ECG is widely used in a graded exercise test usually performed on a treadmill. Almost all the significant ST segment changes, however, can be demonstrated in leads I and V3 to V6. Horizontal or downsloping ST segment junctional (J point) depression of ≥ 1 mm is the typical ischemic response in stress testing (in all leads except aVR) and is the most generally accepted positive response for ischemia. Slow upsloping ST segments is also generally considered to be an abnormal response. A slow upsloping ST depression using 1.5 mm depressing at 80 ms after the J point is accepted as a reasonable criterion for a positive response (Fig. 15A, 15B and Fig. 33).

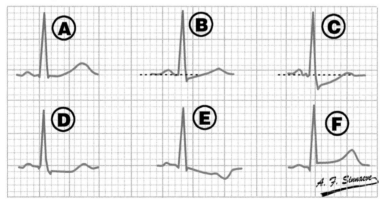

Fig. 33 *Various ST segment patterns produced by exercise: (A) Normal (B) Junctional depression that returns to baseline within 80 ms (C) junctional depression that remains below baseline at 80 ms (D) Horizontal ST depression (E) downsloping ST depression; (F) ST elevation*

CORONARY ARTERY DISEASE AND ACUTE CORONARY SYNDROMES 16

Exercise induction of complete right or left bundle branch block is generally nonspecific. There are many false positive results such as treatment with digoxin, left bundle branch block and left ventricular hypertrophy.

ST segment depression occasionally begins only after exercise. The diagnostic and prognostic significance of such delayed response is generally similar to those occurring during exercise; however, when the onset of the ST abnormalities is delayed by more than 2 to 3 min. into recovery, a false positive response may be present.

Stress-induced ST segment depression is probably caused largely by reduction of perfusion to the subendocardium, the zone most vulnerable to ischemia. Overall, test sensitivity is most often found to lie in the 60 to 70% range.

ST segment elevation

Some patients exhibit ST segment elevation of ≥ 1 mm. In the absence of prior MI, this finding is uncommon but implies severe transmural ischemia of a greater severity than that associated with ST depression. Exercise-induced ST segment elevation is seen most commonly in patients with previous MI. Patients with anterior MI are more likely to have exercise-induced ST segment elevation than are those with inferior MI. The ST elevation almost always occurs in the leads with abnormal Q waves. This response is associated with a left ventricular wall motion abnormality in the corresponding site.

> **In general, the distribution of leads manifesting ST segment depression does not appear to be helpful in localizing the obstructive coronary lesions.**

Arrhythmias in acute myocardial infarction

Supraventricular tachyarrhythmias include sinus tachycardia, premature contractions paroxysmal supraventricular tachycardia, atrial flutter, and atrial fibrillation (AF). AF occurs in 6 to 21% of patients. Many factors can precipitate AF. They include atrial ischemia or infarction, right ventricular MI, pericarditis, severe left ventricular dysfunction and hypokalemia.

Accelerated junctional rhythms

An accelerated junctional rhythm results from increased automaticity of the junctional tissue. The rate is 60–130 bpm. This type of dysrhythmia is most common in inferior MI.

Bradyarrhythmias

These include sinus bradycardia and junctional bradycardia. These disturbances are less common than AV blocks.

Atrioventricular (AV) and intraventricular conduction blocks

These include (1) first-degree AV block, second-degree AV block, and third-degree AV block; (2) intraventricular blocks, including left anterior fascicular block, right bundle branch block (RBBB), and left bundle branch block (LBBB). These conduction disturbances are best understood with a knowledge of the blood supply to the conduction system (Fig. 34).

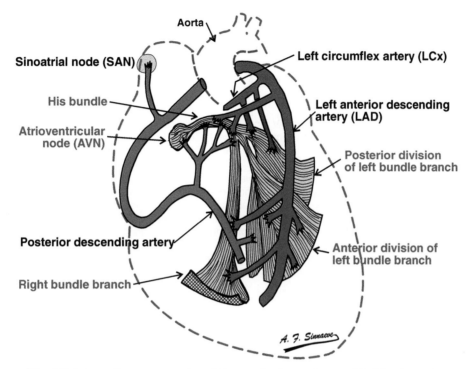

Fig. 34 *Schematic representation of the conduction system and its blood supply*

The AV conduction system (the AV node, the bundle of His, and the bundle branches) is perfused by the right coronary artery (RCA) and the left anterior descending coronary artery (LAD); the AV node and the proximal part of the bundle of His are perfused by the RCA, while the distal part of the bundle of His, the right bundle branch, and the anterior fascicle of the left bundle branch are supplied by the septal branches of the LAD. The posterior fascicle of the left bundle branch is supplied by septal branches from both the LAD and the RCA.

AV nodal conduction disturbances

Conduction abnormalities occur more frequently than sinus node disease or sinus node conduction disturbances. Conduction disturbances at the level of the AV node occur in inferior MI. Second-degree type I (Wenckebach) block may follow first-degree AV block. Type I block may progress to 2:1 AV block, higher degrees of AV block and complete AV block. The QRS remains narrow in most cases. All the conduction disturbances (including complete AV block) are transient with normal AV conduction returning 3–7 days later. AV nodal block after inferior MI is rare

Conduction disturbances below the AV node

The development of conduction disturbances below the AV node is a specific marker for a proximal occlusion of the left anterior descending artery (LAD) and therefore indicates a large jeopardized area of the left ventricle. Therefore conduction disturbances below the AV node carry a poor prognosis. The most common conduction abnormality is right bundle branch block (RBBB) which occurs with an LAD occlusion proximal to the first septal branch with or without left anterior hemiblock. This disturbance is much more common than complete left bundle branch block. When RBBB is the result of the MI, the prognosis is very poor but when the RBBB is preexisting, the hospital mortality rate appears no different from that of patients without RBBB. Infranodal AV conduction disturbances may present with Mobitz type II second-degree AV block (not seen in inferior MI), higher degrees of AV block and complete AV block on the basis of trifascicular block.

CORONARY ARTERY DISEASE AND ACUTE CORONARY SYNDROMES 17

The mortality of patients with complete AV block is very high. Alternating bundle branch block may also occur. Rarely infranodal block presents with a type I (Wenckebach) form of second-degree AV block.

Ventricular arrhythmias

Ventricular arrhythmias include premature ventricular complexes (PVCs), accelerated idioventricular rhythm, ventricular tachycardia, and ventricular fibrillation. An accelerated idioventricular rhythm is seen in as many as 20% of patients. It is a ventricular rhythm characterized by a wide QRS complex with a regular escape rate faster than the atrial rate, but less than 100 bpm. AV dissociation is frequent. Most episodes are short and terminate spontaneously. They occur with equal frequency in anterior and inferior infarctions. If untreated it does not increase the incidence of ventricular fibrillation or death. Idioventricular rhythm may occur more frequently in patients who develop early reperfusion than in others though it should be considered as neither sensitive nor specific for reperfusion

Cardiac ischemia : ECG example 1

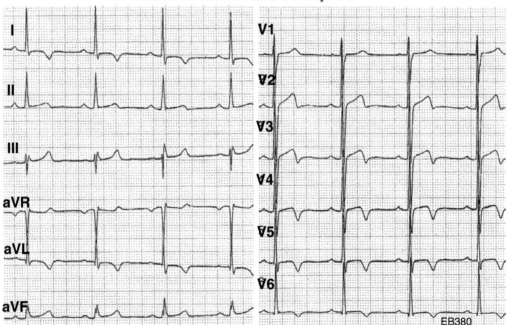

Normal sinus rate at 55 bpm, T wave inversion in I, aVL, V2 to V6 due to ischemia in a patient who presented with unstable angina. Note the terminal inversion in V2 and V3, which occurs typically with ischemia. If these abnormalities are new, the pattern suggests severe ischemia in the distribution of the proximal left anterior descending artery.

Cardiac ischemia : ECG example 2

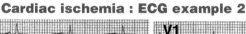

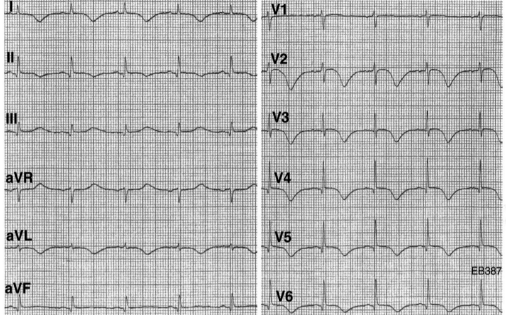

EB387

Normal sinus rate at 75 bpm in a patient with cardiac ischemia. Prominent T wave inversion in I, aVL, V2 to V6. There is also 1 mm ST elevation in V2 to V6. There are small q waves in III and aVF. This pattern may indicate a progressing ST elevation MI. If no MI evolves the abnormalities are due to severe ischemia (unstable angina).

Cardiac ischemia : ECG example 3

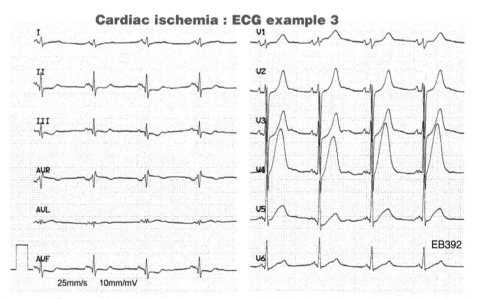

25mm/s   10mm/mV

EB392

Hyperacute T waves V2 to V4 indicating severe acute ischemia or the earliest manifestation of an anterior MI. The ECG evolution and biomarkers will make the diagnosis. There is ST depression inferolaterally. The pattern in the precordial leads is likely to progress to an acute ST elevation MI.

Cardiac ischemia : ECG example 4

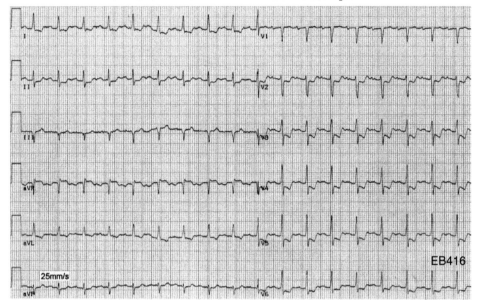

Post-exercise test showing ischemia. Sinus tachycardia at 125 bpm and marked ST and T wave depression in V2 to V6, I and aVL as well as ST elevation in aVR all consistent with ischemia.

Cardiac ischemia : ECG example 5

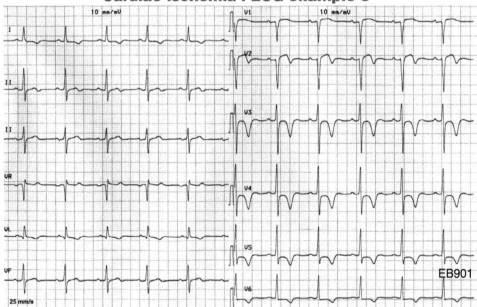

Cardiac ischemia at rest. Sinus rate 70 bpm, ST elevation in V1 and V2, and marked T wave inversion in V2 to V6, I and aVL. The ECG is consistent with ischemia or an early anterior MI. Serial ECGs and biomarkers will make the diagnosis. In the presence of negative biomarker elevation, this pattern is consistent with severe ischemia involving the proximal left anterior descending artery.

Cardiac ischemia : ECG example 6

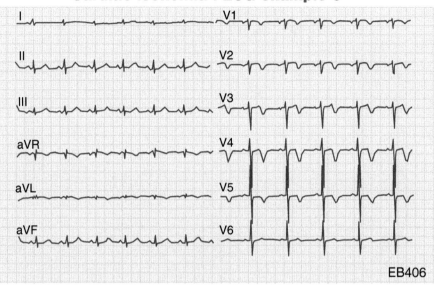

EB406

High risk patient with unstable angina due to stenosis of the proximal left atrial descending artery.
There is T wave inversion in V1 to V5 when the patient was pain free.

Cardiac ischemia : ECG example 7

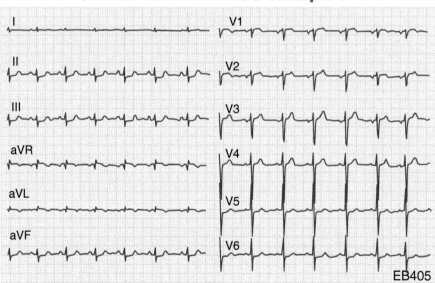

EB405

This ECG was recorded from the same high risk patient as in case 6.
Pseudonormalization during pain.

Inferior myocardial infarction : ECG example 8

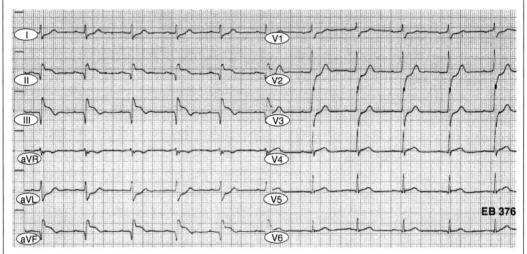

EB 376

Sinus rhythm, acute inferior MI with ST elevation in the inferior leads (III > II suggestive of occlusion of the right coronary artery). Leads II, III and aVF show pathologic Q waves. The R/S ratio in V1 is 1.

Inferior myocardial infarction : ECG example 9

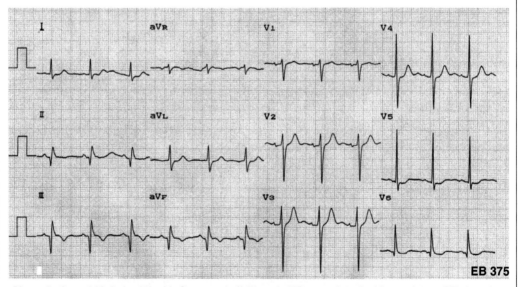

EB 375

Sinus rhythm, old inferior MI with Q waves in II, III and aVF associated with persistent ST elevation. There are nonspecific ST-T wave abnormalities in V5 and V6.

Inferior myocardial infarction : ECG example 10

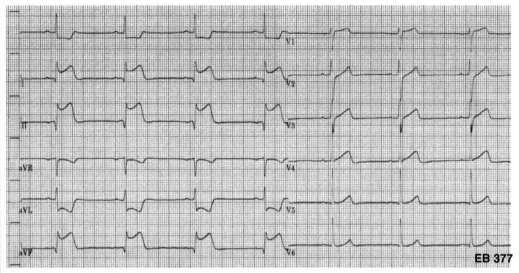

EB 377

Sinus rhythm at 48 bpm, acute inferior MI with ST elevation in II, III, and aVF, (III > II), marked ST depression in I and aVL. The pattern suggests occlusion of the proximal right coronary artery. Note the slight ST elevation in V1 which may be due to a right ventricular infarct.

Inferior myocardial infarction : ECG example 11

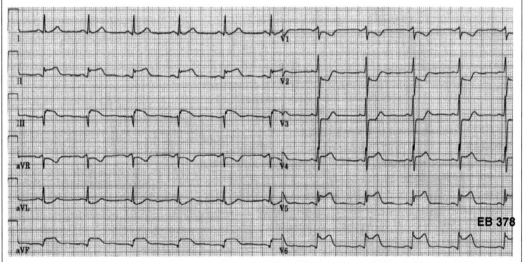

EB 378

Normal sinus rhythm at 68 bpm. Acute inferolateral MI, ST elevation in II, III, aVF, V5 and V6 as well as ST depression in V1 to V3. ST elevation III > II is consistent with occlusion of the right coronary artery. The ST depression in the precordial leads V1 to V3 indicates a large MI with possible involvement of the posterior wall of the left ventricle. With an inferior MI ST-T wave changes in V1 to V3 indicate a large inferior MI but one cannot postulate the presence of a posterior MI or ischemia though both are likely. Lateral involvement is shown in the ST elevation in V5 and V6. Q waves eventually appeared in all inferior leads.

Inferior myocardial infarction : ECG example 12

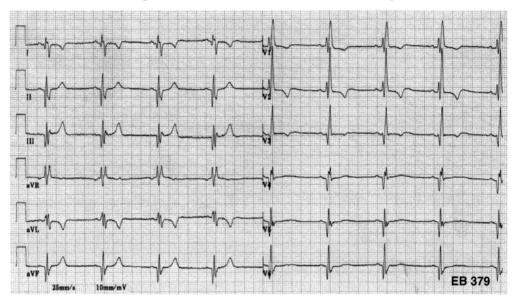

EB 379

Normal sinus rhythm at 60 bpm, complete right bundle branch block, Q waves in II, III, aVF and V4 to V6 consistent with an old inferolateral MI. There is also a low amplitude r wave in V3 which may represent an additional anterior MI. Complete right bundle branch block does not affect the initial forces and therefore does not conceal Q waves of MI.

Inferior myocardial infarction : ECG example 13

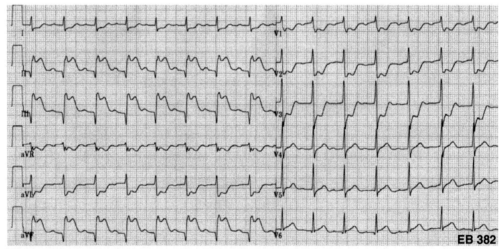

EB 382

Sinus tachycardia at 100 bpm, acute inferior MI with ST elevation in II, III, and aVF and ST III > II consistent with occlusion of the right coronary artery. The marked ST depression in V1 to V3 suggests that the MI is large.

Inferior myocardial infarction : ECG example 14

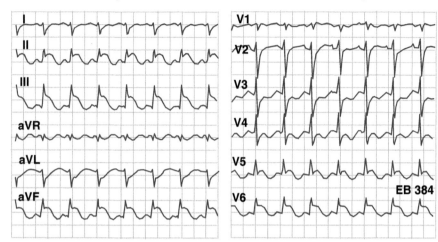

EB 384

Acute inferolateral MI in a cocaine addict. There is right axis deviation, ST elevation in II, III, aVF and V6 and to a lesser extent in V5. There is ST depression and T wave depression in V3 and V4. Lead V1 shows incomplete right bundle branch block. Coronary angiography revealed normal coronary arteries.

Inferior MI with right ventricular infarction : ECG example 15

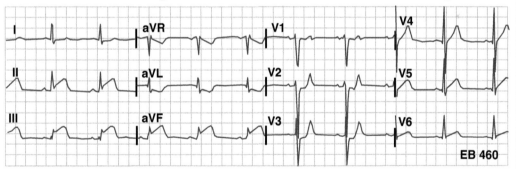

EB 460

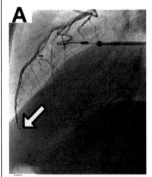 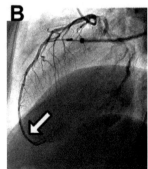

Sinus rhythm.
ST elevation in leads II, III and aVF.
Reciprocal ST depression in aVL.
Slight ST depression in leads V1 to V3.
Acute inferior MI due to occlusion of the left descending artery that curves over the apex.
(A) Coronary angiogram showing distal occlusion of the left descending artery.
(B) The left descending artery after percutaneous coronary intervention.

An apical infarct due to occlusion of the distal left descending artery (which curves around the apex) may result in an ECG suggesting separate inferior MI and anteroseptal MI when there is only one MI.

Inferior myocardial infarction : ECG example 16

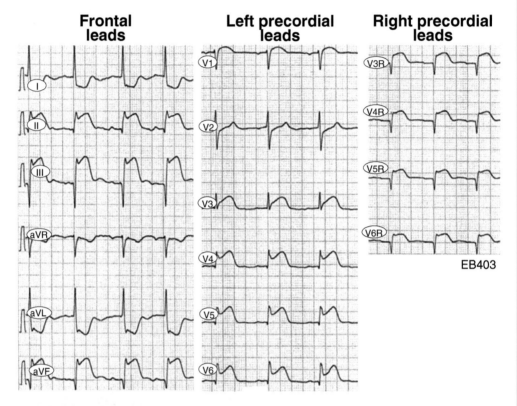

Frontal leads

I

II

III

aVR

aVL

aVF

Left precordial leads

V1

V2

V3

V4

V5

V6

Right precordial leads

V3R

V4R

V5R

V6R

EB403

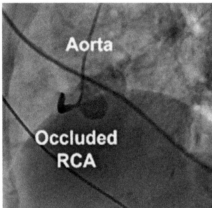

Aorta

Occluded RCA

Normal sinus rhythm at 70 bpm, ST elevation in II, III, and aVF with III > II suggesting a right coronary occlusion. Marked ST depression in I and aVL which are consistent with a lesion in the proximal right coronary artery. There is also slight ST elevation in V1 suggesting the presence of a right ventricular infarct. Leads V3R and V4R show ST elevation > 1 mm indicating the presence of a right ventricular infarct. The patient presented with total occlusion of the proximal portion of a dominant right coronary artery (see coronary angiogram).

RCA = right coronary artery

Posterolateral myocardial infarction : ECG example 17

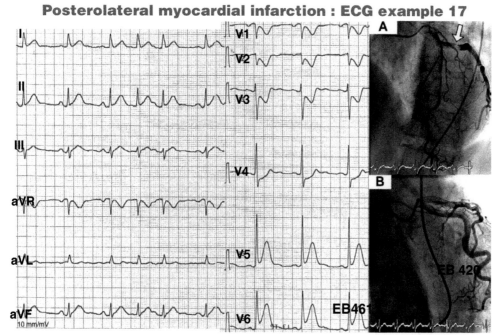

Sinus rhythm and atrial extrasystoles. Acute posterolateral MI. ST elevation in leads V5 and V6. ST depression in leads V1 to V3 which appears to be due to posterior ischemia or MI in this setting. Panel A: Coronary angiogram showing occlusive thrombus (arrow) in the proximal part of of the left circumflex artery (LCx). Panel B: Post PCI and stenting of the LCx.

Posterior myocardial infarction : ECG example 18

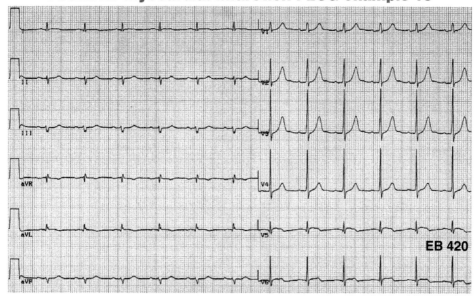

Normal sinus rhythm. Posterior MI with left anterior hemiblock. There is a slight ST elevation in V5 and V6 which may represent lateral injury. Lead V1 shows a dominant R wave due to a recent posterior MI.

Lateral myocardial infarction : ECG example 19

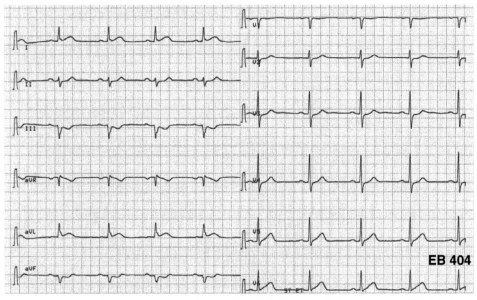

EB 404

Sinus bradycardia. Acute lateral MI with slight ST elevation in leads I and aVL due to a proximal occlusion of a left circumflex coronary artery (as seen in the coronary angiogram).

Infero-posterolateral myocardial infarction : ECG example 20

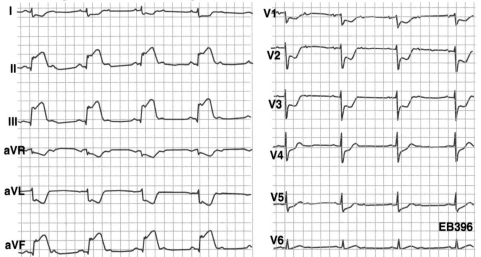

EB396

Acute infero-posterolateral MI. Sinus P waves at a rate of 96 bpm. Ventricular rate at 48 bpm due to second degree AV block. Pardee curve (ST elevation) in the inferior leads II, III, aVF. The ST elevation in lead III being larger than in lead II points to an occlusion of the right coronary artery (RCA). Reciprocal depression in leads I and aVL. The ST depression is greater in aVL than in lead I as lead aVL is more opposed to lead III.

ST depression in V1 to V3 as an expression of posterior ischemia due to occlusion of a dominant RCA. This occlusion of RCA supplying the AV node artery is responsible for the 2nd degree AV block with 2:1 conduction.

Posterior myocardial infarction : ECG example 21

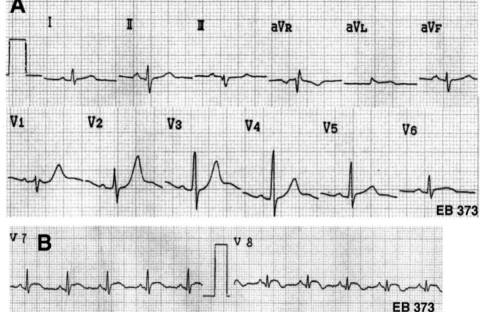

EB 373

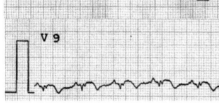

EB 373

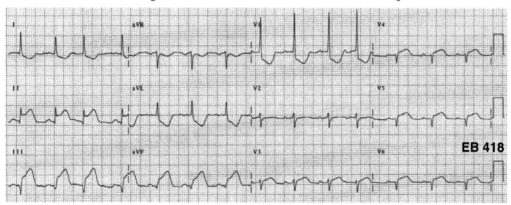

Posterior MI. Normal sinus rhythm with subtle ST elevation in V6 (see panel A). Panel B shows the ECG V7 to V9. Leads V7 to V9 show an acute posterior MI with ST elevation in V7 to V9. There is no evidence of an inferior MI in the inferior leads. The R wave in V2 is slightly larger than the S wave.

Posterior myocardial infarction : ECG example 22

EB 418

Normal sinus rhythm with acute inferolateral MI. There is ST elevation in II, III, aVF, V3 to V6. There are Q waves in II, III, aVF, V5 and V6. There is a tiny r wave in V4. The strikingly tall R wave in V1 was due to an additional acute posterior MI.

Anterior myocardial infarction : ECG example 23

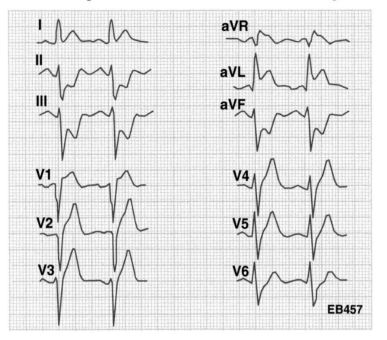

Acute anterior MI involving occlusion of the left anterior descending artery (LAD) proximal to the first septal and first diagonal branches. The ST elevation in aVL indicates an LAD occlusion proximal to the first diagonal branch and the prominent ST elevation in V1 reflects an LAD occlusion proximal to the first septal branch. There is also left anterior hemiblock.

Anterior myocardial infarction : ECG example 24

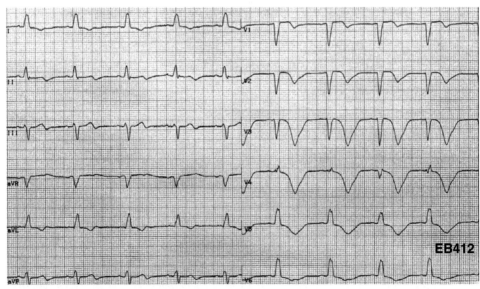

Sinus rhythm (57 bpm). Old anteroseptal MI with anterior ischemia with giant negative T waves from V2 to V5.

Anterior myocardial infarction : ECG example 25

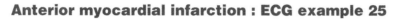

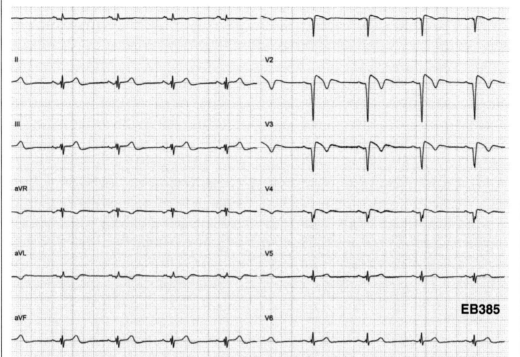

EB385

Old MI with QS waves in leads V1 to V4 and persistent ST elevation consistent with a left ventricular aneurysm.

Anterior myocardial infarction : ECG example 26

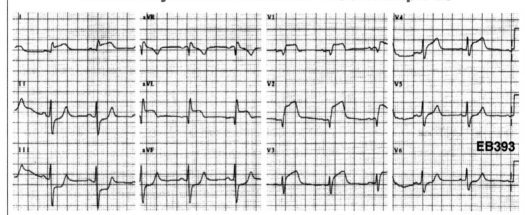

EB393

Extensive anterior myocardial infarction due to a proximal occlusion of the left anterior descending artery; consistent with occlusion of the left anterior descending artery proximal to the first septal and first diagonal branches.

Anterior myocardial infarction : ECG example 27

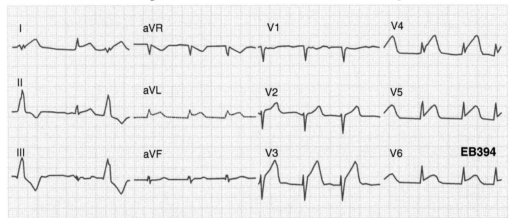

Acute anterior MI due to an occlusion of the left anterior descending artery, distal to the first septal perforator and distal to the first diagonal branch. The ST elevation is predominantly in leads V3 to V6. There is also an ST elevation in leads I and II. There are single premature complexes in leads I, II and III.

Anterior myocardial infarction : ECG example 28

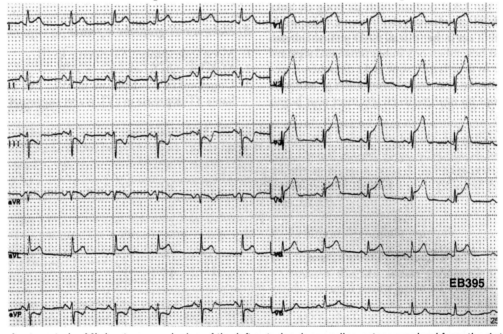

Acute anterior MI due to an occlusion of the left anterior descending artery proximal from the 1st diagonal branch and distal from the 1st septal perforator branch. The diagnosis of anterior MI is based on the ST elevation in V2 to V5. The severity and localization of the MI is based on the evaluation of the frontal leads. The ST depression in the inferior leads II, III and aVF points to a superiorly directed ischemia vector. The ST depression is most pronounced in lead III. Also note the ST elevation in aVL and to a lesser degree in lead I.

Anterior myocardial infarction : ECG example 29

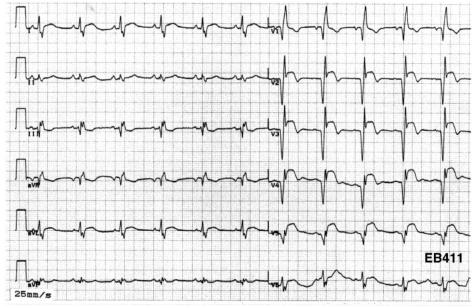

EB411

25mm/s

Sinus rhythm 71 bpm. Old anteroseptal MI. Persistent ST elevation (V2 to V5) as expression of ventricular aneurysm. Complete right bundle branch block (QRS duration 160ms) with initial Q wave due to the MI.

Anterior myocardial infarction : ECG example 30

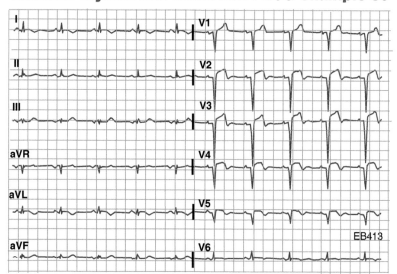

EB413

Sinus rhythm at 69 bpm. Old anterior myocardial infarction with q waves in leads V1 to V5. Persistent ST elevation and terminal negative T waves in leads V1 to V6 due to a left ventricular aneurysm.

Anterior myocardial infarction : ECG example 31

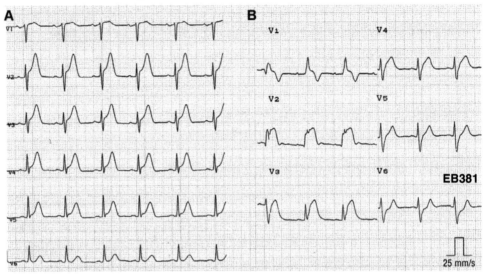

Both ECGs (A & B) are recorded in a patient with a proximal stenosis of the left anterior descending artery. **Panel A** is recorded during an anginal attack. There is a pseudo-normalization of the ECG during pain. The tall and broad T waves are a sign of ischemia. **Panel B**: the diagnosis of proximal left anterior descending artery stenosis was not recognized in this patient and no reperfusion was undertaken. The patient developed an extensive anterior MI with an acquired right bundle branch block and left anterior hemiblock. The development of complete right bundle branch block (which is not rate-dependent or intermittent) reflects a large infarct with a poor prognosis, a situation aggravated by the association of left anterior hemiblock which appeared after the ECG was recorded).

Anterior myocardial infarction : ECG example 32

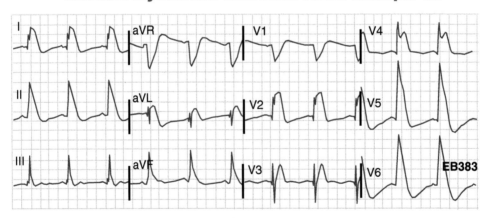

Sinus rhythm at 69 bpm. Acute extensive anterior MI due to occlusion of a left main stem in a patient with a dominant left circumflex artery (LCx). Massive ST elevation

Anterior myocardial infarction : ECG example 33

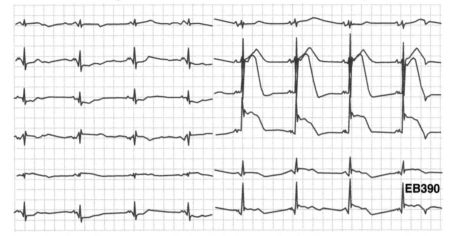

EB390

Sinus bradycardia at 54 bpm. Left atrial abnormality (enlargement or conduction delay). Broad P waves in lead II. Possible old MI : q waves in the inferior leads. Acute anterior ischemia with striking ST elevation in the precordial leads (V2 to V4) and to a lesser degree in leads V5, V6 and aVL. The ECG was recorded 6 hours post resuscitation of ventricular fibrillation.

Anterior myocardial infarction : ECG example 34

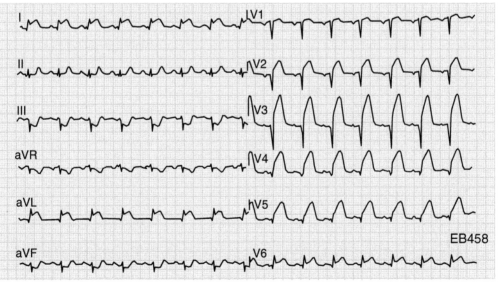

EB458

Acute anterior MI due to occlusion of the left anterior descending artery proximal to the first diagonal branch. ST elevation in all precordial leads. ST elevation in lead I and ST depression in leads III and aVF due to a superiorly oriented ischemia vector.

Anterior myocardial infarction : ECG example 35

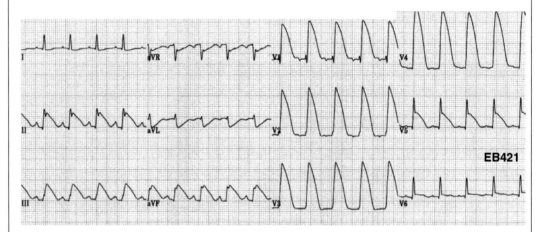

EB421

Sinus tachycardia. Anterior and inferoapical MI beyond apex.
Massive ST elevation in V1 to V5 as well as in the inferior leads suggests proximal occlusion of a large left anterior descending artery which is wrapped around the left ventricular apex or occlusion of a left main coronary artery.

Anterior myocardial infarction : ECG example 36

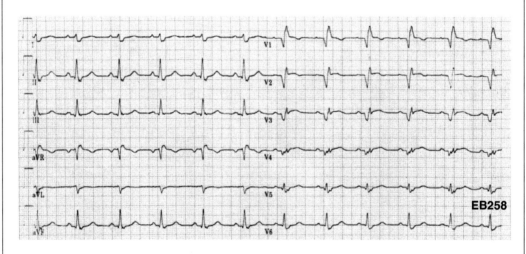

EB258

Sinus rhythm. Anteroseptal MI and recent right bundle branch block.
Note that complete right bundle branch block does not mask an anterior MI.

Anterior myocardial infarction : ECG example 37

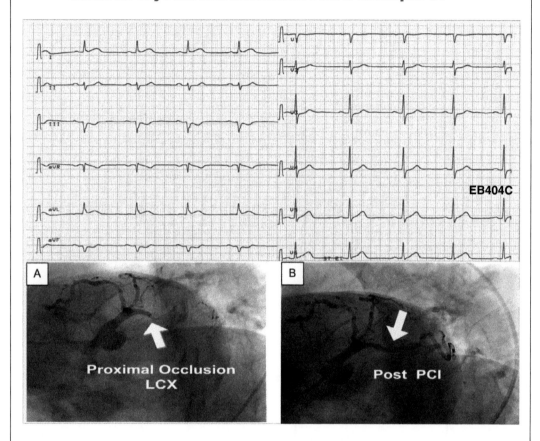

EB404C

A Proximal Occlusion LCX

B Post PCI

Sinus rhythm at 56 bpm. High lateral MI with posterior ischemia. There is only a slight ST elevation in the anterolateral leads aVL, I and V6. A slight ST depression is visible in leads V2 and V3 due to posterior ischemia.
Panel A: Coronary angiogram showing a proximal occlusion of the left circumflex artery (LCx).
Panel B: Coronary angiogram after percutaneous coronary intervention (PCI).

Myocardial infarction and left bundle branch block : ECG example 38

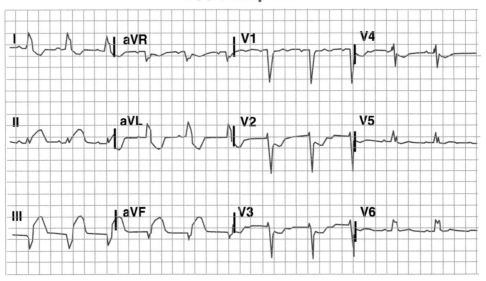

Sinus rhythm. ECG meeting all 3 independent criteria for the diagnosis of inferior MI with left bundle branch block. The ECG shows at least 1 mm concordant ST elevation in lead II, at least 1 mm ST depression in V2 and V3 as well as discordant ST elevation of at least 5 mm in leads III and aVF.

Myocardial infarction and left bundle branch block : ECG example 39

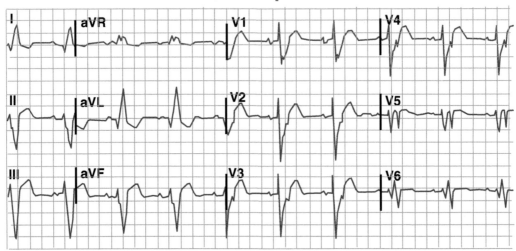

ECG pattern of MI after development of complete left bundle branch block.
There are many signs of anterior MI : tall initial positive deflection (R wave) in lead V1, Cabrera's sign in leads V2 to V4, q wave leads I and aVL, and poor r wave progression in leads V4 to V6.

Myocardial infarction and left bundle branch block : ECG example 40

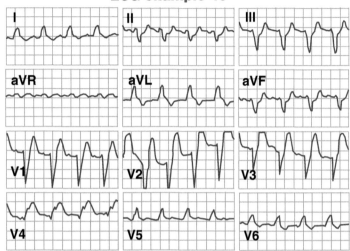

Sinus rhythm with left bundle branch block and an acute anterolateral MI. There is obvious concordant ST elevation in aVL which is less prominent in lead I. The right precordial leads V1 to V4 show marked discordant ST elevation. The striking ST elevation in lead V4 is not seen in uncomplicated left bundle branch block.

Paced rhythm with myocardial infarction : ECG example 41

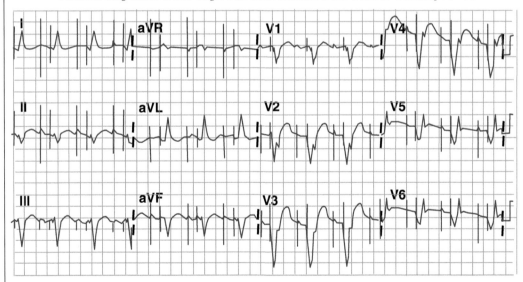

Paced rhythm. 12-lead ECG showing old anteroseptal myocardial infarction during unipolar DDD pacing in a patient with complete AV block. The ventricular stimulus does not obscure nor contribute to the qR pattern in leads I, aVL and V6. Leads V2 to V4 show Cabrera's sign and a variant in lead V5. The lack of an underlying rhythm because of complete AV block excluded the presence of ventricular fusion, which should always be excluded in this situation.

Atar S, Barbagelata A, Birnbaum Y. Electrocardiographic diagnosis of ST-elevation myocardial infarction. Cardiol Clin. 2006;24:343-65.

Atar S, Barbagelata A, Birnbaum Y. Electrocardiographic markers of reperfusion in ST-elevation myocardial infarction. Cardiol Clin. 2006;24:367-76.

Birnbaum Y, Wilson JM, Fiol M, de Luna AB, Eskola M, Nikus K. ECG diagnosis and classification of acute coronary syndromes. Ann Noninvasive Electrocardiol. 2014;19:4-14.

Hurst RT, Prasad A, Askew JW 3rd, Sengupta PP, Tajik AJ. Takotsubo cardiomyopathy: a unique cardiomyopathy with variable ventricular morphology. JACC Cardiovasc Imaging. 2010;3:641-9.

Kakouros N, Cokkinos DV. Right ventricular myocardial infarction: pathophysiology, diagnosis, and management. Postgrad Med J. 2010;86:719-28.

Nikus K, Birnbaum Y, Eskola M, Sclarovsky S, Zhong-Qun Z, Pahlm O. Updated electrocardiographic classification of acute coronary syndromes. Curr Cardiol Rev. 2014;10:229-36.

Sgarbossa EB, Birnbaum Y, Parrillo JE. Electrocardiographic diagnosis of acute myocardial infarction: Current concepts for the clinician. Am Heart J. 2001;141:507-17.

Thygesen K, Alpert JS, Jaffe AS, Simoons ML, Chaitman BR, White HD; Joint ESC/ACCF/AHA/WHF Task Force for the Universal Definition of Myocardial Infarction, Katus HA, Lindahl B, Morrow DA, Clemmensen PM, Johanson P, Hod H, Third universal definition of myocardial infarction. Circulation. 2012;126:2020-35.

Wellens HJ. The ECG in localizing the culprit lesion in acute inferior myocardial infarction: a plea for lead V4R? Europace. 2009;11:1421-2.

White HD, Thygesen K, Alpert JS, Jaffe AS. Clinical implications of the Third Universal Definition of Myocardial Infarction. Heart. 2014;100:424-32.

ST segment elevation

Birnbaum Y, Bayés de Luna A, Fiol M, Nikus K, Macfarlane P, Gorgels A, Sionis A, Cinca J, Barrabes JA, Pahlm O, Sclarovsky S, Wellens H, Gettes L. Common pitfalls in the interpretation of electrocardiograms from patients with acute coronary syndromes with narrow QRS: a consensus report. J Electrocardiol. 2012;45:463-75.

Huang HD, Birnbaum Y. ST elevation: differentiation between ST elevation myocardial infarction and nonischemic ST elevation. J Electrocardiol. 2011;44:494.e1-494.e12.

Jayroe JB, Spodick DH, Nikus K, Madias J, Fiol M, De Luna AB, Goldwasser D, Clemmensen P, Fu Y, Gorgels AP, Sclarovsky S, Kligfield PD, Wagner GS, Maynard C, Birnbaum Y. Differentiating ST elevation myocardial infarction and nonischemic causes of ST elevation by analyzing the presenting electrocardiogram. Am J Card;2009:103:301-6.

Nikus K, Pahlm O, Wagner G, Birnbaum Y, Cinca J, Clemmensen P, Eskola M, Fiol M, Goldwasser D, Gorgels A, Sclarovsky S, Stern S, Wellens H, Zareba W, de Luna AB. Electrocardiographic classification of acute coronary syndromes: a review by a committee of the International Society for Holter and Non-Invasive Electrocardiology. J Electrocardiol. 2010;43:91-103.

Pollak P, Brady W. Electrocardiographic patterns mimicking ST segment elevation myocardial infarction. Cardiol Clin. 2012;30:601-15.

Wang K, Asinger RW, Marriott HJ. ST-segment elevation in conditions other than acute myocardial infarction. N Engl J Med. 2003;349:2128-35.

Wei EY, Hira RS, Huang HD, Wilson JM, Elayda MA, Sherron SR, Birnbaum Y. Pitfalls in diagnosing ST elevation among patients with acute myocardial infarction. J Electrocardiol. 2013;46:653-59.

Early repolarization

Antzelevitch C, Yan GX. J wave syndromes. Heart Rhythm. 2010;7:549-58.

De Ambroggi L, Sorgente A, De Ambroggi G. Early repolarization pattern: innocent finding or marker of risk? J Electrocardiol. 2013;46:297-301.

Junttila MJ, Sager SJ, Tikkanen JT, Anttonen O, Huikuri HV, Myerburg RJ. Clinical significance of variants of J-points and J-waves: early repolarization patterns and risk. Eur Heart J. 2012;33:2639-43.

Obeyesekere MN, Klein GJ, Nattel S, Leong-Sit P, Gula LJ, Skanes AC, Yee R, Krahn AD. A clinical approach to early repolarization. Circulation. 2013;127:1620-9.

Pérez-Riera AR, Abreu LC, Yanowitz F, Barros RB, Femenía F, McIntyre WF, Baranchuk A. "Benign" early repolarization versus malignant early abnormalities: clinical-electrocardiographic distinction and genetic basis. Cardiol J. 2012;19:337-46.

Stern S. Clinical aspects of the early repolarization syndrome: a 2011 update. Ann Noninvasive Electrocardiol. 2011;16:192-5.

CHAPTER 9

ACUTE PERICARDITIS

* Clinical stages
* Other conditions with similar features
* Differential diagnosis
* Early repolarization

ECG from Basics to Essentials: Step by Step. First Edition. Roland X. Stroobandt, S. Serge Barold and Alfons F. Sinnaeve.
Published 2016 © 2016 by John Wiley & Sons, Ltd. Companion Website: www.wiley.com/go/stroobandt/ecg

ACUTE PERICARDITIS 1

ECG changes in acute pericarditis mainly indicate inflammation of the epicardium (the layer directly surrounding the heart). The ECG is useful in the diagnosis of acute pericarditis, with abnormalities found in approximately 90% of cases. Not all cases of pericarditis include each of the four stages shown below. In fact, all four stages are present in only 50% of patients or less.

Stage I:

The most sensitive ECG change characteristic of acute pericarditis is ST segment elevation, which reflects the abnormal repolarization that develops secondary to pericardial inflammation. The ST elevation occurs during the first few days of pericardial inflammation and is mainly characterized by diffuse upward concavity (saddle-shaped). ST segment elevation is usually less than 5 mm with concordance of the T wave. ST elevation involves the limb leads and precordial leads with reciprocal ST segment depression only in aVR and V1. This limited change in aVR and V1 represents a lack of substantial reciprocal changes corresponding to the extensive ST elevation. PR segment depression that may be subtle (1 mm or so) may occur in all the leads except aVR and V1 where the PR segment may be elevated. The PR changes are thought to be due to atrial wall injury.

Thus, the PR and ST changes are opposite in direction. The PR changes are very specific and may be earliest manifestation of pericarditis. The ECG may show low voltage (i.e. decreased amplitude of the QRS complexes) and there are no Q waves. This stage may last up to two weeks.

Stage II:

Normalization of ST and PR deviations; T wave flattening. This stage lasts from days to several weeks.

Stage III:

Diffuse T wave inversion. This stage begins at the end of the second or third week and lasts several weeks (these changes may not be present in all patients).

Stage IV:

Gradual resolution of T wave inversion that may last up to three months. Alternatively T waves may become indefinitely inverted.

The development of a pericardial effusion may cause low QRS voltage and excessive cardiac mobility may cause total electrical alternans.

1. The ST segment elevation in acute pericarditis is usually "concave", compared with the "convex" appearance of the ST segment in the acute injury stage of a myocardial infarction (MI).
2. The widespread ST segment elevation does not correspond with any specific arterial territory, which usually occurs with acute MI.
3. Reciprocal changes are absent in acute pericarditis, but frequent with acute MI.

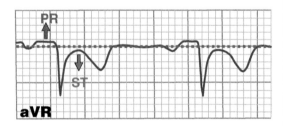

aVR

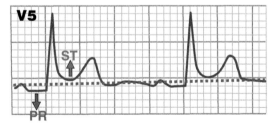

V5

DIFFERENTIAL DIAGNOSIS

Other conditions may have ECG features similar to those of acute pericarditis. These conditions most commonly include myocardial infarction and early repolarization. The ST segment elevation that occurs during acute pericarditis is usually "concave", compared with the "convex" appearance of the ST segment that occurs during the acute injury stage of a myocardial infarction. The widespread ST segment elevation does not correspond with any specific arterial territory, which usually occurs with territorial distribution in acute myocardial infarction. Also, obvious reciprocal changes are absent in acute pericarditis, although they are frequently found with acute myocardial infarction. Another feature that may aid in differentiating acute pericarditis from acute myocardial infarction is the absence of T wave inversion at the time of ST segment elevation in pericarditis. Such a change classically occurs with acute myocardial infarction where T wave inversions appear before the ST segments return to baseline. Acute myocardial infarction may generate Q waves or loss of R wave voltage in the precordial leads.

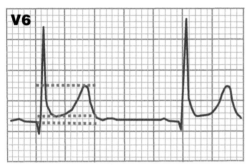

ST segment height = 1 mm
T wave height = 6 mm
ST / T wave ratio = 0.16
ST / T < 0.25 is consistent with ER

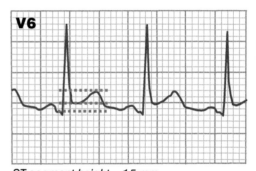

ST segment height = 1.5 mm
T wave height = 3.5 mm
ST / T wave ratio = 0.43
ST / T > 0.25 is consistent with pericarditis

Early repolarization (ER) is a normal variant that does not evolve with the stages of acute pericarditis. Early repolarization is distinguished by ST segment elevation limited to the precordial leads, elevation of the ST segment in V1, an isoelectric ST segment in lead V6 and notching of the terminal aspect of the QRS complex. A useful measurement in differentiating acute pericarditis from early repolarization is the ST / T ratio in lead V6. This is calculated by dividing the millimeters of ST segment elevation by the millimeters to the tallest point of the T wave. Each value is measured from the isoelectric point. With an ST / T ratio greater than 0.25 in lead V6, acute pericarditis is almost always present. An ST / T ratio smaller than 0.25 suggest the early repolarization variant.

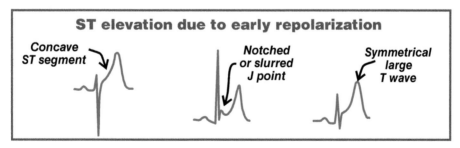

The J point is the point at which there is an abrupt transition from the QRS complex to the ST segment. Deviation of the J point from the isoelectric line causes a J-deflection. Early repolarization is a variant seen in approximately 2 to 5% of the general population, with predominance in young men especially in athletes and people of African-American descent.

ACUTE PERICARDITIS 2

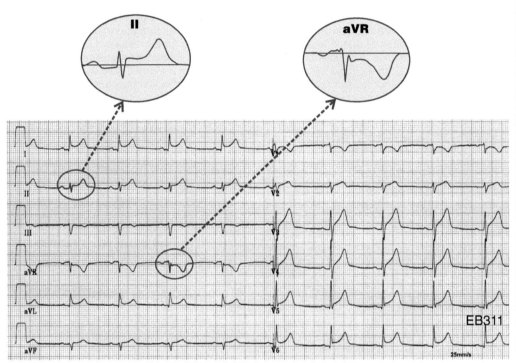

Pericarditis with PR elevation in aVR and PR depression in lead II

Early repolarization is characterized by elevation of the J point or the ST segment itself at the beginning of the ST segment (onset of ventricular repolarization) seen in 2 contiguous leads. Sometimes, this is accompanied by relatively prominent and peaked concordant T waves. There may be slurring of the terminal QRS (the transition from the QRS to the ST segment) or notching (a positive deflection inscribed on the terminal QRS). Notching and slurring at the J point is highly suggestive of early repolarization variant.

The pattern of ST elevation varies in degree, morphology, and location and may be dynamic waxing and waning over time. The ST segment is concave up (cup-like and also referred to as rapidly ascending). The ST elevation (up to 3 mm or so) is more likely in the lateral precordial leads V3 to V6. Although ST changes may be observed diffusely in many leads (normally 1 mm or less in the limb leads), approximately one-half of patients with precordial lead findings have no ST deviations in the limb leads. ST changes may transiently return to the baseline when the J point is minimally elevated with a prominent T wave. Bradycardia enhances the early repolarization pattern. Although so-called "early repolarization" has been considered a completely benign finding for many years, prognosis may vary according to the morphology of the ST segment or which leads are affected.

A pattern of ST segment elevation similar to early repolarization may be seen in patients with myocardial infarction.

Early repolarization has recently been found to be associated with an increased risk of cardiac death from ventricular fibrillation. Early repolarization may be important in patients with syncope, family history of sudden death or even in the presence of ventricular tachyarrhythmias. At present, we have no way of finding the asymptomatic patients at risk for sudden death. Nothing is required in such individuals.

Acute myocarditis can cause diffuse ST segment elevation, as does pericarditis. Furthermore, at times the prominent ST segment elevation of acute myocarditis can simulate acute myocardial infarction.

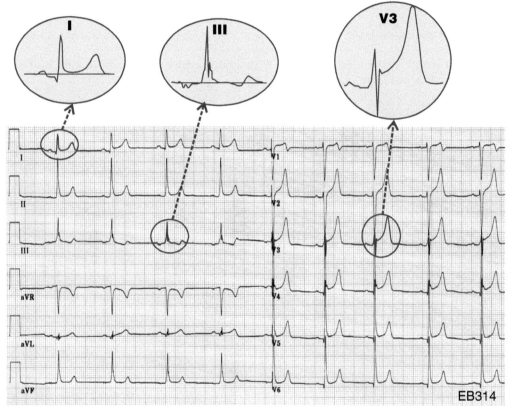

EB314

Early repolarization with concave ST segment elevation, notched J point and symmetrical large T waves.

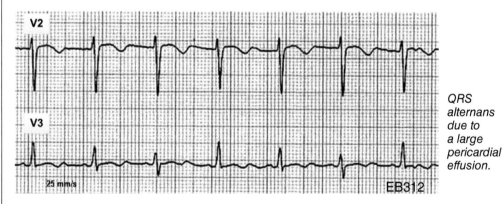

EB312

QRS alternans due to a large pericardial effusion.

Ariyarajah V, Spodick DH. Acute pericarditis: diagnostic cues and common electrocardiographic manifestations. Cardiol Rev. 2007;15:24-30.

Pollak P, Brady W. Electrocardiographic patterns mimicking ST segment elevation myocardial infarction. Cardiol Clin. 2012;30:601-15.

Punja M, Mark DG, McCoy JV, Javan R, Pines JM, Brady W. Electrocardiographic manifestations of cardiac infectious-inflammatory disorders. Am J Emerg Med. 2010;28:364-77.

CHAPTER 10

THE ECG IN EXTRACARDIAC DISEASE

* Pulmonary diseases and cor pulmonale
    ◦ Right atrial enlargement
    ◦ Chronic obstructive pulmonary disease
    ◦ Pulmonary embolism
* Hypothermia
* Diseases of the central nervous system
* Acute pancreatitis
* Hypothyroidism and hyperthyroidism
* Electrocardiography in athletes

ECG from Basics to Essentials: Step by Step. First Edition. Roland X. Stroobandt, S. Serge Barold and Alfons F. Sinnaeve.
Published 2016 © 2016 by John Wiley & Sons, Ltd. Companion Website: [insert url, once provided]

THE ECG IN EXTRACARDIAC DISEASE 1

PULMONARY DISEASES and COR PULMONALE

Cor pulmonale is defined as an alteration in the structure and function of the right ventricle caused by a primary disorder of the pulmonary system. Cor pulmonale usually presents chronically, but two conditions can cause acute cor pulmonale: pulmonary embolism (more common) and acute respiratory distress syndrome (ARDS). In chronic cor pulmonale, right ventricular hypertrophy (RVH) is generally seen. Acute cor pulmonale causes mainly right ventricular dilatation. In massive pulmonary embolism cor pulmonale is due to the sudden increase in pulmonary vascular resistance.

ECG is neither a sensitive nor a specific tool for diagnosing right atrial enlargement, RVH, or pulmonary hypertension. The ECG will be normal in mild cases of RVH. However, the ECG abnormalities may support the patient's clinical evaluation and may prevent the changes on the ECG from being wrongly attributed to other conditions, such as cardiac ischemia.

Right atrial enlargement

The electrocardiographic changes suggesting right atrial enlargement often correlate poorly with the clinical and pathologic findings. Right atrial enlargement is associated with chronic obstructive pulmonary disease, pulmonary hypertension, and congenital heart disease. Right atrial hypertrophy or dilatation generates tall P waves in the anterior and inferior leads, though the overall duration of the P wave is not usually prolonged. A tall P wave (height at least 2.5 mm) in leads II, III and aVF is known as a *P pulmonale*. Right atrial enlargement is mostly associated with right ventricular hypertrophy, a combination that may be reflected in the ECG. The ECG features of right atrial enlargement may be present without coexisting evidence of RVH. P pulmonale may appear transiently and without the manifestations of RVH in patients with acute pulmonary embolism.

Chronic obstructive pulmonary disease

In chronic obstructive pulmonary disease (COPD), hyperinflation of the lungs leads to depression of the diaphragm, a vertical heart position with associated clockwise rotation of the heart (the right ventricle is more anterior and the left ventricle more posterior). This clockwise rotation causes the transitional zone (defined as the progression of rS to qR in the chest leads) to shift towards the left with persistence of an rS pattern as far as V5 or even V6. This may give rise to a "pseudoinfarct" pattern, poor R wave progression or even Q waves as in anterior myocardial infarction. The complete absence of R waves in leads V1 to V3 is known as the "SV1-SV2-SV3" pattern. The amplitude of the QRS complexes may be small as the hyperinflated lungs are poor electrical conductors especially in the left precordial leads (V4 to V6). There may be right axis deviation and right ventricular hypertrophy. Left axis deviation is less common. Right atrial hypertrophy or dilatation is associated with tall P waves. A tall P wave (P pulmonale) may be the most frequent ECG abnormality in COPD. Right atrial enlargement and right ventricular hypertrophy (sometimes indicated by right bundle branch block) are manifestations of cor pulmonale. Typical arrhythmias are atrial fibrillation, atrial flutter and multifocal atrial tachycardia which is a rapid, irregular atrial tachycardia with at least 3 distinct P wave morphologies (associated with increased mortality in patients with COPD). Multifocal atrial tachycardia is typical of COPD and is often confused with atrial flutter.

Pulmonary embolism

Pulmonary embolism (PE) is one of the most commonly missed diagnoses leading to mortality in hospitalized patients. This is often due to the nonspecific signs and symptoms of pulmonary embolism. There are no pathognomonic ECG changes for the diagnosis or its exclusion. No isolated ECG abnormality is definitely associated with PE and the ECG can occasionally be normal. ECG changes are all fairly insensitive for the diagnosis of PE. ECG changes appear when pulmonary embolism is sufficiently large to cause right ventricular dilatation. A large embolus or multiple smaller emboli will cause acute pulmonary hypertension. Rather it is the constellation of ECG abnormalities that helps one to suspect the diagnosis of PE. The commonest ECG abnormality is sinus tachycardia. ECG abnormalities are often transient and sequential ECGs should be recorded. The ECG abnormalities resolve with appropriate therapy. ECG findings noted during the acute phase of pulmonary embolism can include any number of the following:

* Right shift of QRS axis
* Right axis deviation
* "S1Q3T3" - prominent S in lead I, Q and inverted T in lead III
* Right bundle branch block, complete or incomplete, often resolving after the acute phase
* Clockwise rotation: shift of the R/S transition point toward V6, persistent S wave in V6
* ST elevation in V1 and aVR
* Tall R wave in V1
* Generalized low-amplitude QRS (less than 5 mm in the inferior leads)
* Arrhythmias: sinus tachycardia, atrial fibrillation/flutter. New onset of atrial fibrillation is important.
* Right ventricular strain pattern: T wave inversions in V1 to V3, sometimes extending to V4. Simultaneous T wave inversions in the inferior (II, III, aVF) and right precordial (V1 to V3) leads.
* Right atrial enlargement (P pulmonale): peaked P waves in lead II (> 2 mm in height) in the absence of ECG evidence of right ventricular hypertrophy.

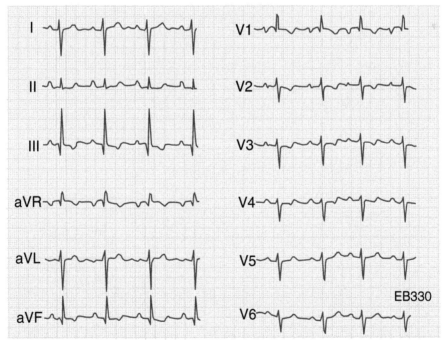

*Acute Pulmonary Embolism. Sinus rhythm - RR = about 880 ms; HR = about 69 bpm;
P pulmonale P wave > 2.5 mV; right axis deviation: QRS axis at +125°; deep S wave in I & aVL;
qR in III & aVF; S1Q3T3 syndrome; incomplete RBBB; negative T wave in V1 & V2.*

THE ECG IN EXTRACARDIAC DISEASE 2

HYPOTHERMIA

Hypothermia can be accidental or medically induced. Therapeutic hypothermia is used to protect the brain of comatose patients with anoxic brain injury following resuscitation from prehospital witnessed cardiac arrest and cardiopulmonary resuscitation.

Elderly people are particularly at risk during the winter months as they often live alone in inadequately heated rooms. The Osborn wave, also known as the J wave, is the most striking ECG feature. It is a "hump-like" deflection between the QRS complex and the early part of the ST segment. The amplitude and the duration of the wave increase with decreasing body temperature. With rewarming, the amplitude decreases but the J wave abnormality can persist 12 to 24 h after restoration of body temperature. Ventricular arrhythmias are the most common mechanism of death in hypothermia. They seem to be more common during rewarming as the body temperature rises through the 28–32 °C range. The Osborn wave is caused by a more prominent potassium current caused by a transmural voltage gradient created by the presence of a prominent action potential notch in the epicardium but not in the endocardium. The Osborn wave is not specific for hypothermia, as it may be seen in hypercalcemia, certain CNS lesions and as a normal variant.

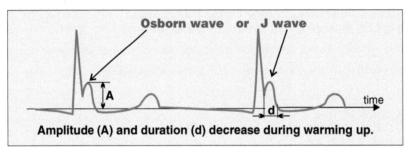

Amplitude (A) and duration (d) decrease during warming up.

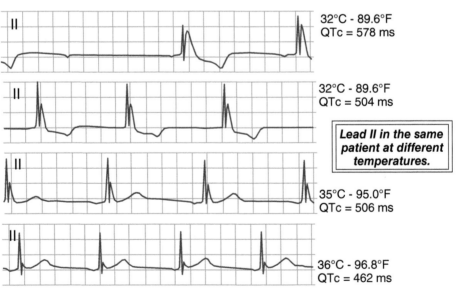

II — 32°C - 89.6°F QTc = 578 ms

II — 32°C - 89.6°F QTc = 504 ms

Lead II in the same patient at different temperatures.

II — 35°C - 95.0°F QTc = 506 ms

II — 36°C - 96.8°F QTc = 462 ms

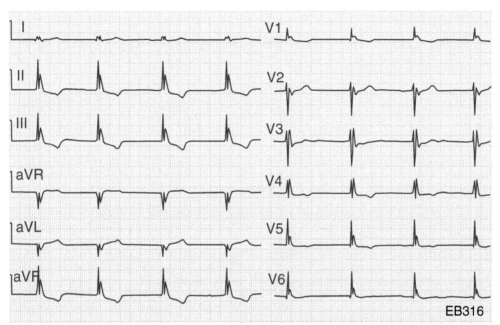

EB316

Patient treated with hypothermia (temp. 32°C - 89.6°F) after resuscitation of out-of-hospital cardiac arrest. Sinus bradycardia 49 bpm. The P waves are hardly visible. First degree AV block: PR = 360 ms. Prominent Osborn waves visible in all leads.

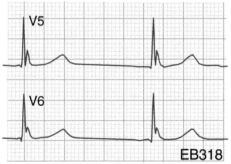

EB318

Same patient with hypothermia at 35°C - 95°F

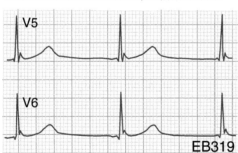

EB319

Same patient with hypothermia at 36°C - 96.8°F

Note. The medical benefit of hypothermia was first discovered in the 19th century when a surgeon in Napoleon's army noticed that wounded soldiers that were put close to a camp-fire expired earlier than those who were not rewarmed...

THE ECG IN EXTRACARDIAC DISEASE 3

DISEASES OF THE CENTRAL NERVOUS SYSTEM

The association of specific ECG changes with intracranial disease has been recognized for over 50 years. ECG abnormalities occur most often in patients with subarachnoid hemorrhage, but also have been described in cases of ischemic stroke, intracranial hemorrhage, head trauma, neurosurgical procedures, and intracranial space-occupying tumors.

The most striking ECG changes are usually associated with subarachnoid hemorrhage. The abnormalities are less pronounced in patients with a nonhemorrhagic stroke. Cerebrovascular disorders mainly cause abnormalities of ventricular repolarization. There is no specific abnormality. The most common findings are depressed ST segments, flat or inverted T waves, prominent U waves (> 1 mm), and prolongation of the QTc interval. Q waves may also occur. The ECG changes also include symmetrically large peaked T waves and giant, wide "roller coaster" inverted T waves that reflect myocardial ischemia unrelated to the traditional form of coronary artery disease. Prolonged QT intervals are uncommonly associated with torsades de pointes (polymorphic ventricular tachycardia). The ECG changes in disease of the autonomic nervous system sometimes cannot be differentiated from those noted in acute coronary syndrome. The ECG abnormalities are often transient but may persist as long as 8 weeks. Many patients with ECG changes have no clinical evidence of myocardial damage.

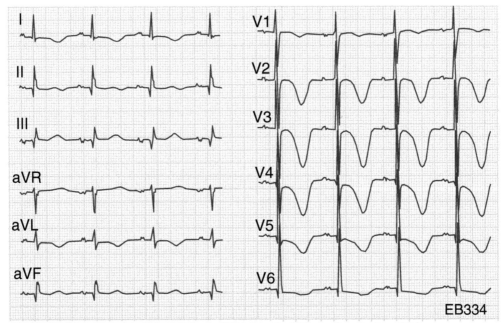

EB334

Patient with subarachnoid hemorrhage. RR interval = 960 ms; heart rate = 63 bpm; measured QT = 450 ms ; corrected QTc = 460 ms . Marked T wave inversions in the absence of coronary artery disease.

The pathophysiology of these ECG abnormalities is not entirely clear. Clinical and experimental data suggest that some kind of neurologically mediated myocardial injury exists especially in subarachnoid hemorrhage. The ECG abnormalities do not represent a manifestation of coexisting coronary artery disease. It is likely that the ECG changes reflect transient electrophysiologic changes in the heart presumably from reflex mechanisms related to a general disturbance of the autonomic system. Autopsy studies of the heart in patients who died following acute stroke have shown widespread myocardial necrosis and hemorrhagic lesions that were detected near the nerve endings suggesting a possible neurogenic origin.

ACUTE PANCREATITIS

Acute pancreatitis may be associated with ST segment elevation imitating acute myocardial infarction. Other abnormalities include nonspecific T wave changes, sinus tachycardia, QT prolongation and intraventricular conduction disturbances. The mechanism of these changes is obscure. It could be the result of metabolites, reflexes, coronary spasm or the effect of proteolytic enzymes causing myocardial necrosis.

HYPOTHYROIDISM

No changes may occur. However possible changes include: sinus bradycardia, a prolonged PR and QT interval, low P, T and QRS amplitude, ST deviation or T wave flattening/inversions across most or all leads, atrioventricular and intraventricular conduction disturbances such as right bundle branch block. A pericardial effusion which may occur in up to 30% of the patients may be responsible for the ECG changes.

HYPERTHYROIDISM

ECG manifestations of hyperthyroidism are common, although no abnormality is pathognomonic. Sinus tachycardia is the most common cardiac arrhythmia. Atrial fibrillation occurs in 25% of hyperthyroid patients and usually is associated with a rapid ventricular response. Evaluation for the presence of underlying structural heart disease in the presence of atrial fibrillation, always requires ruling out hyperthyroidism. Intraventricular conduction disturbances, most commonly a left anterior fascicular block or right bundle branch block, occur in a small proportion of hyperthyroid patients without underlying heart disease. Nonspecific ST segment/T wave abnormalities also are noted in 25% of patients. Atrial flutter, supraventricular tachycardia, and ventricular tachycardia are uncommon.

ELECTROCARDIOGRAPHY IN ATHLETES

Increased QRS voltage

Isolated increases in QRS voltage are common. Such voltage correlates poorly with left ventricular mass in young athletes. In the absence of other markers suggesting actual left ventricular hypertrophy (axis changes, ST-T wave changes in repolarization, atrial abnormalities, increased QRS width), high QRS voltage is not a sufficient reason in isolation to refer an athlete for further evaluation.

Incomplete right bundle branch block

Incomplete right bundle branch block is common in the athlete (36–50%). It occurs most often in athletes engaged in endurance sport. The conduction disorder is probably due to right ventricular enlargement.

Early repolarization

The finding of ST elevation in V3 to V6 with an elevated J point and a peaked upright T wave is common (50–80% of resting ECGs) but it seems to regress with age and when training declines and often changes or disappears during a bout of exercise or with increasing heart rate. The magnitude of ST elevation is modulated by autonomic influences and changes from time to time. ST elevation > 2 mm seems to be unusual even in athletes. The most common pattern in the Caucasian population consists of ST elevation of the QRS-ST junction (J point) of at least 0.1 mm from baseline often associated with notching or slurring of the terminal portion of the QRS complex. It is most often localized in the precordial leads. The ST elevation shows an upward concavity and ends in a positive T wave.

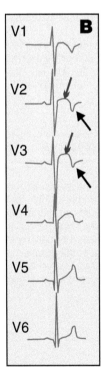

In athletes of African origin, the pattern consists of ST elevation with an upward convexity followed by inversion of the T wave in leads V2 to V4. This pattern must be differentiated from Brugada syndrome. Early repolarization in asymptomatic young people or athletes is not predictive of malignant ventricular tachyarrhythmias despite the findings that early repolarization is more frequent in patients with "idiopathic" malignant ventricular tachyarrhythmias than in patients without the early repolarization pattern.

Precordial early repolarization in two healthy athletes
A. *ST segment elevation with upward concavity (blue arrows), followed by a positive T wave (black arrows)*
B. *ST segment elevation with upward convexity (blue arrows), followed by a negative T wave (black arrows)*

Adapted from Corrado et al. - European Heart Journal 2010; 31 : 243-259

Manifestation of increased vagal tone

Sinus bradycardia, prolonged PR interval, and Wenckebach second-degree AV block are common in athletes as a result of the high resting vagal tone. These findings are related to increased parasympathetic tone and decreased resting sympathetic tone. Further evaluation is not required for sinus bradycardia as low as 30 bpm (with sinus arrhythmia, some RR intervals prolong to 3 seconds) or a prolonged PR interval up to 0.30 s should not prompt further workup. These abnormalities often resolve with exercise, confirming their functional origin.

Axis

The axis of the QRS complex is greatly dependent on age: it begins rightward at birth and shifts leftward with age. As most screened athletes are at an age when the axis is still in transition, right-axis deviation is a common finding. In older populations, right-axis deviation is rare and generally associated with pulmonary disease. Left-axis deviation is the most common abnormal ECG finding in the 30 to 40 age group.

In athletes, mild right-axis deviation should not trigger further evaluation unless there is a history of pulmonary disease or systemic hypertension. For isolated axis deviation an acceptable range lies between –30 and +115 degrees.

T wave inversion

T wave inversion (TWI) has similar prevalence among athletes and sedentary controls, suggesting that it is not a training-related phenomenon. TWI ≥ 2 mm in two adjacent leads is rare. Cardiomyopathy should be ruled out. TWI is more common in black athletes. In athletes not of African origin, TWI ≥ 1 mm in leads III, aVR, V1 and V2 should lead to further evaluation. In athletes of African origin, TWI after ST elevation in V2 to V4 does not need investigation whereas inferior or lateral lead TWI warrants follow-up.

ST depression

ST depression is rare in athletes and always deserves further workup. The mechanism is unknown. Heart disease should be ruled out if the ST depression is accompanied by T wave inversion.

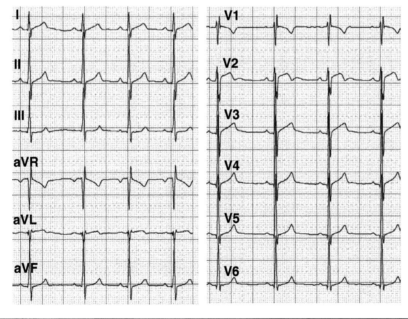

ECG of a 25-year-old soccer player of Caucasian origin.
Sinus rhythm at 61 bpm;
PR = 156 ms;
QRS axis = 74°;
QTc = 423 ms;
incomplete right bundle branch block.

Further Reading

Khairy P, Marsolais P. Pancreatitis with electrocardiographic changes mimicking acute myocardial infarction. Can J Gastroenterol. 2001;15:522-6.

Slovis C, Jenkins R. ABC of clinical electrocardiography: Conditions not primarily affecting the heart. BMJ. 2002;324(7349):1320-3.

Sommargren CE. Electrocardiographic abnormalities in patients with subarachnoid hemorrhage. Am J Crit Care. 2002;11:48-56.

Van Mieghem C, Sabbe M, Knockaert D. The clinical value of the ECG in noncardiac conditions. Chest. 2004;125:1561-76.

Wald DA. ECG manifestations of selected metabolic and endocrine disorders. Emerg Med Clin North Am. 2006;24:145-57.

Yegneswaran B, Kostis JB, Pitchumoni CS. Cardiovascular manifestations of acute pancreatitis. J Crit Care. 2011;26:225. e11-8.

ECG in athletes

Drezner JA, Ackerman MJ, Cannon BC, Corrado D, Heidbuchel H, Prutkin JM, Salerno JC, Anderson J, Ashley E, Asplund CA, Baggish AL, Börjesson M, DiFiori JP, Fischbach P, Froelicher V, Harmon KG, Marek J, Owens DS, Paul S, Pelliccia A, Schmied CM, Sharma S, Stein R, Vetter VL, Wilson MG. Abnormal electrocardiographic findings in athletes: recognising changes suggestive of primary electrical disease. Br J Sports Med. 2013;47:153-67.

Drezner JA, Ashley E, Baggish AL, Börjesson M, Corrado D, Owens DS, Patel A, Pelliccia A, Vetter VL, Ackerman MJ, Anderson J, Asplund CA, Cannon BC, DiFiori J, Fischbach P, Froelicher V, Harmon KG, Heidbuchel H, Marek J, Paul S, Prutkin JM, Salerno JC, Schmied CM, Sharma S, Stein R, Wilson M. Abnormal electrocardiographic findings in athletes: recognising changes suggestive of cardiomyopathy. Br J Sports Med. 2013;47:137-52.

Drezner JA, Ackerman MJ, Anderson J, Ashley E, Asplund CA, Baggish AL, Börjesson M, Cannon BC, Corrado D, DiFiori JP, Fischbach P, Froelicher V, Harmon KG, Heidbuchel H, Marek J, Owens DS, Paul S, Pelliccia A, Prutkin JM, Salerno JC, Schmied CM, Sharma S, Stein R, Vetter VL, Wilson MG. Electrocardiographic interpretation in athletes: the 'Seattle criteria'. Br J Sports Med. 2013;47:122-4.

CHAPTER 11

SINUS NODE DYSFUNCTION

* Sinus rhythms - sinus tachycardia and sinus bradycardia
* Sinoatrial block
* Sinoatrial Wenckebach and sinoatrial 2:1 block
* Wandering atrial pacemaker
* AV junctional rhythm

ECG from Basics to Essentials: Step by Step. First Edition. Roland X. Stroobandt, S. Serge Barold and Alfons F. Sinnaeve.
Published 2016 © 2016 by John Wiley & Sons, Ltd. Companion Website: www.wiley.com/go/stroobandt/ecg

SINUS RHYTHMS

Sinus Tachycardia (> 100 bpm)

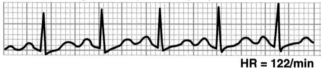

HR = 122/min

PR interval :
   slightly shorter
QT interval :
   slightly shorter

Sinus Bradycardia (< 60 bpm)

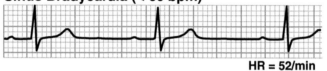

HR = 52/min

PR interval :
   slightly longer
   or normal
QT interval :
   slightly longer

SINOATRIAL BLOCK

Sinoatrial block: **The sinus node continues to discharge at regular intervals but some impulses cannot exit from the sinus node or are considerably delayed. Like AV block, sinoatrial block manifests the patterns of first-, second- or third-degree block.**

1st degree SA block

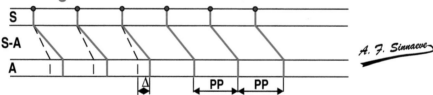

A. F. Sinnaeve

Since the P waves are regular, the ECG looks normal and 1st degree SA cannot be seen.

2nd degree SA block (exit block)

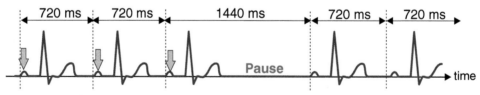

As a rule the sinus pauses exhibit long P-P intervals that are exact multiples of the basic and shorter P-P intervals.
This form is sometimes described as type II SA exit block.

2nd degree type I SA block (Wenckebach)

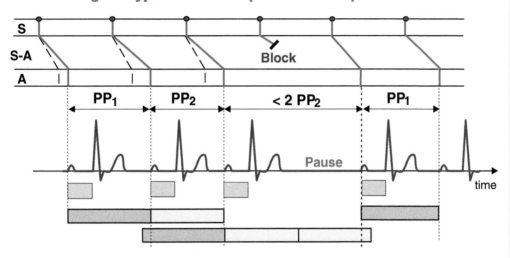

This abnormality causes a gradual decrease in the sinus PP intervals (and in the RR intervals because the PR interval remains constant) or group beating. The Wenckebach phenomenon is in the sinoatrial junction and not in the AV node.

This apparent gradual increase in the sinus rate is then followed by sinus pause. The Wenckebach phenomenon is not recognized by its face but its footsteps, in this case the gradual shortening of the PP intervals.

3rd degree SA block (exit block)

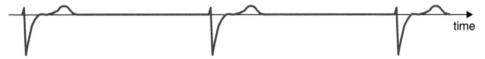

This may be present when there is a slow junctional rhythm and no P waves can be seen.

NOTE : Sinus Pause or Sinus Arrest

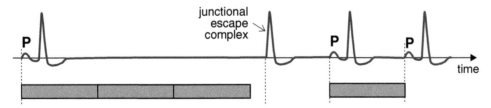

This is a disorder of impulse formation. The pauses show long PP intervals that are not exact multiples of the shorter basic PP interval representing sinus rhythm.

SINOATRIAL BLOCKS

Normal sinoatrial conduction (baseline)

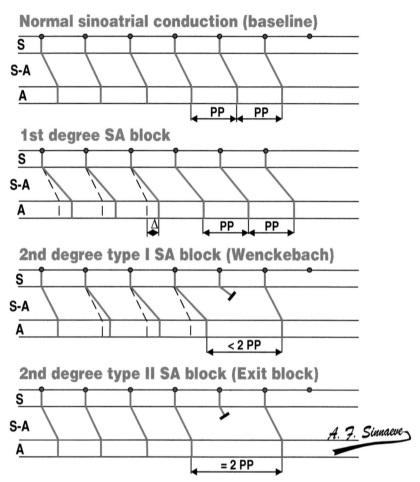

1st degree SA block

2nd degree type I SA block (Wenckebach)

2nd degree type II SA block (Exit block)

A. F. Sinnaeve

S : sinus node ; S-A : sinoatrial junction ; A : atrial tissue ;
PP : interval between consecutive P waves ; Δ : conduction delay

Neither SA node activity (discharge) nor conduction from the SA node to the atrium can be recorded. Neither 1st nor 3rd degree SA blocks can be diagnosed from the ECG. In 1st degree sinus node block the ECG may show sinus rhythm or sinus bradycardia. Only 2nd degree SA block can be diagnosed from ECG.

Abnormalities of SA node function are either due to failure to form impulses or caused by failure to conduct them.

1st degree SA block
the ECG looks normal

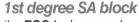

2nd degree type I SA block (Wenckebach)
progressive shortening of the PP interval followed by a pause which is shorter than 2 x the shortest PP interval (occurring immediately before the pause)

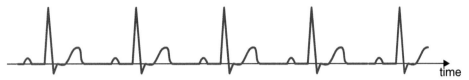

2nd degree type II SA block (Exit block)
a group of constant PP intervals is followed by a pause of exactly 2 regular PP intervals

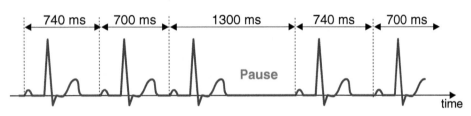

Sinus pause or sinus arrest: the pause is less than 2 x PP interval
a group of constant PP intervals is followed by a pause less than 2 regular PP intervals or longer than 2 PP intervals but not a multiple of the basic PP interval

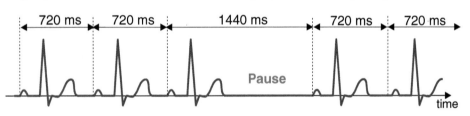

When a pause is not an exact multiple of the PP interval, it is customary to label it as sinus arrest regardless of the mechanism. In other words this diagnosis might ignore a possible combination of 1st-degree and 2nd-degree conduction abnormality involving exit of an impulse from the sinoatrial junction rather than failure of the SA node to generate an impulse.

LADDER DIAGRAM – SA 5:4 WENCKEBACH

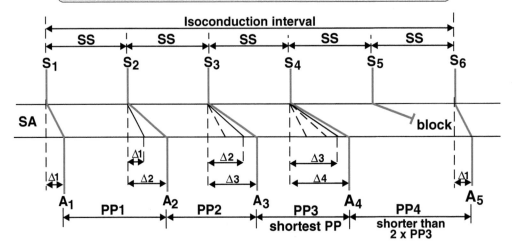

Δ = Sinoatrial delay; increment of delay reduces each interval i.e.
$\{(\Delta2 - \Delta1) > (\Delta3 - \Delta2) > (\Delta4 - \Delta3)\}$

Isoconduction interval = duration of a whole Wenckebach cycle

SS = interval between 2 consecutive pulses of the sinus node

PP = interval between 2 P waves as seen on the ECG

Number of SS intervals: n = next integer greater than $\dfrac{\text{isoconduction interval}}{\text{shortest PP}}$

Duration of the SS interval: $SS = \dfrac{\text{isoconduction interval}}{n}$

EXAMPLE

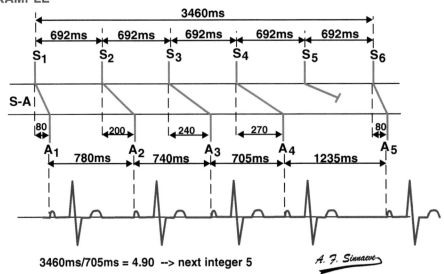

3460ms/705ms = 4.90 --> next integer 5

SS interval = 3460ms/5 = 692ms

A. F. Sinnaeve

Sinoatrial Wenckebach

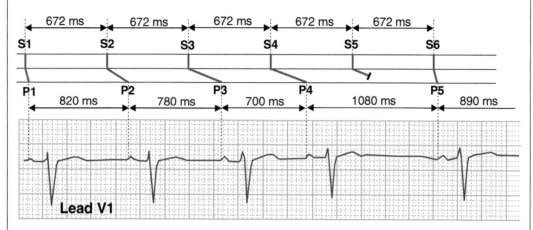

Sudden absence of a P-QRS sequence, progressive shortening of the P-P interval, P-P interval pause < 2x pre-pause interval, post-pause interval > pre-pause interval

> **Note the difference between the two types of pauses (missing QRS complex).**
> * **With a sinoatrial Wenckebach the pause of the P waves is not exactly two times the SS interval and the RR interval is not constant.**
> * **With a sinoatrial block the basic PP interval remains constant and the pause is a multiple of that basic interval.**

Sinoatrial 2:1 block

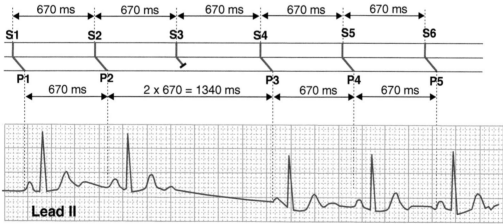

Sudden absence of a P-QRS sequence and the long P-P interval is exactly twice the basic P-P interval

WANDERING ATRIAL PACEMAKER

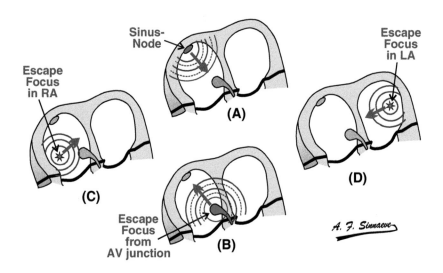

Sinus-Node

Escape Focus in RA

Escape Focus in LA

(A)

(C)

(D)

Escape Focus from AV junction

(B)

A. F. Sinnaeve

Different P wave morphology, different PR intervals, different PP intervals

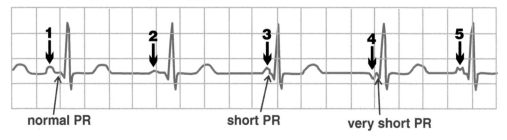

normal PR   short PR   very short PR

DIAGNOSIS

A. Three morphologically different P waves

B. Rate lower than 100 bpm

C. Exclude frequent atrial premature beats

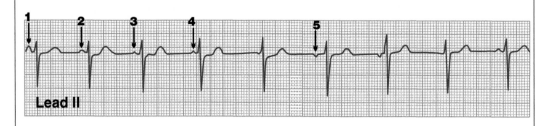

Lead II

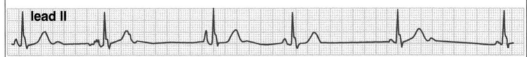

Wandering pacemaker. Note that the pattern consists basically of varying supraventricular escape beats

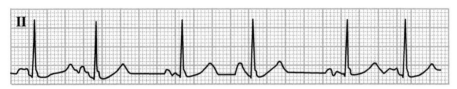

The ECG resembles superficially that of a wandering pacemaker. In fact there are late multifocal atrial premature beats which actively usurp the atrial rhythm. It is not a passive escape mechanism.

Wandering atrial pacemaker (WAP) is an atrial arrhythmia that occurs when the natural pacemaker site shifts passively from the head of the sinoatrial node to more distant sites in the node itself, to other parts of the atria, and/or the AV junction. This shifting of the dominant pacemaker is manifested electrocardiographically by changes in the size, shape and direction of the P waves. The diagnosis of WAP requires 3 morphologically different P waves.

The PR intervals vary according the site of the dominant pacemaker and may be short with AV junctional or low atrial beats as they are located close to the AV node. A wandering atrial pacemaker produces an irregular rhythm with varying RR intervals. The rate is usually between 45 and 100 bpm by definition but the rate is rarely fast. When the rate exceeds 100 bpm, the arrhythmia becomes multifocal atrial tachycardia which is more serious.

A wandering pacemaker is usually caused by varying vagal tone. With increased vagal tone the sinoatrial node slows and permits other pacemaker sites to emerge because their automatic properties are slightly faster for a brief period. After vagal tone decreases the sinus node resumes its natural control of the heart.

A wandering pacemaker is basically benign and often occurs in young people or athletes because of augmented vagal tone. It must be differentiated from sinus rhythm with frequent atrial premature beats where there is a regular underlying rhythm.

AV JUNCTIONAL RHYTHM

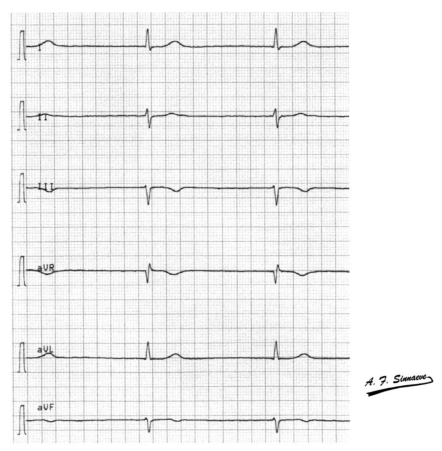

A. F. Sinnaeve

The ECG shows an AV junctional rhythm of 33 bpm. No P waves are visible. The P waves are in all likelihood buried inside the QRS complex.

Together, the bundle of His (down to where it begins to branch), and the AV node are called the AV junction or just "the junction". Cardiac rhythms originating from these areas are called supraventricular rhythms. The regions that constitute the AV junction are divided according to cell types: atrial-nodal (AN) region, nodal (N) region, and the nodal-His (NH) region. The middle N region has no automaticity. The NH part of AV node is the usual site in the AV junction capable of firing spontaneously. AV junctional rhythms were formerly called "AV nodal" or simply "nodal" rhythms. All cells of the conduction system have the potential to generate electrical impulses. Normally the higher frequency of the sinoatrial node will override the other cells of the conduction system. The AV junction has intrinsic automaticity that allows it to initiate depolarizing impulses during periods of significant sinus bradycardia or complete heart block. This escape mechanism usually has a rate of 40–60 bpm (always consider digitalis toxicity when the rate is faster). Junctional rhythms produce a narrow QRS complex because the ventricle is depolarized via the normal conduction pathway. A junctional escape rhythm may occur in the absence of heart disease.

An accelerated junctional rhythm (rate > 60) is a narrow complex rhythm that often supersedes the sinus mechanism which may or may not be slow. Accelerated junctional rhythms may be due to digitalis intoxication or heart disease and are seldom seen in normal individuals. The rate of accelerated junctional rhythms is 60–100 bpm. If the rate is more than 100 bpm, the rhythm is called junctional tachycardia.

AV JUNCTIONAL RHYTHM with ISORHYTHMIC DISSOCIATION

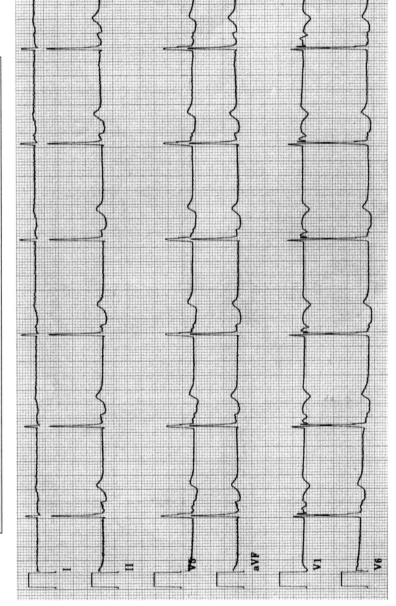

There is a slightly irregular AV junctional rhythm at a rate of about 44 bpm. The atrial rate is similar. The sinus P wave is stuck on the ST segment at the end of the QRS. The constant relationship of atrial and ventricular beats is called isorhythmic dissociation which is a form of AV dissociation. The sinus rate slows with the last beat and the P wave moves away from the QRS. In this patient, at other times, the ventricular rate was faster than the atrial rate. This ruled out AV block where the diagnosis requires a ventricular rate slower than the atrial rate. The P wave is positive in leads II and aVF and therefore retrograde conduction to the atrium is ruled out.

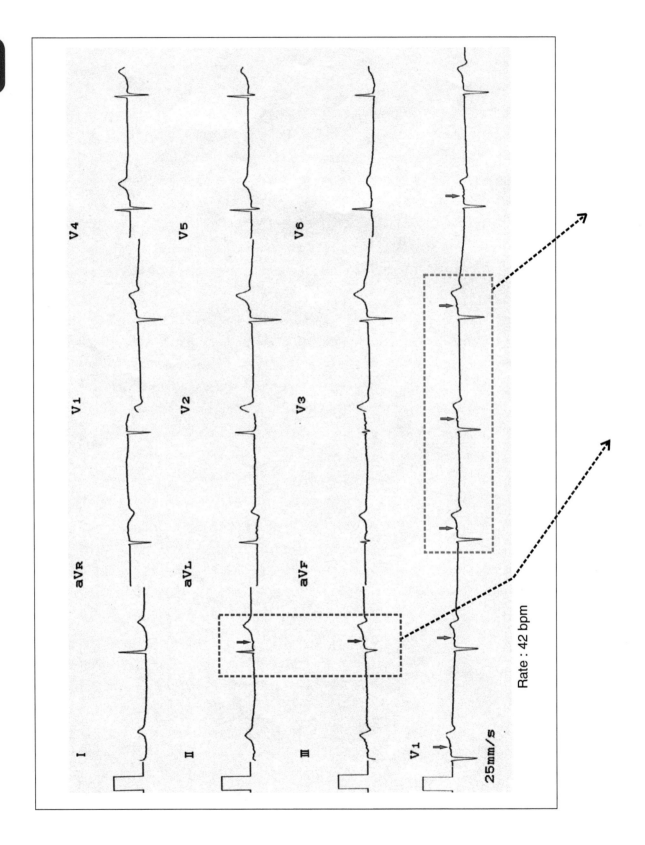

Rate : 42 bpm

AV JUNCTIONAL RHYTHM 2

V1

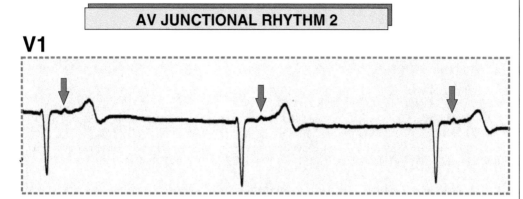

A. F. Sinnaeve

The arrows point to the retrograde P waves

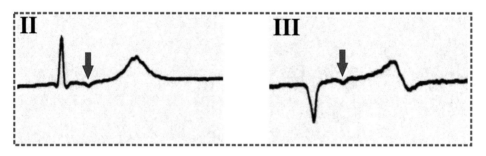

ATRIAL ACTIVITY DURING A JUNCTIONAL RHYTHM

The pattern of atrial activity is similar in all junctional rhythms (escape, accelerated, tachycardia and premature complexes) and the diagnostic criteria similar. AV dissociation will be present if there is no retrograde conduction to the atrium. AV dissociation is often confused with third-degree AV block. It is not AV block and theproof lies in recording long strips to demonstrate capture beats (sinus impulses traversing the AV junction on the way to the ventricle) that will occur earlier than the expected AV junctional beat. The term isorhythmic AV dissociation is used to describe a rhythm where the atrial and ventricular rates are virtuallly similar. However, long rhythm strips should reveal a capture beat.

The key to recognizing a junctional rhythm begins in leads II, III and aVF. Here, the P wave is normally always upright and only negative when the impulse is coming from below the atria. Thus, inverted retrograde P waves in the inferior leads and a narrow QRS immediately indicates that the primary pacemaker has shifted to the AV junction. In the presence of retrograde conduction, the P and QRS relationship may exhibit one of 3 patterns: a visible inverted P wave preceding the QRS in the inferior leads (PR < 0.12 s), an invisible P wave buried within the QRS complex due to simultaneous activation of the atrium and the ventricle, and a visible inverted P wave succeeding the QRS.

Further Reading

Brignole M. Sick sinus syndrome. Clin Geriatr Med. 2002:211-27.

Mangrum JM, DiMarco JP. The evaluation and management of bradycardia. N Engl J Med. 2000;342:703-9.

Semelka M, Gera J, Usman S. Sick sinus syndrome: a review. Am Fam Physician. 2013;87:691-6.

Tse HF, Lau CP. Prevalence and clinical implications of atrial fibrillation episodes detected by pacemaker in patients with sick sinus syndrome. Heart. 2005;91:362-4.

CHAPTER 12

PREMATURE VENTRICULAR COMPLEXES (PVC)

* Definitions
* Unifocal PVC with fully compensatory pause
* Multifocal PVCs
* PVC causing retrograde P wave and noncompensatory pause
* Interpolated PVC and PR prolongation
* Coupling interval
* End-diastolic PVC
* PVCs and the "R on T" phenomenon
* Paired PVCs
* PVC configuration and morphology
* Parasystole
* Accelerated idioventricular rhythm

ECG from Basics to Essentials: Step by Step. First Edition. Roland X. Stroobandt, S. Serge Barold and Alfons F. Sinnaeve.
Published 2016 © 2016 by John Wiley & Sons, Ltd. Companion Website: www.wiley.com/go/stroobandt/ecg

PREMATURE VENTRICULAR COMPLEXES 1

* Premature ventricular complexes (PVC) originate in ectopic foci in the ventricles
* PVCs occur earlier than expected
* They are not preceded by P waves
* The QRS duration of PVCs is larger than 0.12 s because the depolarization front does not follow the normal conduction system (His bundle and bundle branches)
* The T wave is discordant to the QRS complex
* PVCs are followed by a pause that is usually fully compensatory

Unifocal PVC with fully compensatory pause

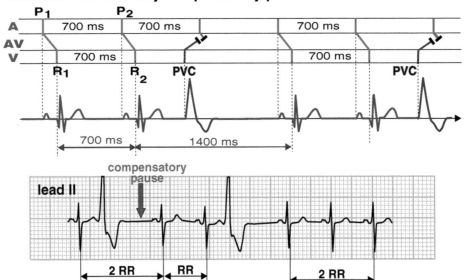

Unifocal PVCs originate in a single location in the ventricles; they are uniform and have identical configuration. On the contrary, multifocal PVCs start at two or more ectopic foci in the ventricles; these PVCs have different configurations

Multifocal PVCs

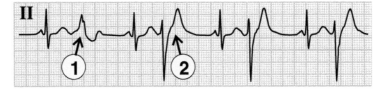

PVC causing a retrograde P wave and noncompensatory pause

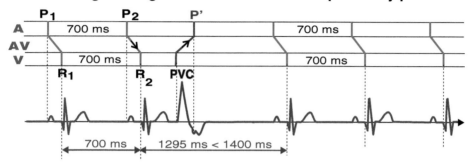

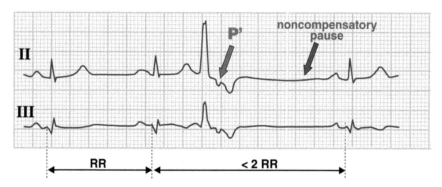

Interpolated PVC and PR prolongation

An interpolated PVC is sandwiched between two consecutive sinus complexes, without causing a pause. The atrium is not retrogradely depolarized and the normal sinus rhythm and its associated ventricular response are completely unperturbed.

However, the PR interval after the PVC may be longer because the impulse from the PVC enters the AV node retrogradely and creates partial refractoriness.

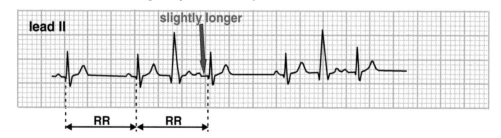

PREMATURE VENTRICULAR COMPLEXES 2

The Coupling Interval

The coupling interval refers to the distance or interval (in ms) between the PVC and the preceding normal QRS complex.

A fixed coupling interval is fairly common for unifocal PVCs originating in the same ectopic focus from which the depolarization wavefront takes the same route.

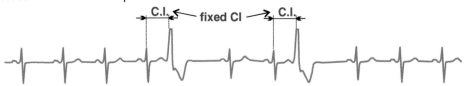

Variable coupling intervals are mostly associated with multifocal PVCs originating from different ectopic foci having different morphologies.

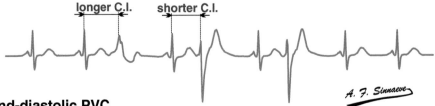

End-diastolic PVC

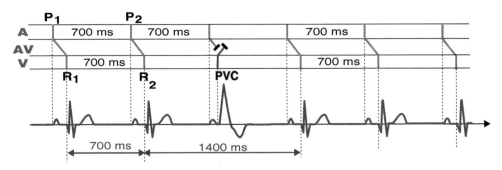

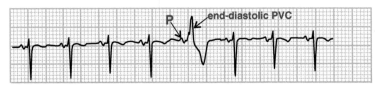

End-diastolic PVCs occur so late that the next P wave is already partially or completely inscribed. This often results in a fusion complex. An end-diastolic PVC always has a long coupling interval. Note that these PVCs may easily be mistaken for aberrantly conducted premature atrial (PAC) or junctional (PJC) complexes. A fusion beat reflects ventricular depolarization from 2 foci (sinus conducted beat and PVC). Its configuration is intermediate between the configuration of a pure supraventricular beat and the configuration of a pure PVC.

PVCs and the "R on T" Phenomenon

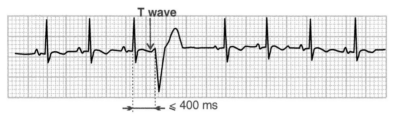

The "R on T" phenomenon describes the occurrence of a PVC beginning at or near the apex of the T wave of the previous complex (the so-called vulnerable period). Such PVCs were originally considered to carry a grave prognosis (being associated with ventricular fibrillation). The R on T PVC is only of importance in patients with an acute myocardial infarction or myocardial ischemia or with long QT intervals where it may be associated with the risk of ventricular fibrillation.

Paired PVCs

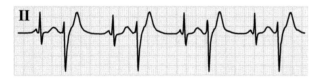

PVCs in bigeminy
the PVCs alternate with normal sinus complexes

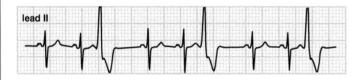

PVCs in trigeminy
a PVC occurs every third complex

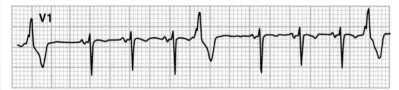

PVC quadrigeminy
every fourth complex is a PVC

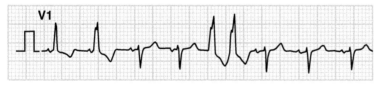

PVCs in couplet
a sequence of two PVCs

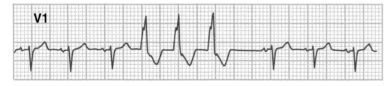

PVCs in triplet
a salvo of three consecutive PVCs (must be differentiated from a run of PVCs or unsustained ventricular tachycardia)

PREMATURE VENTRICULAR COMPLEXES 3

PVC Configuration and Morphology

A PVC may have a morphology that resembles a right or a left bundle branch block depending upon the location of origin. It is assumed that the PVC originates in the left ventricle when it has a positive deflection or tall R wave in lead V1 (right bundle branch block configuration), while a negative complex with a deep S wave in V1 (resembling a left bundle branch block morphology) originates in the right ventricle. A PVC originating in the interventricular septum often has a left bundle branch block morpholgy. However, this is not always a reliable way to identify the site of origin.

Premature Ventricular Complexes (PVC) with Left Bundle
Branch Block Morphology (LBBB)
Two leads (II and V1) from the same patient

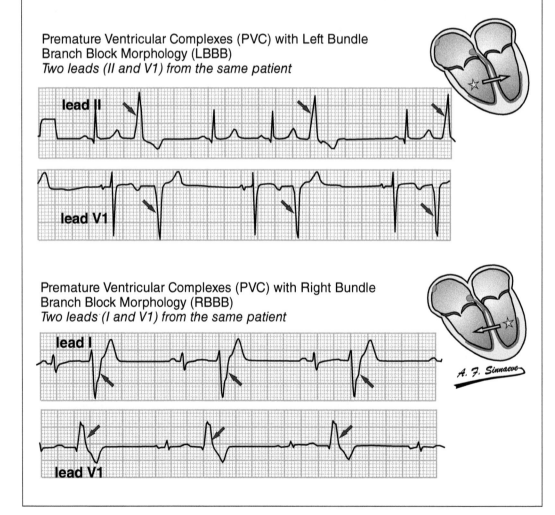

Premature Ventricular Complexes (PVC) with Right Bundle
Branch Block Morphology (RBBB)
Two leads (I and V1) from the same patient

A. F. Sinnaeve

Parasystole

A ventricular parasystolic rhythm refers to an independent ectopic ventricular rhythm whose focus of origin is protected in the sense that impulses coming from the sinus rhythm cannot enter and reset the parasystolic focus (entrance block). Exit block occurs only secondary to refractoriness of ventricular myocardium surrounding the parasystolic focus. Thus, an impulse coming from sinus rhythm can create a field of refractoriness around the parasystolic focus, limiting the rate and timing of its emerging impulses; in other words, the autonomous parasystolic focus can deliver impulses to the myocardium but cannot be reset by impulses originating elsewhere. Accordingly, the ECG shows the classic triad of (1) variable coupling between sinus beats and ectopic QRS complexes, (2) ventricular fusion beats, and (3) a fixed common denominator of interectopic intervals between manifest parasystolic extrasystoles (x2, x3, x4 ... etc).

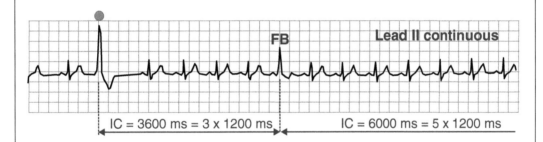

FB   **Lead II continuous**

IC = 3600 ms = 3 x 1200 ms   IC = 6000 ms = 5 x 1200 ms

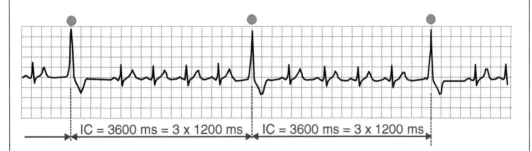

IC = 3600 ms = 3 x 1200 ms   IC = 3600 ms = 3 x 1200 ms

IC = interectopic interval
FB = fusion beat
● = parasystolic extrasystole

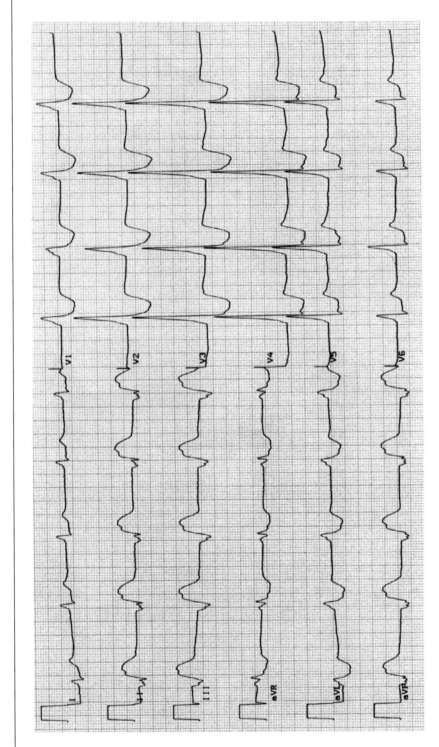

Accelerated idioventricular rhythm (AIVR) at a rate of about 60 bpm. QRS = 0.16–0.18 s. There are no P waves before the QRS complexes. There may be retrograde P waves deforming the ST segment near the peak of the T wave. The tall R wave in lead V1 must not be interpreted as right bundle branch block.

ACCELERATED IDIOVENTRICULAR RHYTHM

Accelerated idioventricular rhythm (AIVR) is defined as an enhanced ectopic ventricular rhythm with at least 3 consecutive ventricular beats faster than normal intrinsic ventricular escape rhythm (> 40 bpm), but slower than ventricular tachycardia (at least 100 bpm). It used to be called slow ventricular tachycardia but this term is inappropriate. It can only emerge when its automatic rate is faster than the sinus rate. It is often a self-limited rhythm. AIVR most often occurs as a marker of successful reperfusion in acute myocardial infarction and rarely occurs in the normal heart. AIVR is often well tolerated and seldom needs any specific treatment. Occasionally it leads to hemodynamic instability due to the loss of AV synchrony or a relatively rapid ventricular rate.

In most cases, the mechanism of AIVR appears to be related to enhanced automaticity in His-Purkinje fibers and/or myocardium caused by a variety of circumstances. When this enhanced automaticity surpasses that of the sinus node, AIVR manifests as the dominant rhythm of the heart. Sinus bradycardia may facilitate the appearance of AIVR. Most AIVRs originate from a single focus.

AIVR should not be diagnosed solely based on ventricular rate. The important diagnostic points are: rate, wide QRS complexes and the absence of P waves preceding the QRS. Misdiagnosis of AIVR as slow ventricular tachycardia or complete heart block can lead to inappropriate therapies with potential complications. AIVR must also be differentiated from bundle branch block. AIVR differs from ventricular tachycardia by additional features such as the gradual onset with a long coupling interval, the end by a gradual decrease of the ventricular rate or increase of the sinus rate. It resolves as sinus rate surpasses the rate of AIVR. AIVR may be associated with frank AV dissociation, retrograde P waves, fusion beats and capture beats. In complete heart block and AV dissociation the atrial rate is faster than the ventricular rate. During AIVR with AV dissociation fusion beats and capture beats provide proof that AV conduction is not compromised. A fusion beat occurs when ventricular depolarization occurs via 2 foci (supraventricular and ventricular). The resultant QRS complex assumes an intermediate configuration from the 2 sites and the QRS may be narrower than the AIVR complexes. A capture beat traverses the AV junction and achieves complete ventricular depolarization so that the QRS is supraventricular and narrow.

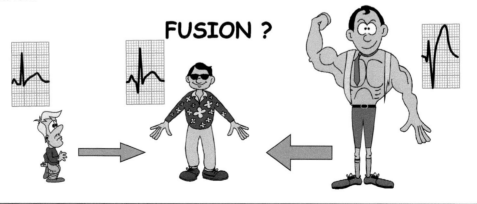

FUSION ?

Further Reading

Adams JC, Srivathsan K, Shen WK. Advances in management of premature ventricular contractions. J Interv Card Electrophysiol. 2012;35:137-49.

Ataklte F, Erqou S, Laukkanen J, Kaptoge S. Meta-analysis of ventricular premature complexes and their relation to cardiac mortality in general populations. Am J Cardiol. 2013;112:1263-70.

Cantillon DJ. Evaluation and management of premature ventricular complexes. Cleve Clin J Med. 2013;80:377-87.

Lee V, Hemingway H, Harb R, Crake T, Lambiase P. The prognostic significance of premature ventricular complexes in adults without clinically apparent heart disease: a meta-analysis and systematic review. Heart. 2012;98:1290-8.

Lee GK, Klarich KW, Grogan M, Cha YM. Premature ventricular contraction-induced cardiomyopathy: a treatable condition. Circ Arrhythm Electrophysiol. 2012;5:229-36.

Nair GM, Nery PB, Redpath CJ, Birnie DH. Ventricular arrhythmias in patients with heart failure secondary to reduced ejection fraction: a current perspective. Curr Opin Cardiol. 2014;29:152-9.

CHAPTER 13

ATRIOVENTRICULAR BLOCK

* Normal conduction
* First-degree AV block
* Second-degree AV block type I and type II
* 2:1 and advanced second-degree AV block
* Complete or 3rd-degree AV block
* AV block with narrow or wide QRS complexes
* Unifascicular, bifascicular and trifascicular blocks
* Overview of 2nd-degree AV block
* ECG pitfalls in the diagnosis of 2nd-degree AV block

ECG from Basics to Essentials: Step by Step. First Edition. Roland X. Stroobandt, S. Serge Barold and Alfons F. Sinnaeve.
Published 2016 © 2016 by John Wiley & Sons, Ltd. Companion Website: www.wiley.com/go/stroobandt/ecg

ATRIOVENTRICULAR BLOCK 1

NORMAL CONDUCTION

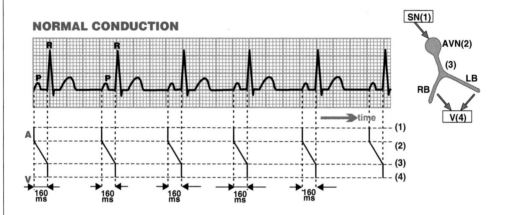

1st degree AV BLOCK

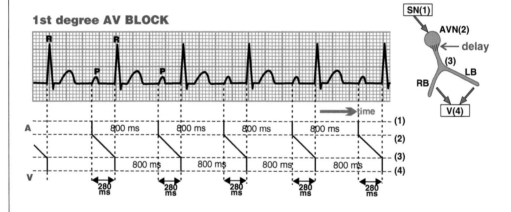

2nd degree AV BLOCK type I (Wenckebach or Mobitz 1)

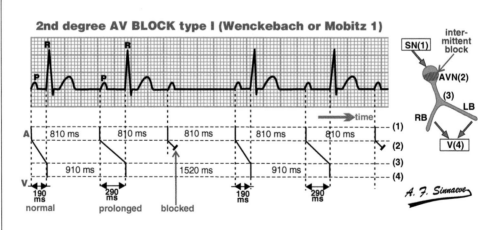

A. F. Sinnaeve

There are three types of **AV block** based on the severity of the conduction abnormality:

☞ **First-degree AV block**

☞ **Second-degree AV block**
      * Mobitz type I (also called AV Wenckebach)
      * Mobitz type II
      * 2:1 fixed-ratio AV block
      * High-grade (also called advanced) 2nd degree AV block

☞ **Third-degree or complete AV block**

1st DEGREE AV BLOCK

1. The PR interval is prolonged > 200 ms or 0.20 s
2. Every P-wave is followed by a QRS complex

The PR interval represents the time from the onset of atrial depolarization to the onset of ventricular depolarization as seen on the ECG.

Activation originating in the sinus node can be delayed anywhere between the atria and the ventricles (including AV node, His bundle, bundle branches and fascicles) although the prolongation is almost always due to slowing of conduction within the AV node.

2nd DEGREE AV BLOCK (Mobitz type I or Wenckebach)

1. **The diagnosis requires the presence of sinus rhythm (which may be regular or irregular) and at least 2 consecutive conducted P waves (thus excluding 2:1 AV block).**
2. **Progressive prolongation of the PR interval before a nonconducted P wave (i.e. before a missing QRS complex).**
3. **Two or more consecutive P waves are conducted but only a single P wave is blocked.**
4. **The PR interval always shortens immediately after the pause i.e. in the first conducted P wave.**

---

* Long sequences often generate atypical behavior of the PR intervals. The greatest increment of the PR interval may not always occur in the second PR interval.
* The conduction ratio is the ratio of the total number of P waves to the number of P waves that are conducted. Thus, a 4:3 Wenckebach means that of 4 consecutive P waves only 3 are conducted and the 4th is blocked.

ATRIOVENTRICULAR BLOCK 2

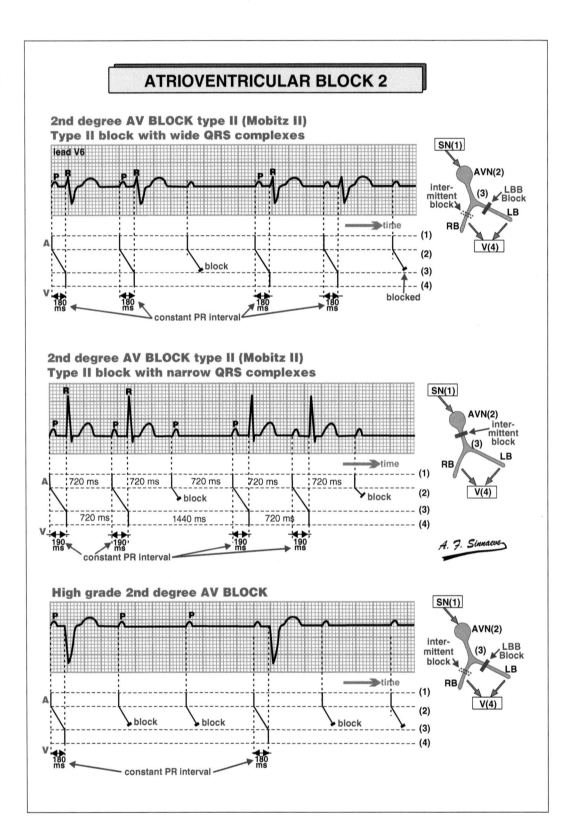

2nd degree AV BLOCK type II (Mobitz II)
Type II block with wide QRS complexes

lead V6

block

blocked

180 ms · 180 ms · 180 ms · 180 ms

constant PR interval

SN(1) · AVN(2) · intermittent block · (3) · LBB Block · LB · RB · V(4)

2nd degree AV BLOCK type II (Mobitz II)
Type II block with narrow QRS complexes

720 ms · 720 ms · 720 ms · 720 ms · 720 ms

block · block

720 ms · 1440 ms · 720 ms

190 ms · 190 ms · 190 ms · 190 ms

constant PR interval

SN(1) · AVN(2) · intermittent block · (3) · LB · RB · V(4)

A. F. Sinnaeve

High grade 2nd degree AV BLOCK

block · block · block

180 ms · 180 ms

constant PR interval

SN(1) · AVN(2) · intermittent block · (3) · LBB Block · LB · RB · V(4)

2nd DEGREE AV BLOCK (Mobitz type II)

1. Two or more consecutive P waves are conducted; only single P waves are blocked (this requirement excludes 2:1 AV block).
2. The PR interval remains constant before and after the blocked P wave. (The PR interval may be normal or prolonged, but does not vary.)
3. The R-R intervals are constant because the sinus rate is constant, i.e. the P-P intervals are stable (the R-R interval is twice as long if a P wave is blocked).

* *Type II block is always infranodal.*
* The QRS complex is mostly wide (65–80%) but may be occasionally narrow (if the block occurs in the His bundle).
* A vagal surge can cause simultaneous sinus slowing and AV nodal block superficially resembling type II block. Therefore stability of the sinus rate is an important criterion for the diagnosis of type II block.
* Diagnosis of type II block may not be possible if there is sinus slowing, but is possible with an increasing sinus rate.

HIGH GRADE 2nd DEGREE AV BLOCK

1. Two or more consecutive P waves are blocked.
2. High grade AV block with narrow QRS complexes may be nodal or infranodal. When the QRS complexes are wide, the block is almost always infranodal.

* The conduction ratio refers to the number of P waves that are blocked before a P wave is conducted ; e.g. a 3:1 ratio means that of three consecutive P waves, only one is conducted.
* High grade 2nd degree AV block might be defined as an AV block with a blocking ratio of 3:1 or higher (3:1 , 4:1 , ...)

ATRIOVENTRICULAR BLOCK 3

Fixed-ratio 2:1 AV BLOCK

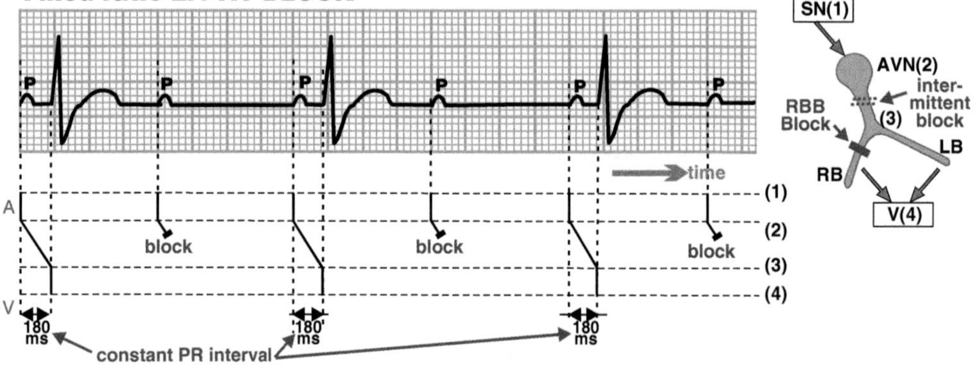

P   P   P   P   P   P

→ time

A ──────────────────────── (1)
block   block   block
────────────────────────── (2)
────────────────────────── (3)
V ──────────────────────── (4)

180 ms   180 ms   180 ms

constant PR interval

SN(1)
AVN(2)
inter-mittent block
RBB Block   (3)
RB   LB
V(4)

Complete or 3rd degree AV BLOCK with narrow QRS complexes

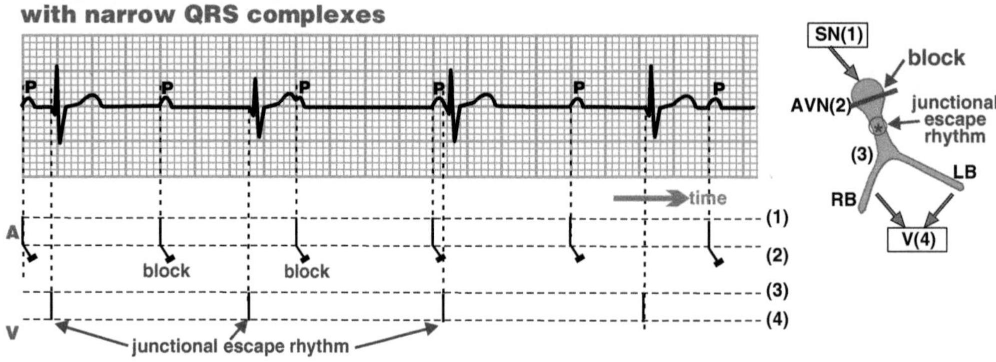

P   P   P   P   P   P

→ time

A ──────────────────────── (1)
block   block
────────────────────────── (2)
────────────────────────── (3)
V ──────────────────────── (4)

junctional escape rhythm

SN(1)
block
AVN(2)   junctional escape rhythm
(3)   LB
RB
V(4)

A. F. Sinnaeve

Complete or 3rd degree AV BLOCK with wide QRS complexes

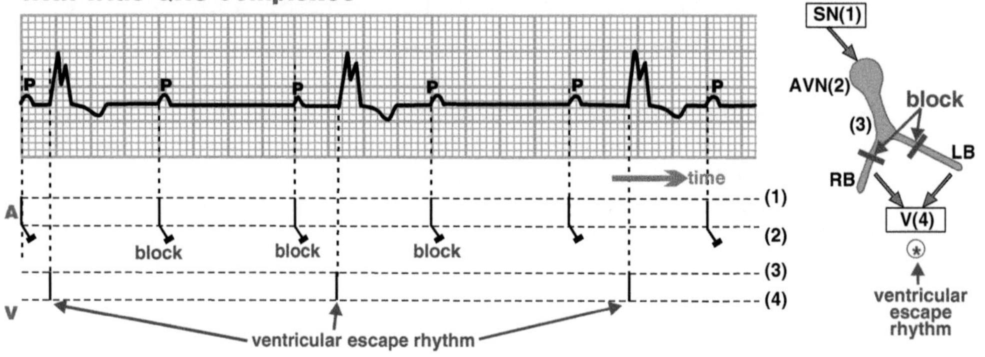

P   P   P   P   P   P

→ time

A ──────────────────────── (1)
block   block   block
────────────────────────── (2)
────────────────────────── (3)
V ──────────────────────── (4)

ventricular escape rhythm

SN(1)
AVN(2)
block
(3)   LB
RB
V(4)
ventricular escape rhythm

FIXED-RATIO 2:1 AV BLOCK

1. Every other P wave is conducted, alternating with every other blocked P wave.
2. 2:1 block cannot be classified as type I or type II because only a single P wave is conducted (two conducted P waves are needed to evaluate the behavior of the PR interval).

* QRS complexes may be wide or narrow.
* Barring myocardial infarction, sustained 2:1 block with a wide QRS complex occurs in the His-Purkinje system in 80% of cases (with 20% in the AV node).
* As the PR interval looks constant, 2:1 AV block is often mistaken for type II block.

COMPLETE or 3rd DEGREE AV BLOCK

1. Third degree AV block is the complete absence of conduction of electrical impulses from the atria to the ventricles.
2. Unless an escape rhythm comes to the rescue, the ventricles will remain asystolic. Only P waves will be present on the ECG causing lightheadedness, syncope or sudden death.
3. The escape rhythm is completely independent of the sinus rhythm. P waves and QRS complexes are completely dissociated.
4. QRS complexes can be narrow or wide, depending upon the location of the block and the origin of the escape rhythm.

The atrial rate must be faster than the ventricular rate !

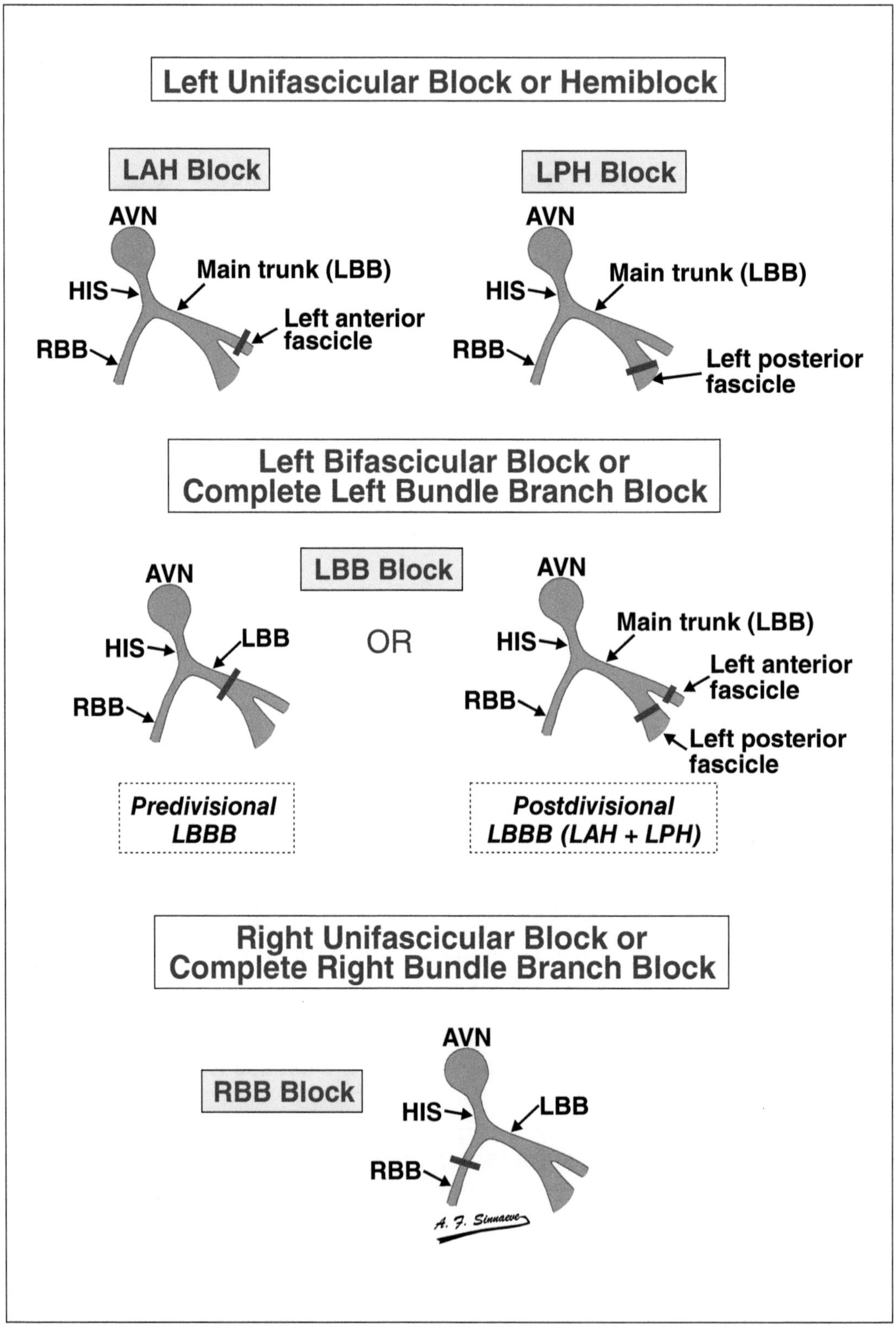

Left Unifascicular Block or Hemiblock

LAH Block

AVN

HIS →

Main trunk (LBB)

Left anterior fascicle

RBB →

LPH Block

AVN

HIS →

Main trunk (LBB)

RBB →

Left posterior fascicle

Left Bifascicular Block or Complete Left Bundle Branch Block

LBB Block

AVN

HIS →

LBB

RBB →

OR

AVN

HIS →

Main trunk (LBB)

Left anterior fascicle

RBB →

Left posterior fascicle

Predivisional LBBB

Postdivisional LBBB (LAH + LPH)

Right Unifascicular Block or Complete Right Bundle Branch Block

AVN

RBB Block

HIS →

LBB

RBB →

A. J. Sinnaeve

Complete AV Block

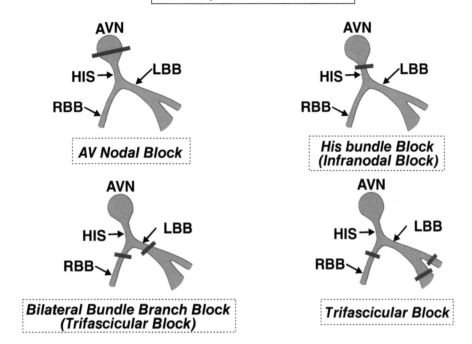

Bilateral bundle branch block such as RBBB alternating with LBBB or vice versa (even recorded at different times) in the same patient constitutes trifascicular block.

The terms complete AV block and trifascicular block are not synonymous. Trifascicular block (or conduction abnormality) may exist without complete AV block in a situation that eventually progresses to complete AV block, e.g. RBBB with alternating LAH and LPH.

It is a common error to label bifascicular block with 1st-degree AV block as trifascicular block because the block can be either in the AV node (outside the His-Purkinje system) or in the His bundle or in all three fascicles.

All conduction disorders in the His-Purkinje system may be permanent, transient, intermittent (rate-independent) or rate-dependent usually precipitated by tachycardia (phase 3 block) and rarely by bradycardia (phase 4 block).

Abbreviations : AVN = atrioventricular node ; LAH = left anterior hemiblock ; LBB = left bundle branch ; LBBB = left bundle branch block ; LPH = left posterior hemiblock ; RBB = right bundle branch ; RBBB = right bundle branch block

OVERVIEW OF 2ND-DEGREE AV BLOCK

Diagrammatic representation of various forms of second-degree AV block. The 3 levels represent activation of the atria (A), the AV junction (AV) and the ventricles (V). All noted values are in ms.

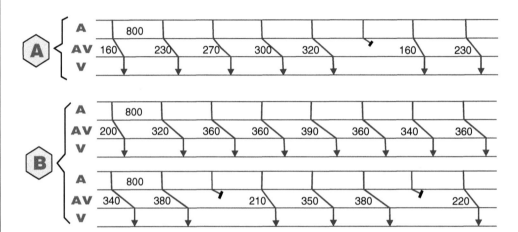

(A) Classic type I AV block. (B) Relatively long and atypical type I sequence. Note the irregular fluctuations of the PR intervals before the dropped beat.

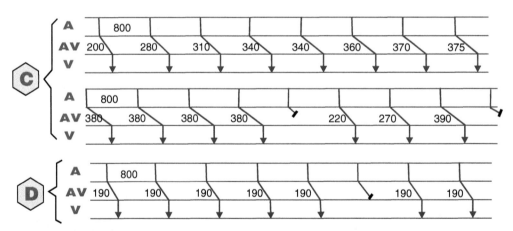

(C) Relatively long and atypical type I sequence with several constant PR intervals before a dropped beat. Note the shorter PR interval after the blocked P wave. This pattern should not be called type II AV block. It is essential to examine all PR intervals in long rhythm strips and not merely several PR intervals preceding a blocked impulse. (D) True type II AV block. Every atrial impulse successfully traverses the AV node which is not afforded a long recovery time as occurs in type I AV block. Note that the PR interval after the blocked beat is unchanged.

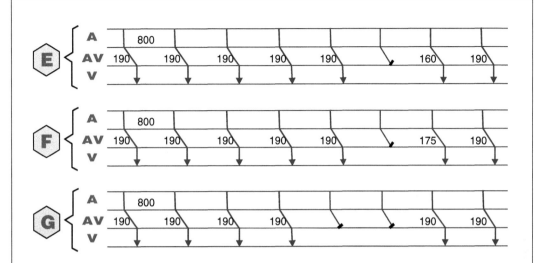

(E) Dropped beat followed by a 30 ms shortening of the PR interval. This pattern should not be called type II AV block. It may be a type I AV block or unclassifiable if shortening of the PR interval is due to an AV junctional escape beat. (F) Type II AV block according to some of the old definitions that allow a 20 ms shortening of the post block PR interval. This is now generally labeled as a type I block with very small increments in conduction. (G) Advanced second-degree AV block (failure of conduction of 2 consecutive P waves without warning). All PR intervals are constant including the first one after the block. This suggests infranodal block.

Illustrative example 1

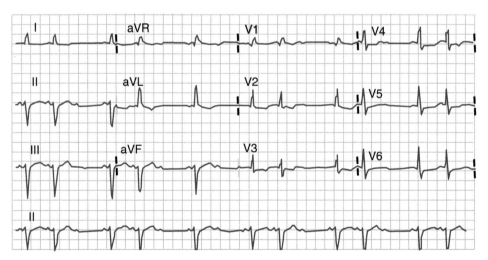

Sinus rhythm; left anterior hemiblock (marked left axis deviation); complete right bundle branch block consistent with bifascicular block.
There is Mobitz type II 2nd-degree AV block (3:2 block) and 2:1 AV block. The PR intervals are constant before and after the blocked P waves.

OVERVIEW OF 2ND-DEGREE AV BLOCK

Illustrative example 2

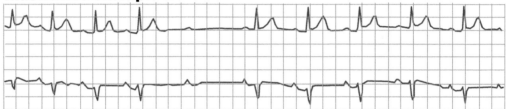

Type I variant. The PR intervals are constant before the blocked beat. There is sinus slowing at the time of the nonconducted P wave. Sinus slowing with concomitant AV block is typical of a vagal effect. The PR interval after the block is shorter than those before the block. Such recordings should not be misinterpreted as type II block.

Illustrative example 3

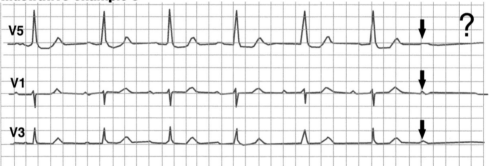

2nd-degree AV block. The PR intervals are constant before the blocked atrial impulse. This should not be misinterpreted as type II block because there is no PR interval for examination after the blocked P wave. This pattern is best described as unclassifiable.

Illustrative example 4

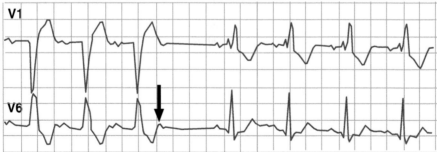

Alternating bundle branch block. The ECG starts with left bundle branch block. A slightly premature atrial impulse (arrow) precipitates right bundle branch block. The longer PR interval during left bundle branch conduction points to a more severely damaged right bundle branch. Alternating bundle branch block is an indication for pacemaker implantation.

Illustrative example 5

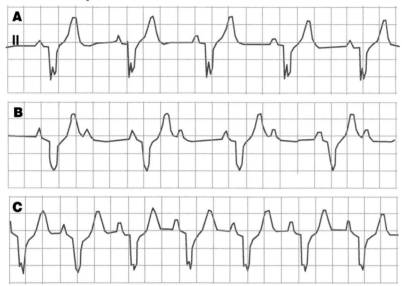

Development of 2:1 AV block induced by exercise shown in a 3-lead ECG. Holter recordings were unremarkable. (A) The ECG showed sinus rhythm at 60 bpm, complete right bundle branch block and left anterior hemiblock. There was no evidence of AV block. (B) During treadmill testing the patient developed an 2:1 AV block. (C) Recovery with return of 1:1 AV conduction. AV block on exercise is typical of infranodal block.

Illustrative example 6

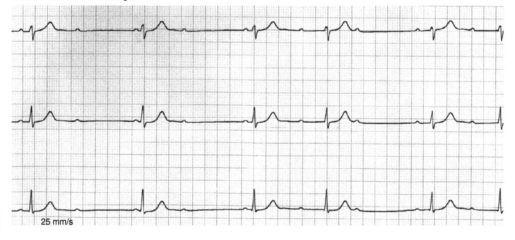

Normal sinus rhythm with a high-degree of AV block. Some of the beats exhibit a very long PR interval. These beats are most probably conducted across the AV node with marked delay and are associated with shortening of the RR interval. Sudden shortening of the RR intervals during complete AV block suggests intermittent AV conduction rather than an irregularity of an idioventricular rhythm.

OVERVIEW OF 2ND-DEGREE AV BLOCK

Illustrative example 7

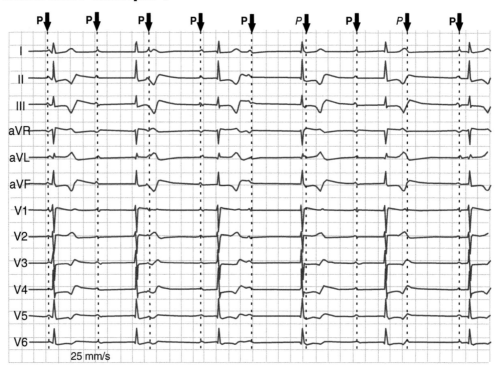

Complete AV block. There is AV dissociation and the atrial rate is faster than the ventricular rate. The idioventricular rhythm is regular at 45 bpm.

Illustrative example 8

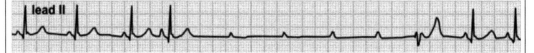

Bradycardia-dependent (phase 4) AV block sometimes called "paroxysmal block". There is sinus rhythm (73 bpm) on the left. An atrial premature beat precipitates paroxysmal AV block with prolonged ventricular asystole during which the sinus rhythm increases to about 83 bpm. During 1:1 AV conduction the ECG was normal with narrow QRS complexes. This type of AV block is always due to disease of the His-Purkinje system. The latter acquires the property of spontaneous depolarization. During long pauses the abnormal site becomes less responsive to subsequent impulses which are therefore blocked. This type of AV block must be differentiated from vagally-mediated AV block.

ECG Pitfalls in the Diagnosis of 2nd-Degree AV Block

* Nonconducted atrial premature beats masquerading as AV block.

* What appears to be narrow QRS type II block may be a type I variant.

* Failure to suspect type I block in the presence of miniscule increments of the PR interval.

* Atypical type I sequences mistaken for type II block.

* Making the diagnosis of type II block without seeing a truly conducted first postblock P wave ("shortage" of PR intervals).

* Type I AV block can be physiologic in athletes (resulting from heavy physical training) and occasionally in young individuals.

* Type I AV block can be physiologic during sleep in individuals with high vagal tone.

* Failure to suspect vagally-induced AV block, i.e. vomiting.

* Poor correlation between narrow QRS type I block and symptoms.

* Beliefs that all type I blocks are AV nodal because type I block with a wide QRS can sometimes be infranodal.

* Failure to realize that type I and type II almost never occur in the same ECG or Holter recording especially if the QRS is narrow. Therefore the presence of type I block strongly suggests that the tracings resembling type II block are in effect type I blocks with very small increments of the PR interval.

Further Reading

Barold SS, Hayes DL. Second-degree atrioventricular block: a reappraisal. Mayo Clin Proc. 2001;76:44-57.

Barold SS. Lingering misconceptions about type I second-degree atrioventricular block. Am J Cardiol. 2001;88:1018-20.

Barold SS. 2:1 Atrioventricular block: order from chaos. Am J Emerg Med. 2001;19:214-17.

Barold SS, Stroobandt RX, A.F. Sınnaeve, E. Andrıes, B. Herweg . Reappraisal of the traditional Wenckebach phenomenon with a modified ladder diagram. Ann Noninvasive Electrocardiol. 2012: 17:3-7.

Barold SS, Jaïs P, Shah DC, Takahashi A, Haïssaguerre M, Clémenty J. Exercise-induced second-degree AV block: is it type I or type II? J Cardiovasc Electrophysiol. 1997;8:1084-6.

Barra SN, Providência R, Paiva L, Nascimento J, Marques AL. A review on advanced atrioventricular block in young or middle-aged adults. Pacing Clin Electrophysiol. 2012;35:1395-405.

Lee S, Wellens HJ, Josephson ME. Paroxysmal atrioventricular block. Heart Rhythm. 2009;6:1229-34.

Wang K, Benditt DG. AV dissociation, an inevitable response. Ann Noninvasive Electrocardiol. 2011;227-31.

CHAPTER 14

ATRIAL RHYTHM DISORDERS

* Atrial flutter definition and reentry
* Atrial flutter diagnosis
* Atrial flutter and ventricular rate
* Atypical atrial flutter
* Atrial fibrillation definition and classification
* Long-short rule – Ashman phenomenon
* Pathophysiology and principles of therapy
* Carotid sinus massage
* Sick sinus syndrome – bradycardia-tachycardia syndrome
* Supraventricular tachyarrhythmias
    ◦ Tachycardias related to the sinoatrial node
    ◦ Atrial tachycardias
* Atrioventricular nodal reentrant tachycardia
* Atrioventricular reentrant tachycardia (AVRT)
    ◦ Accessory pathways and delta waves
    ◦ Orthodromic and antidromic AVRT
* Permanent junctional reciprocating tachycardia (PJRT)

ECG from Basics to Essentials: Step by Step. First Edition. Roland X. Stroobandt, S. Serge Barold and Alfons F. Sinnaeve.
Published 2016 © 2016 by John Wiley & Sons, Ltd. Companion Website: www.wiley.com/go/stroobandt/ecg

ATRIAL FLUTTER 1

Atrial flutter (AFL) is a very fast atrial rhythm (240–300 bpm). The atrial flutter rate may be slower (even < 200 bpm) in the presence of pharmacologic therapy or marked conduction delay within the atria. The atrial rhythm is regular and organized. Occasionally it may coexist with atrial fibrillation and is then called atrial flutter-fibrillation.

The common type of AFL is a macro-reentrant phenomenon in the right atrium in contrast to atrial fibrillation which is never sustained by macro-reentry.

There are two types of common flutter: anticlockwise and clockwise. They both engage the same macro-reentrant pathway in the right atrium but in opposite directions. The anticlockwise form constitutes about 90% of all atrial flutters and is by far more common than the clockwise form of common atrial flutter (AFL).

Schematic representation of reentry circuits

Anticlockwise

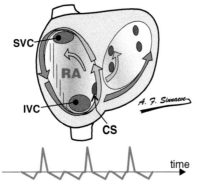

negative flutter waves in the
inferior leads (leads II, III, aVF)

Clockwise

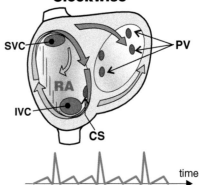

positive flutter waves in the
inferior leads (leads II, III, aVF)

CS = coronary sinus ; IVC = inferior vena cava ; SVC = superior vena cava ; PV = pulmonary veins

Reentry

All **reentrant processes** must have an area of slow conduction for sustaining an arrhythmia. In common AFL the area of slow conduction is in the lower part of the right atrium.

In **anticlockwise** AFL the depolarization front emerges from the site of slow conduction and passes along the posterior wall of the right atrium, then upwards along the atrial septum and then it travels inferiorly along the anterior and lateral wall of the right atrium to its destination point of origin where it reengages the same macro-reentrant pathway in a self-perpetuating fashion.

Clockwise (inverse or reverse) AFL takes the identical depolarization pathway but in the opposite direction.

Common AFL can be cured by catheter ablation of the area or slow conduction in the lower right atrium (cavotricuspid isthmus between the tricuspid orifice and the inferior vena cava). This type of atrial flutter is called isthmus dependent.

ECG of the typical AFL

There is a typical sawtooth appearance without isoelectric segments and without P waves. The flutter waves called "F waves" are inverted in the inferior leads (II, III, aVF) because the activation moves from the inferior to the superior part of the heart. The F waves are positive in lead V1. The positive part of the F wave (craniocaudal) lasts longer and is less visible than the negative portion (inferior to superior). There are no isoelectric segments in the inferior leads. This pattern is highly predictive of anticlockwise atrial flutter.

In clockwise AFL, the flutter waves are reversed (i.e. positive) in the inferior leads and negative in V1. The pattern of clockwise AFL may be impossible to differentiate from that of atypical AFL.

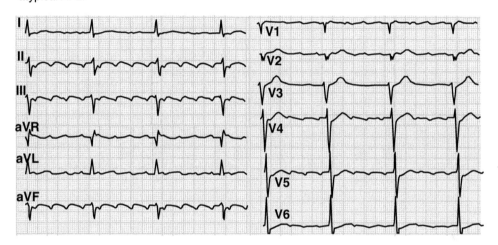

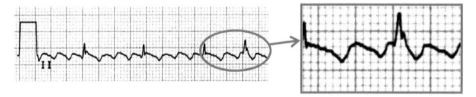

Atrial flutter with varying AV block 2:1, 4:1, etc.
(The atrial rate is 300 bpm and the ventricular rate varies from 150 bpm to 75 bpm)

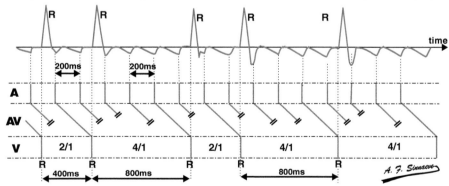

3:1 and 5:1 blocks are possible but are rare.
The diagram shows how the atrial impulses achieve varying degrees of penetration into the AV node

ATRIAL FLUTTER 2

Diagnosis

The diagnosis is usually easy. A common mistake is to call AFL sinus tachycardia at a rate of 150 bpm. It is an important clinical rule that a narrow QRS tachycardia at a rate close to 150 bpm should be considered as being AFL until proven otherwise. With this concept one can then look for the "hidden" F waves on the T wave. AFL must be differentiated from other forms of supraventricular tachycardia. Carotid sinus massage often causes a higher degree of AV block such as 4:1 AV block whereupon the atrial flutter waves are easily recognizable. With the common types of reentrant supraventricular tachycardia, carotid sinus massage may either terminate the tachycardia or have no effect. Multifocal atrial tachycardia and atrial tachycardia with AV block (atrial rate usually < 240 bpm) must be ruled out. If the QRS complex is wide (functional or stable bundle branch block), AFL at a rate of 150 bpm may mimic ventricular tachycardia. Artifacts from tremor (as in Parkinson's disease) may closely resemble AFL. The ECG should then be taken at the highest points on the extremities.

Atrial flutter rate slowed due to the effect of antiarrhythmic drug

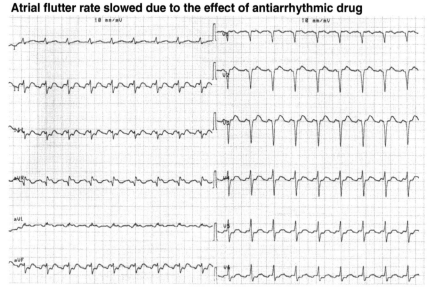

The atrial rate is 220 bpm (slower than classic AFL) and the ventricular rate is 110 bpm. It is important not to mistake this arrhythmia for sinus tachycardia.

Atrial flutter (300 bpm) with 2:1 ventricular response (150 bpm)

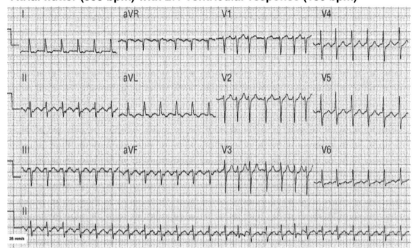

There is mostly 2:1 AV block. The average irregular ventricular rate is about 150 bpm. Note that in AFL with 2:1 block the ventricular rate is almost never perfectly regular. Some atrial impulses are blocked in the AV node. They may travel along the AV node and are then blocked at various levels within the node while others traverse the AV node successfully. The atrial impulses blocked in the body of the AV node influence the conduction of subsequent atrial impulses with resultant variations in AV conduction that cause obvious or subtle irregularity of the ventricular rate.

Effect of Carotid Sinus Massage (CSM) on atrial flutter.
CSM slows the ventricular rate by producing high grade AV block

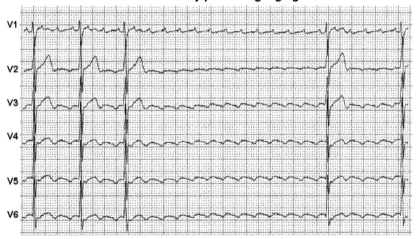

The ECG suggests anticlockwise AFL at a rate of 250 bpm

ATRIAL FLUTTER 3

Ventricular rate

The ventricular rate is usually 150 bpm because of 2:1 AV block (i.e. 2 atrial impulses and 1 ventricular impulse). This is a functional AV block (the tollbooth effect as a safety or protective mechanism) because the normal AV node can conduct the atrial impulses on a 1:1 fashion (300 bpm) only in exceptional circumstances. Such a 1:1 conduction is rare but may occur in patients with an accessory pathway that bypasses the AV node (no protective mechanism as in the AV node) or in states of excessive catecholamine (adrenaline) stimulation or even exercise. Some antiarrhythmic agents can also precipitate 1:1 AV conduction. With medication with drugs that block AV nodal function the degree of functional block may increase to 4:1 AV block or periods of 2:1 AV block may occur with periods of 4:1 block. Conduction ratios of 3:1 or 5:1 are unusual. The ventricular rate may be slow if the patient already has partial or complete AV block.

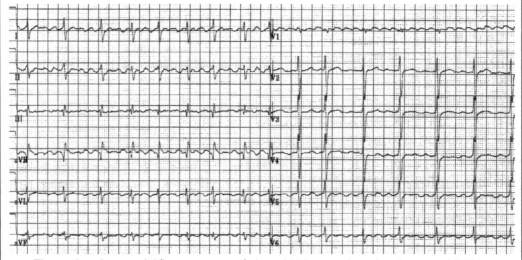

The tracing shows atrial flutter at a rate of about 300 bpm and varying degrees of AV block. Anticlockwise AFL is ruled out by the pattern in lead II where the F waves are positive. This is compatible with clockwise AFL but a nonisthmus-dependent AFL cannot be ruled out.

Atrial flutter with complete AV block

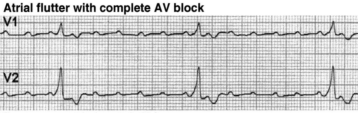

The escape ventricular rate is 33 bpm

Atypical Atrial Flutter

Atypical AFL may occur in many parts of the heart especially the left atrium. AFL may also revolve around a scar from previous cardiac surgery or occur after catheter ablation in the left atrium as for atrial fibrillation. These flutters produce electrocardiographic patterns that usually do not resemble those of common AFL in the right atrium. Indeed, left AFL is often fast, 340–350 bpm, obviously not isthmus-dependent and behaves like atrial fibrillation. Finding the origin and mechanism of these atypical flutters requires an invasive electrophysiologic study.

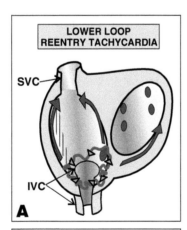

LOWER LOOP
REENTRY TACHYCARDIA

A

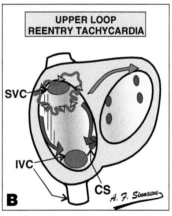

UPPER LOOP
REENTRY TACHYCARDIA

B

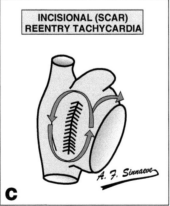

INCISIONAL (SCAR)
REENTRY TACHYCARDIA

C

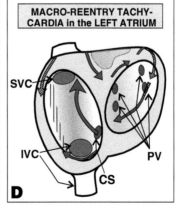

MACRO-REENTRY TACHY-
CARDIA in the LEFT ATRIUM

D

ATRIAL FLUTTER 4

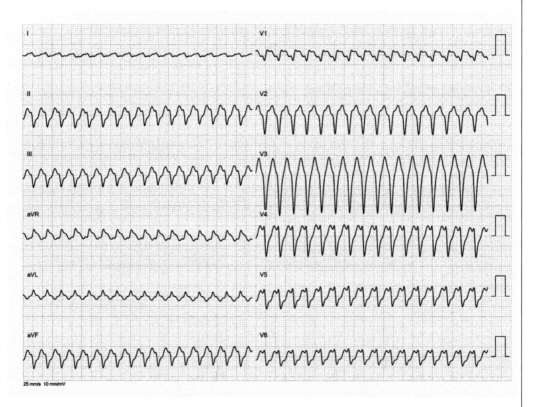

25 mm/s 10 mm/mV

Antiarrhythmic drugs, especially flecainide or propafenone (class 1C), may slow the flutter to 200 +/- 20 bpm. A slower atrial rate can change the usual 2:1 AV block (e.g. when the atrial rate is 300 bpm and the ventricular rate is 150 bpm) to 1:1 AV conduction which seems to be a paradoxical response as far as the ventricular rate is concerned. 1:1 AV conduction may occur if AV nodal blocking drugs are not administered together with antiarrhythmic agents. A 1:1 AV response may be blocked by the administration of AV nodal suppressing agents that delay AV nodal conduction.

1:1 AV conduction of ordinary atrial flutter is rare. The ventricular rate approaches 300 bpm and causes aberrant ventricular conduction thereby mimicking ventricular tachycardia. The commonest cause of 1:1 AV conduction is an accessory pathway (with a short refractory period) as in the Wolff-Parkinson-White syndrome. Other patients with an AV node capable of rapid conduction (due to a bypass tract across part or all of the AV node) may develop 1:1 atrial flutter especially in response to increased sympathetic tone as with exercise. Such patients may have short PR interval in sinus rhythm. Rapid AV conduction may also occur in hyperthyroidism. Very fast ventricular rates close to 300 bpm may lead to syncope, hemodynamic collapse and ventricular fibrillation.

Coronary Care Unit
Keep quiet

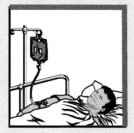

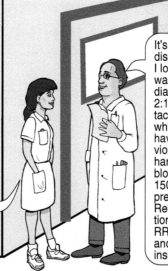

How did you make the diagnosis of atrial flutter from the end of the bed where you could not possibly see the monitored ECG ?

It's simple. I saw the monitor display a rate of 150 and then I looked at the patient. As he was in no distress, I made the diagnosis of atrial flutter with 2:1 AV block. I ruled out sinus tachycardia at a rate of 150 in which case the patient would have been in distress and obviously very sick. On the other hand, atrial flutter with 2:1 AV block and a ventricular rate of 150 (or close to it) may be interpreted as sinus tachycardia. Remember if an atrial deflection occurs in the middle of an RR interval, there is probably another atrial deflection buried inside the QRS complex.

> It is important to remember that the ventricular rate in atrial flutter varies slightly. This is because the atrial impulses achieve varying degrees of penetration in the AV node before being blocked thereby creating different levels of refractoriness which will influence AV conduction of subsequent beats. Therefore an absolutely regular ventricular rate may represent a separate AV regular junctional rhythm as in digitalis toxicity.

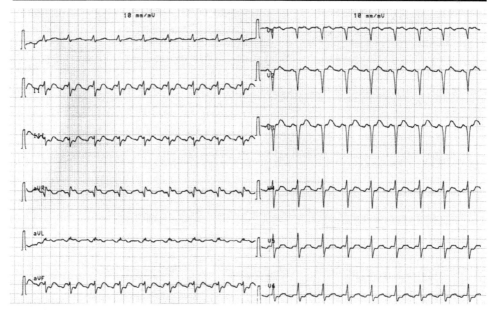

On the other side the ECG shows 1:1 atrial flutter at a rate of 215 bpm in a patient taking flecainide. At this fast ventricular rate the QRS complex is different from the one at a slower rate on the right. The altered QRS morphology is caused by aberrant ventricular conduction at a fast rate. On this page the ECG shows atrial flutter at a rate of 210–215 bpm with 2:1 AV block (ventricular rate of approximately 107 bpm) after administration of an agent that attenuated AV nodal conduction.

ATRIAL FIBRILLATION 1

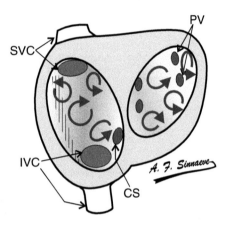

CS: coronary sinus; PV: pulmonary vein;
IVC: inferior vena cava; SVC: superior vena
cava

Compared with atrial flutter in which there is one reentrant circuit and is organized, atrial fibrillation has multiple reentrant circuits and no organization.

Atrial fibrillation (AFib) is the most common arrhythmia and is due to uncoordinated atrial myocardial activity due to multiple reentry circuits associated with deterioration of atrial mechanical activity. In essence the atria quiver with no effective contraction.

AFib has a high incidence in the elderly, increasing with age. Patients can develop AFib secondary to cardiac disease that affects the atria (e.g. congestive heart failure, hypertensive heart disease, rheumatic heart disease, coronary artery disease) but sometimes no cause is found. AFib patients tend to be older, and AFib is more likely to be persistent in the elderly.

In AFib, the normal regular electrical impulses generated by the sinoatrial node are overwhelmed by impulses usually originating in the roots of the pulmonary veins that disorganize the atrial rhythm, creating an irregular atrial rhythm (AFib), leading in turn to irregular conduction of impulses to the ventricles. AFib may occur in episodes lasting from minutes to days ("paroxysmal"), or may be permanent in nature.

Classification scheme for patients with atrial fibrillation

Published guidelines from an American College of Cardiology (ACC)/ American Heart Association (AHA)/ European Society of Cardiology (ESC) Committee of experts on the treatment of patients with atrial fibrillation recommend classification of AFib into the following 3 patterns :

* **Paroxysmal AFib** : Episodes of AFib that terminate spontaneously within 7 days (most episodes last less than 24 hours).
* **Persistent AFib** : Episodes of AFib that last more than 7 days and may require either pharmacologic or electrical intervention to terminate.
* **Permanent AFib** : AFib that has persisted for more than 1 year, because electrical cardioversion has either failed or has not been attempted.

This classification scheme pertains to cases that are not related to a reversible cause of AFib. Paroxysmal AFib is considered to be recurrent when a patient has 2 or more episodes. If recurrent AFib terminates spontaneously, it is designated as paroxysmal. Long-term follow-up of paroxysmal AFib often shows progression to permanent AFib. Persistent AFib is considered persistent, irrespective of whether the arrhythmia is terminated by pharmacologic therapy or electrical cardioversion. Persistent AFib may be either the first presentation of AFib or the result of recurrent episodes of paroxysmal AFib. Patients with persistent AFib also include those with long-standing AFib in whom cardioversion has not been indicated or attempted, often leading to permanent AFib.

Lone atrial fibrillation

In addition to the above scheme, the term "lone atrial fibrillation" has been used to identify AFib in younger patients without structural heart disease, who are at a lower risk for thromboembolism. The definition of lone AFib remains controversial, but it generally refers to paroxysmal, persistent, or permanent AFib in youger patients (< 60 y) who have normal echocardiographic findings.

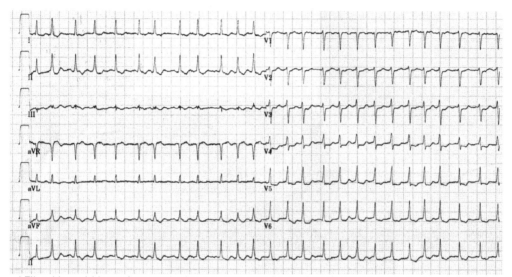

AFib with rapid irregular ventricular rate 150–160 bpm. Note the low amplitude f waves in V1 .

Electrocardiogram

AFib produces a totally irregular rhythm with absence of P waves. There are small irregular "f waves" (350–600 bpm) creating an undulating baseline. A wise observer coined the statement "the tracing never sits still!". Occasionally the baseline is flat, a finding more commonly seen with longstanding AFib. When the baseline is flat, an AV junctional rhythm should be ruled out if the ventricular rate is slow. AFib can coexist with third degree AV block in which case the ventricular rate is slow and the baseline shows a pattern typical of AFib.

In the untreated patient, the ventricular rate is fast and irregular; it may be as fast as 200 bpm though it is usually 140–160 bpm. There is no pattern to the irregularity, so AFib may be described as irregularly irregular. The rate can be close to 300 in patients with a bypass (accessory) tract that does not utilize the AV node for transmission to the ventricles.

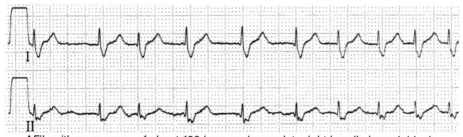

AFib with an average of about 100 bpm and complete right bundle branch block.

ATRIAL FIBRILLATION 2

Atrial fibrillation is an irregularly irregular ventricular rhythm. However, when there is a rapid ventricular response, on the first look the rhythm may appear regular but on closer inspection it is clearly definitely irregular. The irregularity is best ascertained with calipers.

An ECG report of AFib should state whether the ventricular rate is regular or irregular

- Increased morbidity and mortality is due in part to thromboembolic stroke. Disruption of the atrial electromechanical function causes stasis and the development of thrombus most commonly in the left atrial appendage from which it can embolize. AFib increases the risk of a stroke by a factor of 5.
- AFib may precipitate heart failure by loss of the atrial contribution to the cardiac output. AFib is very common in heart failure patients. Acutely, AFib may cause hemodynamic deterioration, left ventricular dysfunction and heart failure.
- Tachycardia-mediated cardiomyopathy is a long-term complication of a fast ventricular rate and may lead to heart failure. The process can often be reversed by slowing the ventricular rate or returning to sinus rhythm.
- AFib is dangerous in patients with an accessory tract capable of conducting rapidly to the ventricle. Such a bypass tract should always be considered when the ventricular rate is 200–300.

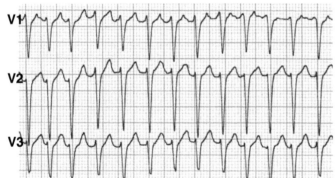

Atrial fibrillation and apparent regular ventricular response. Simultaneous recording of V1 to V3 showing atrial fibrillation and a fast ventricular rate. Note that the ventricular intervals become virtually regular. The irregularity becomes apparent only on close inspection. This is a normal response when the rate is rapid and it should not be misinterpreted as an AV junctional tachycardia.

Regular ventricular rate

1. **Slow rate.** An escape or relatively slow AV junctional rhythm is often caused by digitalis toxicity. The RR intervals may normalize in duration for only a few cycles, merging in and out of the basic irregular ventricular rate. This rhythm is often missed. The regular intervals can be identified with calipers. The rhythm is the reason for stating in an ECG report whether the ventricular rate is regular or irregular.

2. **Fast rate.** AV junctional tachycardia. Also suspect digitalis toxicity.

3. **Wide complex tachycardia.** This is usually ventricular tachycardia if the ventricular rate is regular.

Controlled and uncontrolled ventricular rate with drug therapy.
A controlled ventricular rate (VR) at rest may not be controlled on exercise.
1. At rest : aim for a VR < 80–90 bpm.
2. With activity (e.g. during a brisk walk) aim for VR < 110–115 bpm.

Control the rate and prevent strokes with anticoagulant therapy

How to determine the average ventricular rate ?
1. Count out 6 seconds (30 big squares).
2. Count the number of QRS complexes in that period.
3. Multiply the number of QRS complexes by 10.

Long-Short Rule – Ashman phenomenon

The Ashman phenomenon refers to aberrant ventricular conduction due to a change in QRS cycle length. The long-short rule was first described in 1947 in AFib to explain aberrant conduction (usually with right bundle branch block morphology). Aberrancy was observed when a relatively long cycle was followed by a relatively short cycle. The short cycle ended with the aberrantly conducted beat.
Aberrant conduction depends on the relative refractory period of the components of the conduction system distal to the AV node. The refractory period (recovery time of the conduction system) depends on the heart rate and changes with the RR interval of the preceding cycle. A short RR interval reduces the duration of the refractory period. A longer cycle or slower heart rate lengthens the ensuing refractory period and, if a shorter cycle follows, the beat ending it is likely to be conducted with aberrancy. A right bundle branch block pattern is more common than a left bundle branch block pattern because of the longer refractory period of the right bundle branch. The Ashman phenomenon causes diagnostic confusion with ventricular premature complexes.

Pathophysiology

AFib needs a trigger that induces the arrhythmia and a substrate that sustains it. The pulmonary veins (with a sleeve of atrial tissue) were found to be the focal triggers for many cases of AFib. This has been confirmed by the successful treatment of AFib by catheter ablation of these pulmonary triggers. Other trigger sites with a muscular sleeve around a large vein such as the superior vena cava have been found less commonly and can be eradicated by catheter ablation. The atria acting as a substrate for AFib respond to the rapid firing of the pulmonary veins by creating 4 to 6 wavelets of excitation that meander around the atria. Some of these wavelets may self-organize into a "mother" rotor which then exerts more control over the electrophysiologic process. A self-sustaining rotor can fire at a high frequency resulting in complex patterns of activation. One wonders whether elimination of only a "mother" rotor might prevent AFib. The complex electrophysiologic process that sustains AFib consisting of multiple wavelets, mother waves, fixed or moving rotors, and macro-reentrant circuits present a formidable challenge in the search for a simpler catheter ablation technique.

Principles of therapy

Persistent AFib with an uncontrolled, rapid ventricular heart rate response can cause a dilated cardiomyopathy with poor left ventricular function and left atrial dilatation from electrical remodeling.
AFib may be treated with medications to either slow the ventricular rate by their depressant effect on the AV node by limiting the number of impulses reaching the ventricles ("rate control") or revert the heart rhythm back to normal sinus rhythm ("rhythm control"). Electrical cardioversion can be used to convert AFib to a normal rhythm. Patients with AFib often take anticoagulant therapy to protect them from a stroke as about a third of all strokes are caused by AFib. Catheter ablation of active foci in the pulmonary veins may eliminate the trigger of many types of atrial fibrillation and prevent recurrence.

CAROTID SINUS MASSAGE

Carotid sinus massage is a vagal maneuver that involves rubbing a large part of the arterial wall at the point where the common carotid artery, located in the neck, divides into its two main branches. This is the site of baroreceptors that control the blood pressure. Massage is done for 5 seconds. Both sides are never done at the same time. Carotid sinus massage will slow the sinus rate or heart rate during episodes of atrial flutter or atrial fibrillation by producing AV block. It may also terminate some reentrant supraventricular tachycardias.

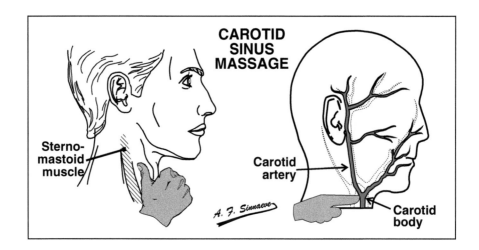

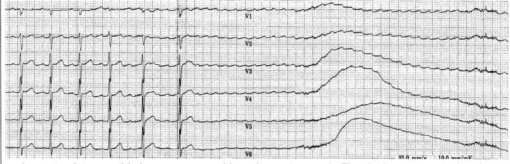

Inappropriate carotid sinus massage with prolonged asystole. The rhythm returned after the patient was told to cough.

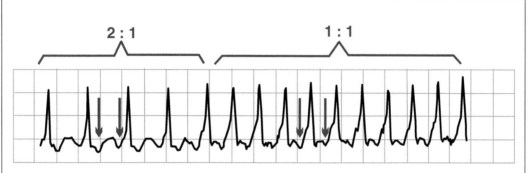

Atrial flutter showing transition from 2:1 to 1:1 flutter

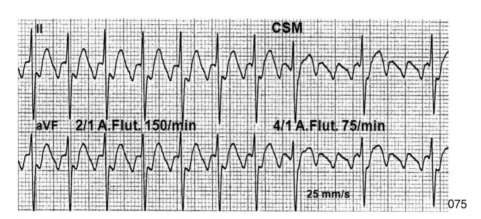

Carotid sinus massage may facilitate diagnosis by slowing the ventricular response and revealing the flutter waves. During CSM there is a transition from 2:1 to 4:1 flutter.

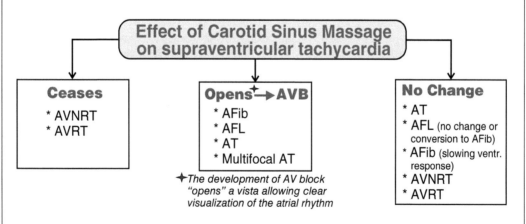

AFib = atrial fibrillation; AFL = atrial flutter; AT = atrial tachycardia; AVRT = atrioventricular reentrant tachycardia; AVNRT = AV nodal reentrant tachycardia

SICK SINUS SYNDROME

Sick sinus syndrome (SSS) is an irreversible dysfunction of the sinus node, atria and a disease that involves much of the conduction system of the heart. The diffuse cardiac involvement of the heart overshadows the terminology that focuses only on the sinoatrial node though SSS is basically a generalized abnormality of cardiac impulse formation and features that may take years to become manifest. SSS commonly affects elderly persons. There are many causes, but it usually is idiopathic. Functional sinus bradycardia due to enhanced vagal tone must be excluded before the diagnosis of SSS can be made.

> **The so-called bradycardia-tachycardia syndrome is a misnomer and should be called tachycardia-bradycardia syndrome since overdrive suppression occurs after tachycardia. In other words bradycardia occurs after tachycardia !**

The manifestations of SSS can be either persistent or just sporadic. The diagnosis of SSS can be difficult because of its nonspecific symptoms and elusive findings on the ECG and even on a 24 hr Holter monitor. SSS has multiple manifestations on the ECG, including sinus bradycardia, sinus arrest, sinoatrial block, atrioventricular conduction disturbances and alternating patterns of bradycardia and tachycardia (bradycardia-tachycardia syndrome). Supraventricular tachyarrhythmias include atrial fibrillation, atrial flutter and supraventricular tachycardia. Atrial fibrillation is the most common tachyarrhythmia in these patients. Overdrive suppression of the sinus node occurs often upon termination of a supraventricular tachyarrhythmia. This may cause a long pause with failure of an AV junctional escape mechanism (as would occur in a normal heart) and syncope according to the duration of the pause. Failure of an appropriate AV junctional escape under these circumstances reflects the presence of abnormalities affecting the AV junction. SSS includes an atrial rate inappropriate for physiologic requirements (chronotropic incompetence). In this respect, exercise testing may be useful in determining the response of the sinus node to physiologic requirements. Occasionally SSS presents as a long pause and severe bradycardia following electrical cardioversion of an atrial tachyarrhythmia. The diagnosis of SSS also includes frequent symptomatic sinus pauses where the cause is iatrogenic and occurs as a consequence of essential long-term drug therapy for which there are no acceptable alternatives.

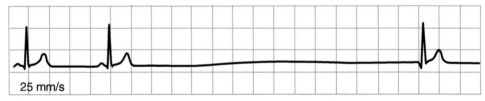

25 mm/s

Sinus rhythm at 75 bpm. Abrupt sinus arrest of 3 s followed by a junctional escape beat

SSS is the most important indication for antibradycardia pacing. The management after pacemaker implantation may be difficult because of recurrent or permanent atrial fibrillation, risk of embolic stroke and anticoagulant therapy. The pacemaker cannot prevent the supraventricular tachyarrhythmias, but facilitates drug therapy by preventing bradycardia.

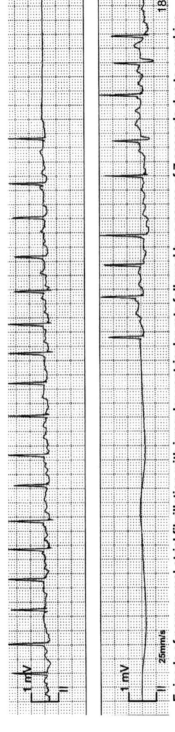

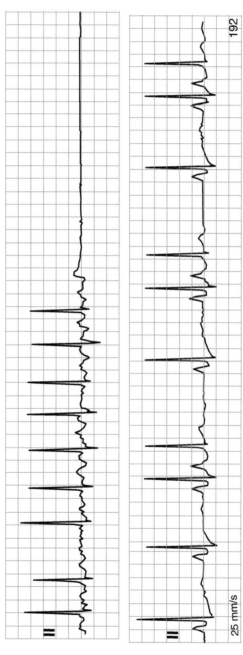

189

Episode of paroxysmal atrial fibrillation with irregular ventricular rate followed by a pause of 7 seconds due to overdrive suppression of the sinus node. There is an unsuccessful attempt to restore sinus rhythm. After the long pause with ventricular asystole, atrial fibrillation resumes.

192

Atrial fibrillation with an irregular ventricular rate. Cessation of the arrhythmia is associated with prolonged sinus arrest (ventricular asystole) of about 5 sec due to overdrive suppression. When sinus rhythm returns frequent atrial premature beats are evident.

SUPRAVENTRICULAR TACHYARRHYTHMIAS 1

Supraventricular tachycardia (SVT) describes any tachyarrhythmia that requires the atrium or the atrioventricular (AV) junction for its initiation and maintenance. It usually has a narrow complex and is a regular and rapid rhythm with exceptions such as atrial fibrillation and multifocal atrial tachycardia which are irregular. Aberrant conduction during SVT results in a wide-complex tachycardia that resembles ventricular tachycardia. SVTs may be classified as atrial or AV dependent according to the site of origin and mechanism.

Atrial tachyarrhythmias include (1) sinus tachycardia, (2) inappropriate sinus tachycardia, (3) sinus node reentrant tachycardia, (4) atrial tachycardia, (5) multifocal atrial tachycardia, (6) atrial flutter, and (7) atrial fibrillation.

AV tachyarrhythmias depend on the AV junction and include (1) AV nodal reentrant tachycardia, (2) AV reentrant tachycardia utilizing an accessory pathway, (3) junctional ectopic tachycardia, and (4) nonparoxysmal junctional tachycardia.

TACHYCARDIAS RELATED TO THE SINOATRIAL NODE

Sinus tachycardia refers to an accelerated sinus rate that is a physiologic response to a stressor. It is characterized by a heart rate faster than 100 bpm and generally involves a regular rhythm.

Inappropriate sinus tachycardia consists of an accelerated sinus rate in the absence of a physiologic stressor. There is an elevated resting heart rate and an exaggerated heart rate response to even minimal exercise. This tachyarrhythmia occurs most commonly in young women without structural heart disease. The underlying mechanism may be hypersensitivity of the sinus node to autonomic influences or an abnormality in the sinus node or both. Inappropriate sinus tachycardia is a diagnosis of exclusion so that causes of appropriate sinus tachycardia must first be excluded.

Sinus node reentrant tachycardia is frequently confused with inappropriate sinus tachycardia. Sinus node reentrant tachycardia is due to a reentry circuit, either in or near the sinus node. Therefore, it has an abrupt onset and offset in contrast to physiologic sinus tachycardia which starts and ends gradually. The heart rate is usually 100–150 bpm. It has an activation sequence similar to that of normal sinus rhythm so that the P waves on the surface ECG appear to be normal. In comparison, atrial tachycardias (focal or reentrant) have a different activation sequence of atrial depolarization resulting in a P wave morphology that differs from that of normal sinus rhythm. The tachycardia is uncommon, usually of no clinical significance (inducible in the electrophysiologic laboratory), but the arrhythmia is on occasion sufficiently recurrent, rapid and sustained to be symptomatic. It can occur in both normal hearts and those with a sick sinoatrial node.

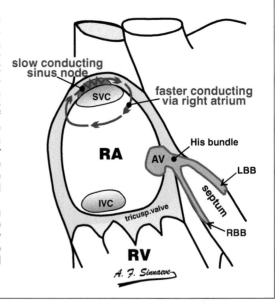

> **Sinus tachycardia, inappropriate sinus tachycardia and sinus node reentrant tachycardia all display a P wave configuration similar to that seen in normal sinus rhythm.**

start CSM

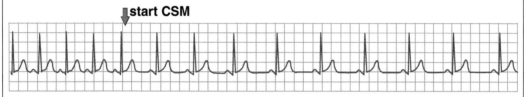

Sinus tachycardia gradually slowed down by carotid sinus massage (CSM) pressure

start CSM

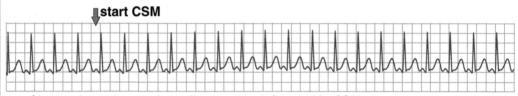

Sinus node reentrant tachycardia cannot be influenced by CSM

ATRIAL TACHYCARDIAS

A number of methods are used to classify atrial tachycardia (AT).

1. Endocardial activation. *(A) Focal atrial tachycardias,* which arises from a localized area in the atria such as the crista terminalis, pulmonary veins, etc. *(B) Reentrant tachycardias* are usually macro-reentrant, and most commonly occur in the setting of structural heart disease, and particularly after surgery involving incisions or scarring in the atria.

2. Pathophysiologic mechanisms are another method for classifying ATs: enhanced automaticity, triggered activity, or reentry.

3. Anatomic classification of atrial tachycardia is based on the location of the arrhythmogenic focus.

Atrial tachycardia (AT) arises in the atria and not in the sinoatrial node. AT (100–250 bpm) can be observed in persons with normal hearts and in those with structurally abnormal hearts. ATs do not require the AV junction, accessory pathways, or ventricular myocardium for initiation and maintenance of the tachycardia. The ECG typically shows a narrow QRS complex (unless bundle branch block aberration occurs). The atrial rhythm is usually regular. The conducted ventricular rhythm is also usually regular but may become irregular, often at higher rates because of variable conduction through the AV node, with conduction patterns such as 2:1, 4:1, a combination of those, or even in the form of second-degree Wenckebach block.

SUPRAVENTRICULAR TACHYARRHYTHMIAS 2

ATRIAL TACHYCARDIAS continued

Focal versus macro-reentrant atrial tachycardia

Focal AT may be initiated by increased automaticity or triggered automaticity or microentry as stated above. A focal AT starts from a point source from which it spreads centrifugally. The mechanism may be difficult to determine from the ECG except for automatic AT. The latter is rare and exhibits a gradual onset (warm-up) and gradual slowing (cooling down) thereby mimicking sinus tachycardia. Triggered ATs and macro-reentrant ATs may have sudden onset and offset. Macro-reentrant AT occurs around a large central obstacle usually centimeters in diameter. The distinction from focal AT may be impossible from the ECG. It can be differentiated from atrial flutter by the presence of discrete P waves and a slower atrial rate (170–220 bpm). In contrast to sinus tachycardia, macro-reentrant AT starts abruptly and the P waves differ from sinus P waves.

P wave morphology

The P wave morphology as observed on the ECG may give clues to the site of origin and mechanism of the atrial tachycardia. In the case of a focal tachycardia, the P wave morphology and axis depend on the location in the atrium from which the tachycardia originates. In the case of macro-reentant circuits the P wave morphology and axis depend on activation patterns. The polarity of the P wave may be difficult to interpret if it is inscribed upon the ST segment or the T wave. The determination of the site of AT origin according to the configuration of the P wave belongs in the realm of the cardiac electrophysiologist armed with a sophisticated algorithm that can define various sites according to P wave morphologies. Briefly, either a negative or biphasic (positive/negative) P wave in lead V1 identifies AT in the right atrium. A positive or biphasic (negative/positive) P wave identifies AT in the left atrium. A positive P wave in the inferior leads suggests a superior focus and a negative P wave suggests an inferior focus.

> Atrial tachycardia can be focal or macro-reentrant. It can be difficult to differentiate these two types from the ECG.

> Always look for a P wave that may be hidden within the QRS complex. Carotid sinus massage may cause AV block (usually 2:1) allowing evaluation of the P wave rate and configuration. It is worth stressing again that the presence or induction of AV block (2:1 A V block; Wenckebach type 1 block) is diagnostically helpful in ruling out reentrant SVT whose reentrant pathway includes the AV node (AV nodal reentrant tachycardia and AV reentrant tachycardia) and establishing the diagnosis of an atrial tachycardia independent of the AV node.

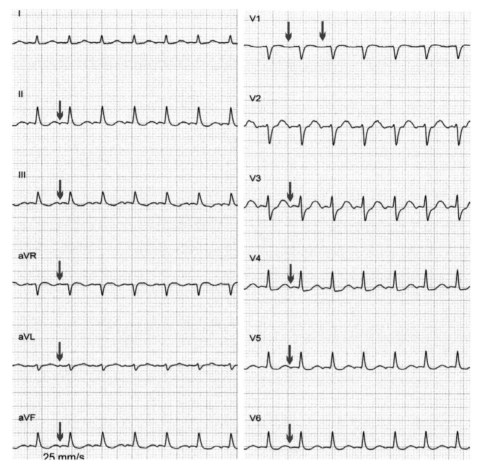

Atrial tachycardia at a rate of 136 bpm. Isoelectric P wave in V1 and negative P waves in V3 to V6 consistent with a right atrial perinodal (close to the AV node) atrial tachycardia.

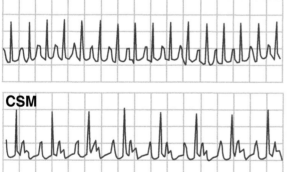

Atrial tachycardia at a rate of about 250 bpm. Carotid sinus massage (CSM) produces a 2:1 atrioventricular block permitting visualization of the P waves.

The diagnosis of any supraventricular tachycardia (SVT) involves measurement of the ventricular rate, assessment of the ventricular rhythm, identification of P, F (flutter) or f (fibrillation) waves, measurement of the atrial rate and establishment of the relation of P waves to the ventricular complexes. The ventricular rate will depend on the degree of atrioventricular block. Increasing atrioventricular block by maneuvres such as carotid sinus massage or administration of intravenous adenosine may slow the ventricular rate to allow visualization of atrial activity. Such maneuvres will not usually stop atrial tachycardia, but may terminate a reentrant SVT involving the atrioventricular node.

SUPRAVENTRICULAR TACHYARRHYTHMIAS 3

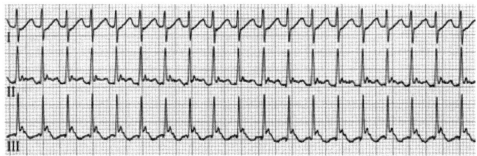

AT 1:1 at a rate of 240 bpm

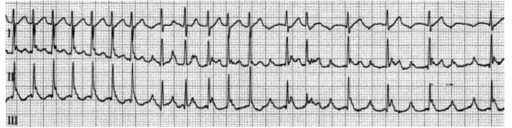

Same patient. Treatment with intravenous beta-blocker transition from 1:1 to 2:1 AV conduction, etc.

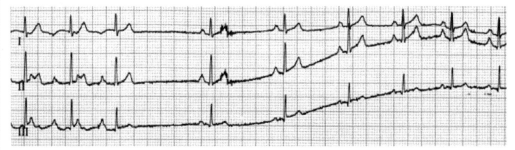

Same patient as above. Return to sinus rhythm

> **Suspect atrial tachycardia if there is a long RP interval (> 50% of the RR interval) or AV block. A long RP interval can also occur in some AV junctional reentrant tachycardias but AV block indicates that the tachycardia must be atrial because it does not depend on the AV junction for its initiation and maintenance.**

ATRIAL TACHYCARDIA WITH AV BLOCK

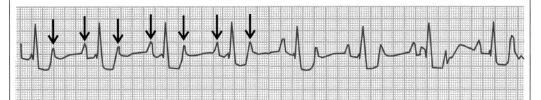

Atrial tachycardia with 2:1 AV block. The atrial rate is 107 bpm.

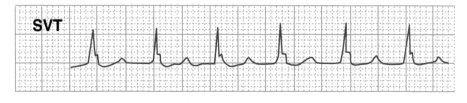

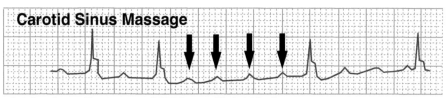

Atrial tachycardia at a rate of 250 bpm with 2:1 block.
Carotid sinus massage increases the degree of AV block permitting the diagnosis but does not terminate the tachycardia.

> **AT with Wenckebach AV block is easily overlooked. The increments of the PR interval may not be visible. The diagnosis is made at seeing a regular AT with occasional prolongation of the RR interval which corresponds to the pause that terminates a Wenckebach response.**

In AT with AV block, the ventricular rate may be irregular if there is varying AV block or Wenckebach AV block but the atrial rate remains constant. Complete AV block in AT is rare. Digitalis toxicity is an important cause of AT with AV block.

> **In AT there is an isoelectric baseline between the P waves in contrast to atrial flutter where there is no isoelectric baseline between the F waves.**

The degree of AV block may increase with carotid sinus pressure or adenosine, a drug that depresses AV conduction. However these maneuvers do not terminate AT. AT may be misdiagnosed as atrial flutter or fibrillation.

> **Atrial fibrillation is irregularly irregular. AT with AV block is regularly irregular as is atrial flutter with varying AV block.**
> **Multifocal atrial tachycardia can also be irregularly irregular.**

SUPRAVENTRICULAR TACHYARRHYTHMIAS 4

Multifocal atrial tachycardia

Multifocal atrial tachycardia (MAT) arises from the atrium and is composed of at least 3 morphologies of the P wave. The mechanism of MAT is unclear but it is probably due to increased automaticity and not reentry. MAT may be related to theophyline a drug used in the therapy of COPD. MAT is not due to digitalis (digoxin) toxicity. Indeed it is contraindicated in this tachyarrhythmia. The definition requires the presence of 3 different and discrete (organized) P waves in the same lead. Atrial activity is well organized and the baseline between the P waves is isoelectric. The P waves are separated by isoelectric intervals. The PP intervals, PR duration and RR intervals are all variable. The rate is 100–250 bpm and the arrhythmia may be intermittent. Other kinds of atrial arrhythmias (such as atrial fibrillation) may precede or follow an episode of MAT. The irregular rhythm is often misinterpreted as atrial fibrillation. The differential diagnosis is crucial because the therapy of AF and MAT differ considerably. MAT with aberrant conduction or preexisting bundle branch block may be misinterpreted as ventricular tachycardia. It must also be differentiated from sinus tachycardia or a slower sinus rhythm and salvos of atrial premature beats. MAT typically occurs in elderly patients with chronic obstructive pulmonary disease.

> **Multifocal atrial tachycardia typically occurs in elderly patients with chronic obstructive pulmonary disease.**

Some experts believe that a rate of 90 bpm with multifocal atrial activity should be treated as MAT in patients with COPD. A rhythm with multifocal activity and a rate < 100 bpm is best called a multifocal atrial rhythm.

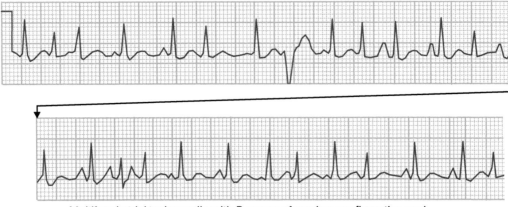

Multifocal atrial tachycardia with P waves of varying configuration and totally irregular ventricular rate.

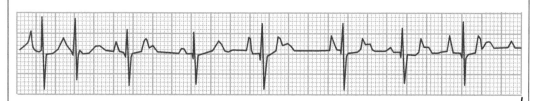

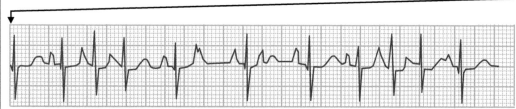

Unusual manifestation of supraventricular tachycardia.
Multifocal atrial tachycardia with varying P wave configuration and irregular ventricular rate. Early P waves are not conducted as the AV node is still refractory, adding to the irregularly irregular response.

Unusual atrial tachycardia

3:2 WB   4:3 atypical WB

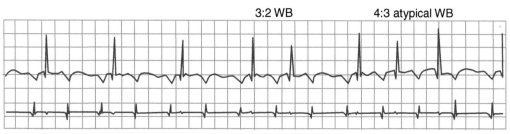

Wenckebach (WB) second degree (type I) AV block.
*Atrial tachycardia with Wenckebach AV block on 2 occasions, once atypical
The bottom tracing is an esophageal recording showing only P waves*

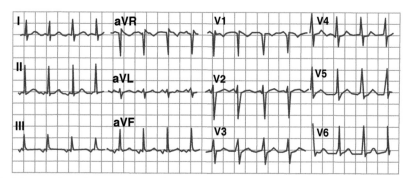

AT with very short PR interval; the P waves give rise to the second QRS that follows it.

ATRIOVENTRICULAR NODAL REENTRANT TACHYCARDIA 1

Atrioventricular nodal reentry tachycardia (AVNRT) is the most common type of reentrant supraventricular tachycardia (SVT) with an incidence of 60% of paroxysmal SVT. The nonspecific term paroxysmal supraventricular tachycardia, paroxysmal atrial tachycardia (PAT) should no longer be used. Current nomenclature is based on the mechanism of reentry. The substrate for AVNRT may be functional rather than anatomic. These arrhythmias occur in young healthy patients and in those with chronic heart disease. It occurs somewhat more commonly in adult females than in males. The rate ranges from 120 to 250 bpm.

A reentrant rhythm involves the presence of an anatomic and functional circuit or 2 distinct pathways that join to form a circle. There is a zone of slow conduction in one pathway and unidirectional block in the other pathway, allowing an electrical impulse to travel down the second pathway and reenter the blocked pathway from the other direction. During AVNRT, the circuit typically involves both a fast and a slow pathway within the region of the AV node.

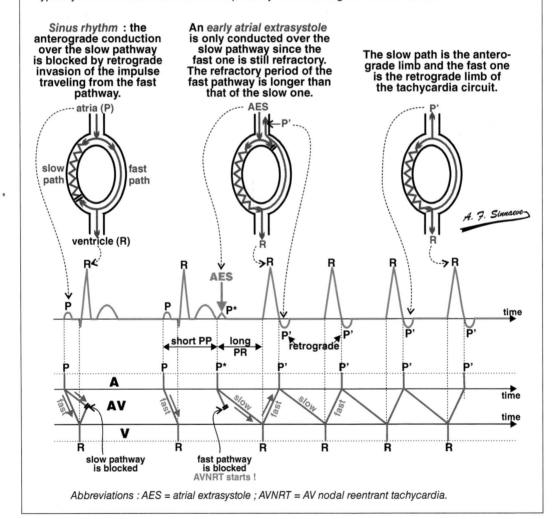

Sinus rhythm : the anterograde conduction over the slow pathway is blocked by retrograde invasion of the impulse traveling from the fast pathway.

An *early atrial extrasystole* is only conducted over the slow pathway since the fast one is still refractory. The refractory period of the fast pathway is longer than that of the slow one.

The slow path is the anterograde limb and the fast one is the retrograde limb of the tachycardia circuit.

A. F. Sinnaeve

Abbreviations : AES = atrial extrasystole ; AVNRT = AV nodal reentrant tachycardia.

In patients with AVNRT, the AV node is functionally divided into 2 longitudinal pathways (with different electrophysiologic characteristics) that form the reentrant circuit. In the normal situation conduction across the AV node to the His-Purkinje system occurs in the fast pathway and conduction in the slow pathway is therefore blocked at the point where the 2 pathways join inferiorly. In the majority of patients, during AVNRT, anterograde conduction occurs to the ventricle over the slow pathway and the retrograde conduction occurs over the fast pathway. The tachycardia is often initiated by an atrial premature complex blocked in the fast pathway according to prematurity and because the fast pathway has a longer refractory period. Consequently the impulse conducts in the slow pathway with a shorter refractory period. Thus the initiating AES has a long PR interval. While the impulse conducts to the ventricle in the slow pathway, the fast pathway recovers (provided the delay in the anterograde conduction is long enough to permit fast pathway recovery) and allows the impulse to be conducted via the fast pathway (when outside its refractory period) back to the atrium and the atrial end of the slow pathway where it completes the circuit.

Less commonly AVNRT is induced by premature ventricular beats. In addition to the above, atypical AV nodal reentry can occur in the opposite direction, with anterograde conduction in the fast pathway and retrograde conduction in the slow pathway. The typical form is slow-fast referring to anterograde and retrograde conduction. This slow-fast form occurs in 90% of clinical AVNRT episodes. In the atypical form, the conduction moves fast-slow i.e. anterogradely in the fast pathway, resulting in a short PR interval and a long RP interval. A third form also occurs where both the anterograde and the retrograde conduction occur through slow pathways (slow-slow).

AVNRT and AVRT (AV reciprocating or orthodromic tachycardia with accessory pathway) are dependent on AV nodal conduction. Sinus node reentry, atrial tachycardia, atrial flutter and atrial fibrillation are independent of AV nodal conduction.

In AVNRT the ventricle and atrium are activated simultaneously. The ventricle is not necessary for the reentrant process. 2:1 block (in the His bundle) may occur rarely. RP interval of AVNRT is less than 70 ms.

Slow-fast form
The QRS complex is generally narrow unless there is aberrant conduction (usually a right bundle branch pattern) or there is a preexisting conduction defect. The P waves are usually embedded in the QRS complex in the typical form and therefore not identifiable. When seen alone, the retrograde P wave is called an echo beat. P waves may be seen at the end of the QRS complex (as if they form part of the QRS) in the form of a pseudo-r' in lead V1 (imitating incomplete right bundle branch block) or a pseudo-s wave in leads II, III, and aVF (reflecting the negative retrograde P waves). These patterns can only be recognized by comparing the ECG during AVNRT with one in sinus rhythm. After the episode, significant ST depression is common as in AVRT and most patients do not have coronary artery disease.

Fast-slow form
In atypical cases the P waves can be clearly seen. The fast-slow AVNRT is thought to use the same pathways as in the typical AVNRT but in reverse direction. In the fast-slow type, the PR can be normal and there is a corresponding long PR interval. The retrograde P waves are inverted in leads II, III, and aVF.

Slow-slow form
The slow-slow variety of AVNRT presents as a long RP tachycardia and resembles the fast-slow form. In the slow-slow type the RP interval depends on the relative conduction time over both pathways. The fast-slow and the slow-slow varieties of AVNRT may resemble sinus tachycardia because a P wave precedes the QRS complex.

ATRIOVENTRICULAR NODAL REENTRANT TACHYCARDIA 2

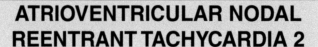

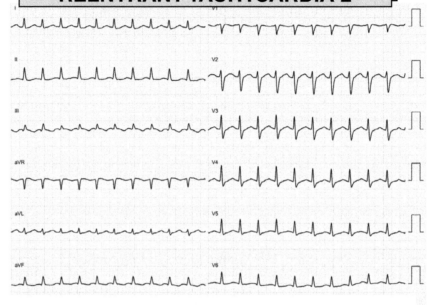

**AVNRT rate about 140 bpm. No P waves are seen.
An electrophysiologic study confirmed the diagnosis.**

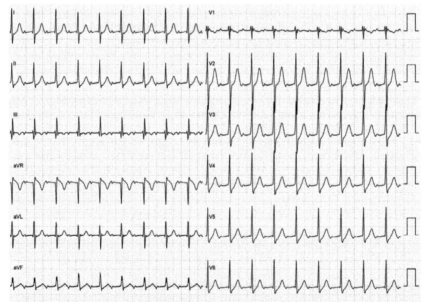

**AVNRT with 2:1 block. The atrial rate is about 220 bpm. The block is in the His bundle
and tends to occur mostly at the onset of tachycardia. AV block rules out AVRT utilizing
an accessory pathway. Note the peculiar terminal S wave in the inferior leads suggesting
the presence of a P wave stuck at the end of the QRS complex.**

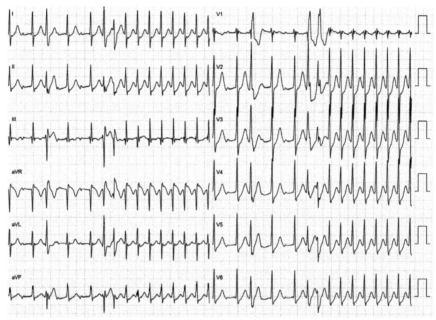

Same patient as previous ECG. The 2:1 AV block is intermittent. Note the relatively long RR interval followed by a short RR interval which terminates with an aberrantly conducted beat with a right bundle branch configuration (Ashman phenomenon).

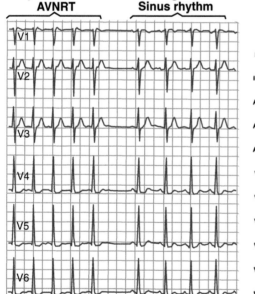

AVNRT rate 136 bpm and sinus rate 107 bpm. Note the terminal portion of lead V1 which shows a pattern consistent with incomplete right bundle branch block. This pattern disappeared in sinus rhythm confirming that the tachycardia is AVNRT.

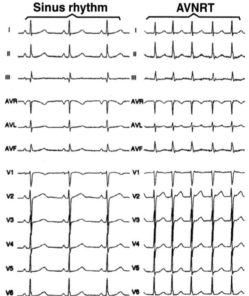

AVNRT showing terminal s waved in leads II, III and aVF during the tachycardia but not in sinus rhythm. Similarly, there is an r' in V1 present only during the tachycardia. These findings reflect the presence of P waves at the end of the QRS and are diagnostic of AVNRT.

ATRIOVENTRICULAR REENTRANT TACHYCARDIA 1

Atrioventricular reentrant tachycardia (AVRT) is the second most common form of paroxysmal supraventricular tachycardia. AVRT is more common in males than in females. Patients with AVRT do not have evidence of structural heart disease but they have accessory pathways, or bypass tracts. Accessory pathways are congenital strands of myocardium that bridge the mitral or tricuspid valves and are capable of conducting electrical activation from atrium to ventricle.

AVRT is the result of two or more conducting pathways: the AV node and one or more bypass tracts. The accessory pathways may conduct impulses in an anterograde manner from atrium to ventricle, a retrograde manner from ventricle to atrium, or in both directions. In classic (or manifest) Wolff-Parkinson-White (WPW) syndrome, anterograde conduction occurs over both the accessory pathway and the normal conduction system during sinus rhythm. The accessory pathway, being faster, depolarizes some of the ventricle early, resulting in a short PR interval and a slurred upstroke to the QRS complex (delta wave). Not all accessory pathways conduct in an anterograde manner. Concealed accessory pathways are not evident during sinus rhythm because they are only capable of retrograde conduction. These occur in about 30-40% of patients with accessory pathways. A large reentry circuit is most commonly established by impulses traveling in an anterograde manner through the AV node and in a retrograde manner through the accessory pathway; this is often called orthodromic AVRT. "Orthodromic" comes from Greek where it means "straight or correct" because ventricular activation is normal. Concealed pathways cannot be detected by standard ECG. Distinction between concealed accessory pathway and AVNRT may be difficult, although a faster rate (>200 per minute) and a retrograde P wave after, rather than within, the QRS complex favor a concealed bypass tract.

Schematic representation of the conduction system and an accessory pathway

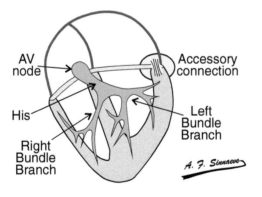

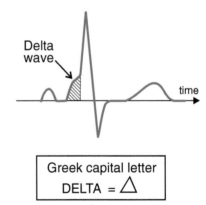

Greek capital letter
DELTA = $\triangle$

Occasionally, the reentrant circuit revolves in the opposite direction, from the atrium to the ventricle via the accessory connection, and returns from the ventricle in the retrograde direction up the normal AV conduction system (called antidromic reciprocating tachycardia and constitutes about 5% of the arrhythmias in WPW syndrome). The QRS complex is wide (maximal preexcitation) because the ventricles are activated abnormally. The bizarre, wide complex tachycardia can be mistaken for ventricular tachycardia.

The reentrant circuit in AVRT is large and involves the atrium and the ventricle. In contrast the circuit is small in AVNRT and does not involve the atrium nor the ventricle. Therefore AV block is incompatible with diagnosis of AVRT.

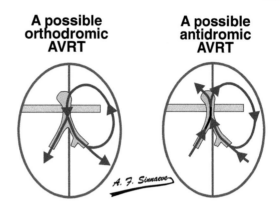

A possible orthodromic AVRT

A possible antidromic AVRT

A. F. Sinnaeve

AVRT : mechanism of an orthodromic reciprocating tachycardia

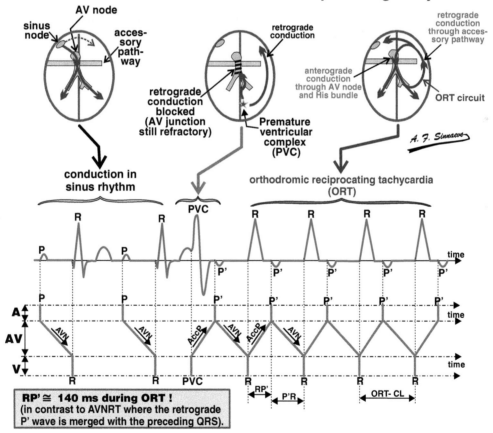

RP' ≅ 140 ms during ORT !
(in contrast to AVNRT where the retrograde P' wave is merged with the preceding QRS).

Abbreviations : AccP = accessory pathway ; AV = atrioventricular ; AVN = AV node ; AVRT = AV reentrant tachycardia ; PVC = premature ventricular complex ; ORT = orthodromic reciprocating tachycardia ; ORT- CL = ORT cycle length

ATRIOVENTRICULAR REENTRANT TACHYCARDIA 2

In patients with 2 accessory AV connections (not uncommon), a reciprocating tachycardia using one accessory connection in the anterograde direction and the other in the retrograde direction may occur. Patients with Wolff-Parkinson-White syndrome can develop atrial fibrillation and atrial flutter. The rapid nondecremental conduction via accessory pathways can result in extremely rapid ventricular rates, which can degenerate into ventricular fibrillation and cause sudden death. Patients with preexcitation syndromes with atrial fibrillation must not be given an AV nodal blocking agent; these agents can further increase conduction via the accessory pathway, which increases the risk of ventricular fibrillation and death.

Tachycardias in WPW syndrome may begin as or degenerate into atrial fibrillation. When atrial flutter or fibrillation occur in patients with WPW, the risk of potentially lethal arrhythmias due to very rapid conduction across accessory pathways must be considered. The risk is especially treacherous in patients with short-refractory period anomalous pathways, since atrial fibrillation may lead to ventricular fibrillation. Conversely an accessory pathway may behave as a bystander during a tachycardia if it does not participate in the mechanism of tachycardia.

Manifestations of orthodromic AV reentrant tachycardia

1. Rate: 170–250 bpm.
2. May be initiated by atrial or ventricular premature beats.
3. In patients with a delta wave in sinus rhythm, the delta wave disappears during tachycardia.
4. The R-P interval is short, usually < 120 ms. This reflects fast retrograde conduction in the accessory pathway. The retrograde P wave occurs after the QRS complex. The relatively short R-P interval may be mistaken for a bump on the T wave. In contrast, in typical AVNRT the P waves are either absent or stuck on the QRS complex.
5. Any evidence of AV block rules out AVRT because the ventricle is an integral part of the reentrant circuit.
6. Alternans of the QRS complex is more common in AVRT than in AVNRT and seems to occur at faster rates. Alternans describes amplitude changes of the QRS complex in alternate beats.
7. Marked ST-T wave abnormalities not due to coronary artery disease occur more frequently than in AVNRT.
8. The P waves are inverted because activation reenters via the accessory pathway. The P wave morphology depends on the site of the accessory pathway. A negative P wave in lead I indicates a left lateral pathway.
9. Functional bundle branch block may reveal the site of the accessory pathway. For example, lengthening of cycle length (slowing of the rate) with functional left bundle branch block (LBBB) indicates that the reentrant circuit has increased in size and the travel time to the ventricular insertion of the accessory pathway has increased. Such an observation during LBBB confirms the left site of the accessory pathway.

> **An increase of the cycle length (slowing of the rate) with the occurrence of bundle branch block (BBB) is diagnostic of an accessory pathway on the same (ipsolateral) side as the BBB.**

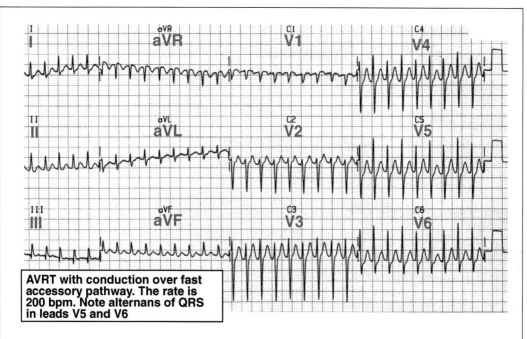

I aVR V1 V4

II aVL V2 V5

III aVF V3 V6

AVRT with conduction over fast accessory pathway. The rate is 200 bpm. Note alternans of QRS in leads V5 and V6

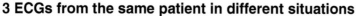

3 ECGs from the same patient in different situations

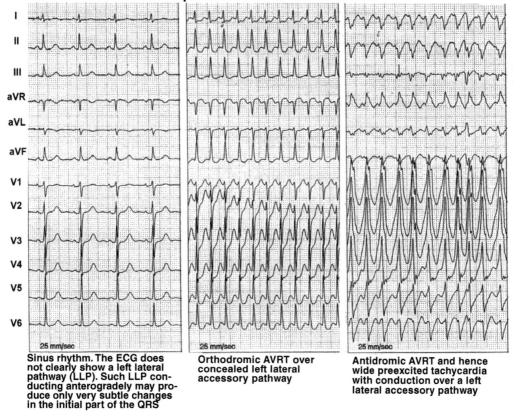

Sinus rhythm. The ECG does not clearly show a left lateral pathway (LLP). Such LLP conducting anterogradely may produce only very subtle changes in the initial part of the QRS

Orthodromic AVRT over concealed left lateral accessory pathway

Antidromic AVRT and hence wide preexcited tachycardia with conduction over a left lateral accessory pathway

ATRIOVENTRICULAR REENTRANT TACHYCARDIA 3

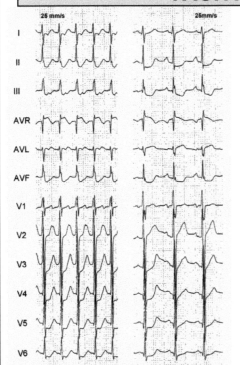

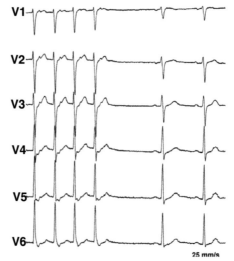

Spontaneous termination of AVRT. The tachycardia terminates with a retrograde P wave indicating that the AV node is the weakest link in the circuit. Note the retrograde P wave away from the QRS complex and RP < PR interval.

Orthodromic AVRT and sinus rhythm in the same patient. A retrograde P wave is seen in lead III away from the QRS complex and RP < PR interval typical of orthodromic tachycardia.

Permanent junctional reciprocating tachycardia (PJRT)

PJRT is basically an orthodromic tachycardia in the setting of a slowly conducting concealed bypass tract (no delta wave or evidence of Wolff-Parkinson-White in sinus rhythm). The QRS complex is narrow and the P waves are easily seen and inverted in the inferior leads. PJRT is rare and occurs mostly in infants and children. It is often incessant with occasional interruption by sinus beats. It does not require a premature beat or PR prolongation for its initiation and may be initiated by a modest increase in the sinus rate. The rate is 90–250 bpm and may vary significantly with autonomic influences. The tachycardia travels anterogradely via the AV node and retrogradely via a slowly conducting accessory pathway (usually postero-septal) that exibits AV nodal properties. This produces a tachycardia with a long RP interval (RP > PR). The chronic uncontrolled heart rate may cause a tachycardia related cardiomyopathy which is usually reversible when the rate becomes controlled. PJRT has been called pseudo-slow-slow tachycardia because of its ECG similarity to the unusual form of AVNRT.

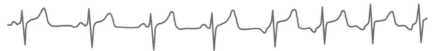

Initiation of PJRT. The PJRT starts when the heart rate increases.

Focal junctional tachycardia

This rare arrhythmia occurs mostly in children with or without congenital heart disease. It is often a diagnosis of exclusion. The tachycardia is paroxysmal because it starts and terminates suddenly. It is regular with a rate of 110–250 bpm. AV dissociation is common but there may be retrograde ventriculoatrial conduction with varying degree of retrograde block. The tachycardia does not require the atrium nor the ventricle for its propagation. When incessant it can cause a tachycardia-dependent cardiomyopathy with heart failure.

Nonparoxysmal junctional tachycardia

Nonparoxysmal junctional tachycardia (also known as accelerated junctional tachycardia) is a benign arrhythmia at a rate of 70–140 bpm. It is a marker for potentially serious heart disease or digitalis intoxication. It may be due to enhanced automaticity or triggered activity. It starts and terminates gradually. It may show AV dissociation or retrograde ventriculoatrial conduction.

Overview of supraventricular tachycardia

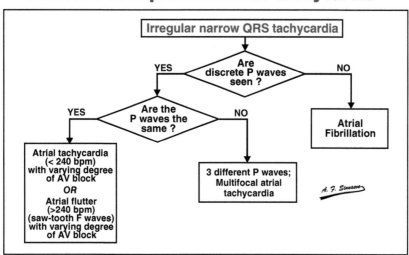

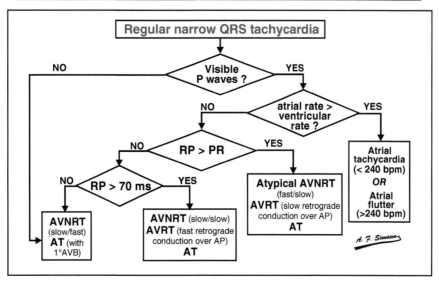

Further Reading

Fox DJ, Tischenko A, Krahn AD, Skanes AC, Gula LJ, Yee RK, Klein GJ. Supraventricular tachycardia: diagnosis and management. Mayo Clin Proc. 2008;83:1400-11.

Goel R, Srivathsan K, Mookadam M. Supraventricular and ventricular arrhythmias. Prim Care. 2013;40:43-71.

González-Torrecilla E, Arenal A, Atienza F, Datino T, Atea LF, Calvo D, Pachón M, Miracle A, Fernández-Avilés F. ECG diagnosis of paroxysmal supraventricular tachycardias in patients without preexcitation. Ann Noninvasive Electrocardiol. 2011;16:85-95.

Kumar UN, Rao RK, Scheinman MM. The 12-lead electrocardiogram in supraventricular tachycardia. Cartd Clin. 2006;24:427-37.

Lee KW, Badhwar N, Scheinman MM. Supraventricular tachycardia–part I. Curr Probl Cardiol. 2008;33:467-546.

CHAPTER 15

VENTRICULAR TACHYCARDIAS

* Ventricular tachycardia
* Electrocardiography of monomorphic ventricular tachycardia
* Brugada algorithm for the diagnosis of wide complex tachycardia
* The Brugada syndrome
* Catecholaminergic polymorphic ventricular tachycardia
* Idiopathic ventricular tachycardia
* Arrhythmogenic right ventricular dysplasia
* Bundle branch reentry
* Long QT syndrome – early afterdepolarization
* Torsades de pointes
* Short QT syndrome
* Polymorphic ventricular tachycardia and cardiac ischemia
* Short-coupled variant of TdP

ECG from Basics to Essentials: Step by Step. First Edition. Roland X. Stroobandt, S. Serge Barold and Alfons F. Sinnaeve.
Published 2016 © 2016 by John Wiley & Sons, Ltd. Companion Website: www.wiley.com/go/stroobandt/ecg

VENTRICULAR TACHYCARDIA 1

Ventricular tachycardia (VT) originates from the ventricles or more specifically below the bundle of His in the AV junction. By definition it consists of 3 or more beats at a rate > 100 bpm and a QRS of at least 0.12 s. In exceptional cases the QRS may be < 0.12 s. VT occurs mostly in the presence of heart disease. It is a potentially life-threatening arrhythmia. VT can be classified in many ways. The mechanism, prognosis and management of VT differs according to the underlying substrate coronary artery disease, mitral valve prolapse, cardiomyopathy, etc.)

① **Duration.**
Sustained for VT > 30 s, and unsustained VT for < 30 s.

② **Electrocardiographic morphology.**
Monomorphic with a regular rate and consistent beat-to-beat QRS morphology or polymorphic with frequent changes in QRS configuration. The latter comprises VT with QT prolongation or without QT prolongation. Bidirectional VT shows alternation of frontal plane axis during VT.

③ **Underlying mechanism especially reentry.**
Reentry takes place in the ventricles or in the bundle branches (bundle branch reentry is usually seen in cardiomyopathy). The commonest cause of VT is post myocardial infarction where reentry is the mechanism. Areas of slow conduction have been identified in the substrate for reentry.

④ **Disease entity.**
Chronic coronary artery disease, congenital heart disease, cardiomyopathy or absence of structural heart disease. Absence of heart disease makes SVT with aberration more likely. The presence of heart disease makes VT more likely. A wide QRS tachycardia in a patient with an old myocardial infarction is almost always VT. Family history of sudden cardiac death suggests conditions such as hypertrophic obstructive cardiomyopathy, congenital long QT syndrome, Brugada syndrome or arrhythmogenic right ventricular dysplasia.

⑤ **Clinical presentation.**
Asymptomatic, hemodynamically stable, hemodynamically unstable, presyncope, syncope, sudden cardiac arrest and sudden cardiac death. With faster heart rates and underlying heart disease loss of consciousness (syncope) or sudden death may occur. Episodes lasting only a few beats may produce no or minimal symptoms. VT rates between 110 and 150 bpm may be tolerated even if sustained for minutes to hours. However, faster rates (>180 bpm) may cause a drop in the blood pressure and low cardiac ouput. It is a misconception that hemodynamically stable patients cannot have VT.

⑥ **Mechanism.**
Reentry, enhanced automaticity and triggered activity. VT related to a scar after myocardial infarction is always due to reentry.

⑦ **Rate.**
Fast, "slow".

⑧ **Site of origin.**
Septal, apical, basal, outflow tract. Right or left ventricle.

⑨ **Relation to exercise.**

⑩ **Inducible by electrophysiologic study.**

⑪ **VT without structural heart disease.**
Inherited syndromes.

Electrocardiography of monomorphic ventricular tachycardia

1. AV dissociation

The finding of atrioventricular (AV) dissociation is one of the most useful practical criteria for the diagnosis of VT. However, retrograde ventriculoatrial (VA) conduction, whether 1:1 or 2:1, or Wenckebach VA conduction occurs in up to 50% of all VT. Retrograde VA conduction is more frequent at slower VT rates. Occasionally a different arrhythmia such as atrial fibrillation is present in the atrium. P waves can be difficult to recognize during a broad QRS tachycardia with AV dissociation. As the ventricular beats may occur so rapidly, P waves may be lost within the QRS complexes. The absence of AV dissociation is not helpful for two reasons: (1) AV dissociation may be present but not obvious on the ECG; (2) some patients have 1:1 retrograde VA conduction.

The use of the Lewis lead can be helpful in detecting the P waves on the ECG. The Lewis lead can be obtained from registration of lead I by placing the right arm electrode to the right, second intercostal space adjacent to the sternum, and the left arm electrode to the right, fourth intercostal space adjacent to the sternum. Voltage should be calibrated at mV = 20 mm. Esophageal leads were used in the past to bring out hidden P waves (from the left atrium).

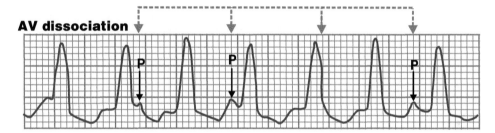

AV dissociation

2. Fusion and capture beats

In patients with slow VT rates occasional conduction from atrium to ventricle over the AV node-bundle branch system may result in "capture" or "fusion" beats. The presence of fusion or capture beats when present are diagnostic of VT and help distinguish supraventricular tachycardia with aberrancy vs. VT. A fusion beat occurs when ventricular depolarization consists of a combination of a conducted supraventricular beat superimposed on a VT beat. The fusion beat is generally narrower than a pure VT beat. A capture beat represents total ventricular depolarization by a conducted supraventricular beat.

Ventricular fusion (F)

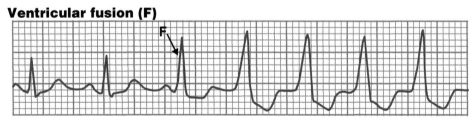

3. Width of the QRS complex

When the arrhythmia arises in the lateral free wall of the ventricle, activation of the ventricles results in a very wide QRS. The QRS complex is less wide when the VT originates in or close to the ventricular septum. QRS width is also influenced by scar tissue (after myocardial infarction), ventricular hypertrophy, cardiomyopathy and drug therapy. A QRS width of more than 0.14 s in right bundle branch block (RBBB) tachycardias and more than 0.16 s during left bundle branch block (LBBB) favor VT in the absence of drugs that may affect QRS duration.

VENTRICULAR TACHYCARDIA 2

4. Frontal plane axis

The presence of a superior axis (especially right superior) in patients with RBBB shaped QRS, very strongly suggests VT. With a LBBB shaped VT, right axis deviation is suggestive of VT.

5. Leads V1 and V6

In RBBB shaped tachycardia, presence of a monophasic or biphasic QRS complex (R, qR, QR, RS) in lead V1 strongly argues for VT while a triphasic (RSR') pattern suggests a supraventricular origin. The triphasic (RsR') pattern of aberrant conduction (2 R peaks) has been called "rabbit's ears". It is aberration if the right ear is larger than the left (rR') and VT (2 R peaks) if the left ear is larger than the right one (Rr'). In a RBBB shaped tachycardia VT is very likely when the R:S ratio is smaller than 1 in V6.

In LBBB shaped VT, lead V1 (and also V2) shows an initially positive QRS with positivity measuring more than 0.03 s; slurring or notching of the downstroke of the S wave; and an interval between the beginning of the QRS and the nadir of the S wave of 0.07 s or more favor VT. A q or Q wave in lead V6 is diagnostic of VT.

QR complexes in VT strongly suggest VT in patients with old myocardial infarction (scar) in the same leads as the Q waves in sinus rhythm.

Typically, conduction delay with uncomplicated RBBB or LBBB shows an RS pattern in at least one of the precordial leads. When there is no RS morphology in any of the precordial leads, VT is very likely.

> **You must know the classic features of uncomplicated RBBB and LBBB before you can recognize the atypical forms produced by VT.**

6. Concordant pattern

When all precordial leads show either negative or positive QRS complexes this is called negative or positive concordance. Negative concordance is highly suggestive of a VT arising in the apical area of the heart. Negative concordance in the precordial leads is almost always VT. Positive concordance may be due either to VT or to SVT using a left posterior accessory atrioventricular pathway for AV conduction.

7. QRS more narrow than in sinus rhythm

When the QRS is more narrow than during sinus rhythm a VT is present. This can only be explained by a ventricular origin close to the intraventricular septum, resulting in more simultaneous activation of the right and left ventricles than during sinus rhythm. Fascicular tachycardia arising from the fascicular system generates a less prolonged QRS duration of 0.14 s or less which is more narrow than classic VT.

> **The ECG differential diagnosis of VT includes supraventricular tachycardia with functional aberration, preexisting bundle branch block, and intraventricular conduction disturbances, or preexcitation.**

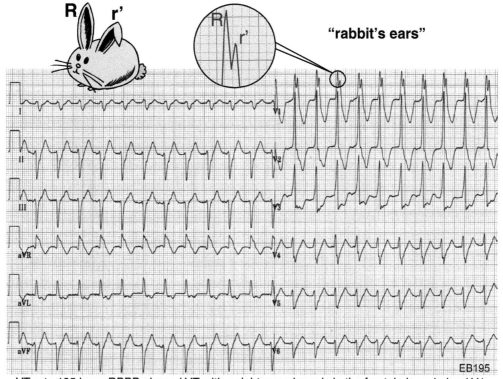

"rabbit's ears"

EB195

VT rate 135 bpm; RBBB-shaped VT with a right superior axis in the frontal plane; In lead V1 the rabbit's ear on the left is larger than the one on the right. The combination of the findings strongly suggests VT.

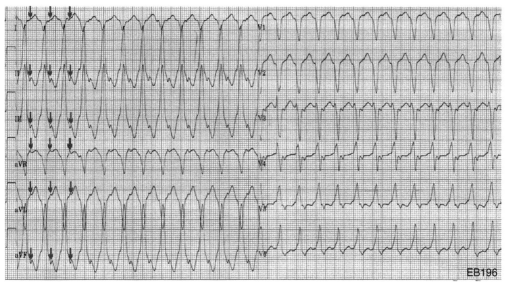

EB196

LBBB-shaped VT (rate = 150 bpm) with right axis deviation in the frontal plane (QRS = 0.16 s). This combination strongly favors VT. There is 1:1 retrograde ventriculoatrial conduction (see arrows).

VENTRICULAR TACHYCARDIA 3

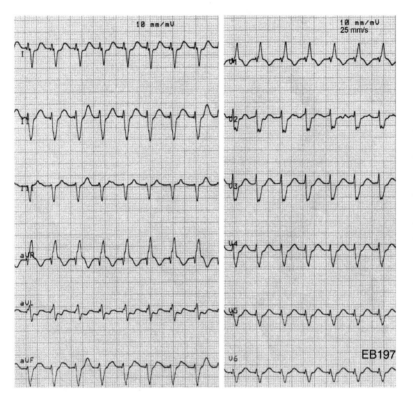

Fascicular VT at a rate of 143 bpm and QRS = 0.13 s. Lead V1 shows the typical pattern of RBBB and the frontal plane axis is in the right superior quadrant. The origin is in all likelihood in the left posterior fascicle.

Brugada algorithm for the diagnosis of wide complex tachycardias

The Brugada criteria were established to distinguish SVT with aberrancy from VT. It is a relatively simple stepwise decision tree-like algorithm to differentiate between SVT with aberration from VT in wide complex tachycardias. The algorithm retains the traditional morphological criteria in its last step (step 4). A negative response to all 4 questions should yield SVT with aberration in almost all cases. Using the Brugada criteria is very useful; the sensitivity and specificity have been found adequate since its original description but not as high as previously thought. Although not foolproof the Brugada algorithm remains the most popular algorithm for the evaluation of wide QRS complex tachycardias.

Limitations of the Brugada algorithm criteria

1. The algorithm was developed without cases of idiopathic VT.
2. Preexcited tachycardias can be falsely diagnosed as VT.
3. Bundle branch reentry tachycardia may be diagnosed as SVT with aberration because it presents with a typical LBBB configuration.

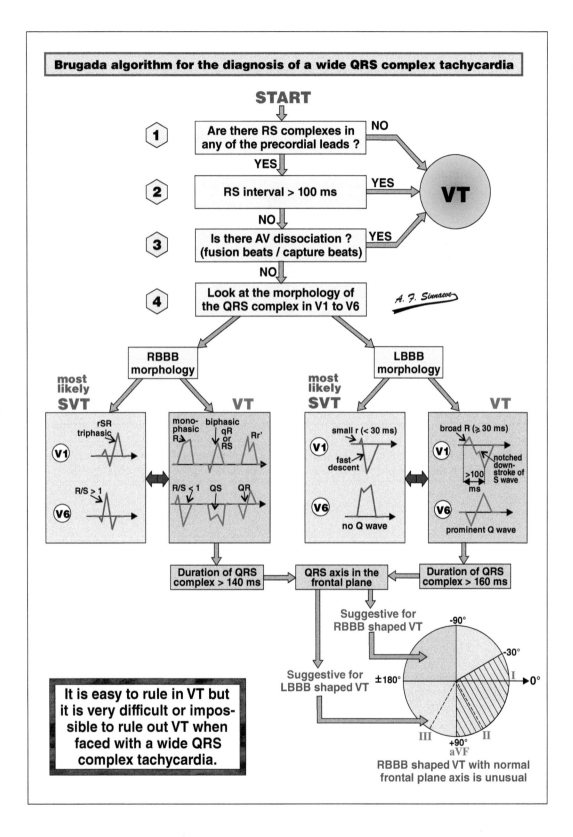

Brugada algorithm for the diagnosis of a wide QRS complex tachycardia

START

1 Are there RS complexes in any of the precordial leads ? — NO

YES

2 RS interval > 100 ms — YES → **VT**

NO

3 Is there AV dissociation ? (fusion beats / capture beats) — YES → VT

NO

4 Look at the morphology of the QRS complex in V1 to V6

A. F. Sinnaeve

RBBB morphology

most likely SVT ... **VT**

- V1: rSR triphasic
- V6: R/S > 1

- V1: mono-phasic R, biphasic qR or RS, Rr'
- V6: R/S < 1, QS, QR

LBBB morphology

most likely SVT ... **VT**

- V1: small r (< 30 ms), fast descent
- V6: no Q wave

- V1: broad R (≥ 30 ms), notched down-stroke of S wave, >100 ms
- V6: prominent Q wave

Duration of QRS complex > 140 ms → QRS axis in the frontal plane ← Duration of QRS complex > 160 ms

Suggestive for RBBB shaped VT

Suggestive for LBBB shaped VT

-90° -30° ±180° 0° I +90° aVF II III

RBBB shaped VT with normal frontal plane axis is unusual

It is easy to rule in VT but it is very difficult or impossible to rule out VT when faced with a wide QRS complex tachycardia.

VENTRICULAR TACHYCARDIA 4

The causes of wide QRS tachycardia include:

1. Ventricular tachycardia

2. Supraventricular tachycardia with bundle branch block either preexisting or due to tachy cardia dependent aberrant conduction, or the effect of antiarrhythmic drugs that slow intraventricular conduction, resulting in marked QRS complex widening

3. Supraventricular tachycardia with conduction of impulses to the ventricles over an accessory pathway (preexcited tachycardia)

The classic diagnostic criteria include a concordant precordial pattern, a sign that can also be expressed as absence of RS (or even rs, Rs, rS) complexes in the precordial leads. Analysis of previous ECGs recorded during sinus rhythm, if available, can provide futher keys to the diagnosis. Some criteria proposed in the past, such as QRS axis or ventricular complex duration, are nowadays no longer considered to the same extent as they were in the past.

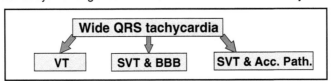

There are multiple approaches and protocols, each having its own pros and cons. No protocol is 100% accurate. In this book we try to to summarize approaches which we consider optimal for the evaluation of patients with wide QRS complex tachycardias.

Age, hemodynamic status, heart rate and regularity of R-R intervals may be misleading and should not be considered in making the diagnosis of VT.

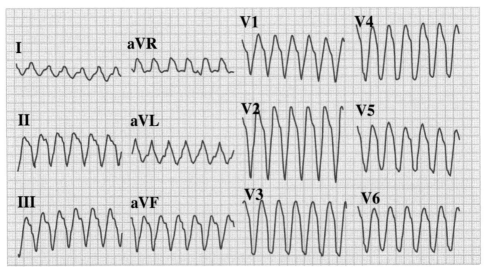

VT at a rate of about 160 bpm, QRS = 200 ms. All the QRS complexes are negative in the precordial leads. This is called negative concordance and is diagnostic for VT. The absence of RS complexes in the precordial leads is also diagnostic for VT.

Scar-related VT

VT is generally a consequence of structural heart disease associated with myocardial scarring. The most common setting for VT is ischemic heart disease, in which scar tissue is the substrate for reentry, but VT can occur in other conditions that create myocardial scar tissue. VT in the setting of ischemic heart disease is predominantly manifest as monomorphic VT, caused by a relatively fixed anatomic substrate for reentrant VT. Although most patients with VT have underlying structural heart abnormalities, monomorphic VT is occasionally observed in patients with structurally normal hearts (idiopathic VT). These VTs often occur during exercise and their clinical features are more consistent with triggered activity or normal automaticity.

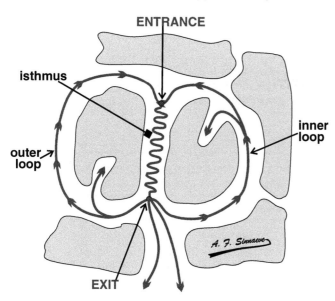

The diagram of reentry is a simplistic representation of a complex process. The reentry circuits can be multiple with shared and separate components. The circuit utilizes the slow conduction properties of a central critical isthmus located in a position intimately related to the scar border zone. The isthmus is protected by anatomic and electrophysiologic barriers. The isthmuses can vary significantly in length and electrophysiologic properties. The electrical activation travels slowly through the isthmus during diastole and forms a silent zone on the surface ECG. The wavefront breaks out of the scar at the exit sites (which may be multiple), activates the ventricle, and reenters the slow conduction critical isthmus at the entrance zone. This produces a "figure of 8" or double loop pattern. One arc moves in a clockwise fashion and the other in a counterclockwise fashion in a pretzel-like configuration. The VT morphology reflects the location of the exit site. Adjacent bystander sites are blind alleys that are purely passive and not essential to the reentry circuit.

Analysis of QRS configuration in V1 and V6.
* Aberration due to functional bundle branch block results in a "typical" bundle branch block morphology.
* VT is associated with "atypical" bundle branch block.
  Complicating factors: previous myocardial infarction can result in an "atypical" form of bundle branch block in the presence of supraventricular tachycardia.

Preexcited tachycardia from an accessory pathway looks like VT. Preexcited tachycardia can be ruled out in the presence of negative precordial concordance (QS complexes in all chest leads) or deep q waves in a precordial lead other than V1.

VENTRICULAR TACHYCARDIA 5

WIDE QRS TACHYCARDIA

DEFINITION :
a regular tachycardia at a rate faster than 100 bpm
with QRS complexes of at least 120 ms.

VENTRICULAR TACHYCARDIA (VT)

SUPRAVENTRICULAR TACHYCARDIA (SVT)
A supraventricular tachycardia (SVT) commonly has a narrow QRS complex because the impulse originates in the atria and follows the normal AV conduction system.

VT

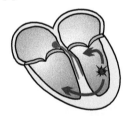

The arrhythmia originates in the ventricle below the bifurcation of the bundle of His.
The impulse does not follow the normal conduction system, hence the activation of both ventricles does not occur simultaneously.

SVT with BBB

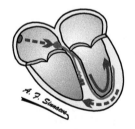

The tachycardia originates in the atria but the impulses are conducted with aberration into the ventricles either due to a preexistent or a rate related bundle branch block.

AVRT (antidromic)

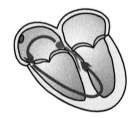

Antidromic AV reciprocating tachycardia (AVRT) with anterograde conduction over a bypass tract and retrograde conduction over the AV node or a second bypass tract.

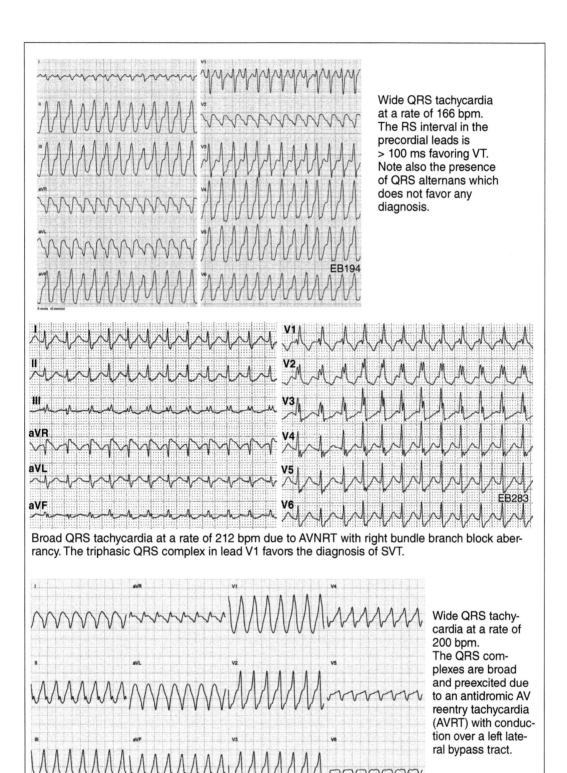

EB194

Wide QRS tachycardia at a rate of 166 bpm. The RS interval in the precordial leads is > 100 ms favoring VT. Note also the presence of QRS alternans which does not favor any diagnosis.

EB283

Broad QRS tachycardia at a rate of 212 bpm due to AVNRT with right bundle branch block aberrancy. The triphasic QRS complex in lead V1 favors the diagnosis of SVT.

25 mm/s 10 mV/mm

EB289

Wide QRS tachycardia at a rate of 200 bpm. The QRS complexes are broad and preexcited due to an antidromic AV reentry tachycardia (AVRT) with conduction over a left lateral bypass tract.

VENTRICULAR TACHYCARDIA 6
Examples of Wide QRS Tachycardias

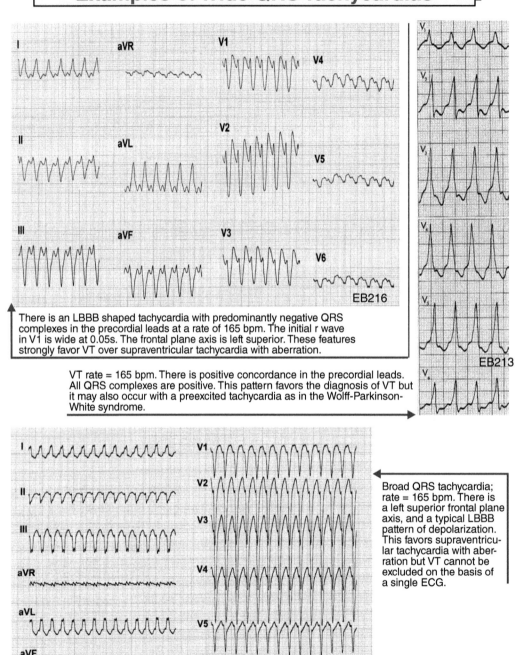

EB216

There is an LBBB shaped tachycardia with predominantly negative QRS complexes in the precordial leads at a rate of 165 bpm. The initial r wave in V1 is wide at 0.05s. The frontal plane axis is left superior. These features strongly favor VT over supraventricular tachycardia with aberration.

VT rate = 165 bpm. There is positive concordance in the precordial leads. All QRS complexes are positive. This pattern favors the diagnosis of VT but it may also occur with a preexcited tachycardia as in the Wolff-Parkinson-White syndrome.

EB213

EB218

Broad QRS tachycardia; rate = 165 bpm. There is a left superior frontal plane axis, and a typical LBBB pattern of depolarization. This favors supraventricular tachycardia with aberration but VT cannot be excluded on the basis of a single ECG.

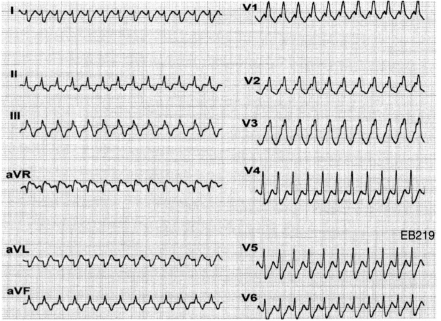

Broad QRS tachycardia with a typical RBBB complex in V1. Rate = 158 bpm. Right axis deviation. This favors supraventricular tachycardia with aberration but VT cannot be excluded on the basis of a single ECG.

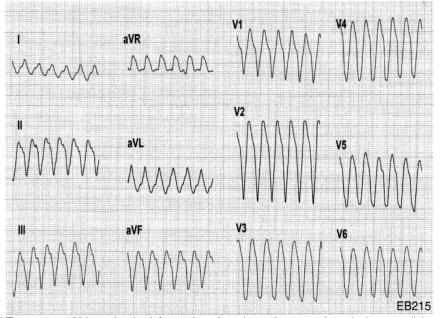

VT at a rate = 180 bpm showing left superior axis and negative concordance in the precordial leads. All precordial leads show a QS (negative) configuration. Such negative concordance (QS pattern in all precordial leads or predominantly negative QRS complexes in all precordial leads) strongly favors VT. In the past such a pattern was considered 100% diagnostic of VT. However, it has now been shown that a QS pattern across the precordial leads can also occur infrequently with aberrantly conducted supraventricular tachycardia.

VENTRICULAR TACHYCARDIA 7
THE BRUGADA SYNDROME

Brugada syndrome is an example of channelopathy, and a genetically determined disease (auto-somal dominant pattern of transmission in about 50% of familial cases) caused by an alteration in the transmembrane ion currents that constitute the cardiac action potential. It is characterized by ST elevation in leads V1 to V3, polymorphic ventricular tachycardia that may lead to syncope, cardiac arrest, or sudden cardiac death. There may be atrial fibrillation in 20% of patients. About 5% of survivors of cardiac arrest have no clinically identified cardiac abnormality. About half of these cases are thought to be due to Brugada syndrome. The context of the cardiac event is important. In many cases, cardiac arrest occurs during sleep or rest. Cases occurring during physical activity are rare. The typical patient with Brugada syndrome is young, male, and otherwise healthy, with normal general medical and cardiovascular physical examinations. In the initial description of Brugada syndrome, the heart was reported to be structurally normal, but this concept has been challenged. Subtle structural abnormalities in the right ventricular outflow tract have been reported.

Type I is the only ECG criterion that is diagnostic of Brugada syndrome. The type I ECG is characte-rized by a J elevation of at least 2 mm (= 0.2 mV), a coved type gradually descending STsegment followed by a negative T wave. Brugada syndrome is definitively diagnosed when a type I ST-segment is observed in more than one right precordial lead (V1 to V3) in the presence or absence of a sodium channel-blocking agent, in combination with an ill-defined form of complete or incomplete right bundle branch block. The ST segment elevation in V1 to V3 is characteristic and different from changes observed in other conditions. Placement of the right precordial leads in a superior position (up to the 2nd intercostal spaces above normal) can increase the sensitivity of the ECG for detecting the Brugada phenotype in some patients, both in the presence or absence of drug challenge. There are many patients with a normal electrocardiogram in whom the syndrome can only be recognized with a drug challenge. There are also patients who remain asymptomatic, despite an ECG with the characteristic type I pattern.

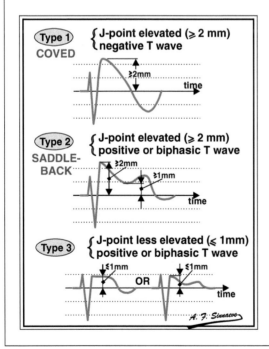

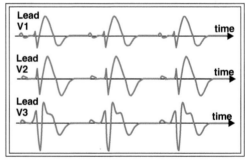

A drug challenge with a sodium channel bloc-ker (procainamide in the US or flecainide or ajmaline in Europe) to unmask Brugada syn-drome should be considered in patients with syncope in whom no obvious cause is found or in patients with cardiac arrest of unknown etiology.

Note that fever amplifies the expression of Brugada syndrome since Na channels are temperature dependent and inactivated faster at a higher temperature.

The ECGs of Brugada patients can change over time from type I to type II and/or normal ECGs and back. All three patterns may be observed sequentially in the same patient or following the introduction of specific drugs.

Individuals with ECGs displaying only one diagnostic right precordial lead have similar clinical profile and arrhythmic risk as Brugada patients with ECGs displaying more than one precordial leads. Revision of the consensus criteria should be considered.

Type II and III ST-segment elevation should not be considered diagnostic of Brugada syndrome because they are nocturnal variants. Type II ST-segment elevation has a saddleback appearance with a high take-off ST-segment elevation of at least 2 mm followed by a through displaying of more than 1 mm ST elevation followed by either a positive or biphasic T wave. Type III ST-segment elevation has either a saddleback or coved appearance with an ST-segment elevation ≤ 1 mm.

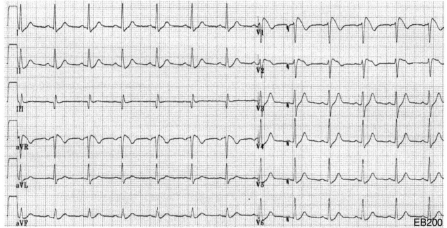

Typical type I Brugada ECG diagnostic of Brugada syndrome. In V1, note the 4 mm elevation of the J point, prominent coved ST elevation with a gradual descent and negative T waves. Lead V2 also shows coved ST elevation > 2 mm.

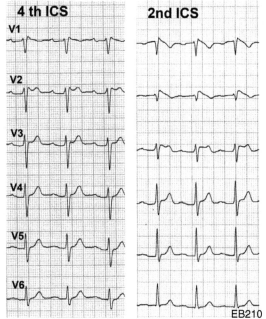

Baseline ECG (V1 and V2 recorded in the 4th intercostal space) is suggestive of Brugada syndrome. Placing the V1 and V2 electrodes at the level of the 2nd interspace reveals the diagnostic pattern of the Brugada syndrome.

Only type I pattern is diagnostic of Brugada syndrome

The ECG is dynamic. The electrocardiographic manifestations of the Brugada syndrome when concealed can be unmasked by sodium channel blockers, a febrile state, or vagotonic agents.

VENTRICULAR TACHYCARDIA 8

Catecholaminergic Polymorphic Ventricular Tachycardia

Catecholaminergic polymorphic ventricular tachycardia (CPVT) is a congenital familial disease that leads to exercise-induced ventricular arrhythmias and/or syncope and carries an increased risk of sudden death. The onset of arrhythmias occurs in the first or second decade of life. There are no structural cardiac abnormalities. Molecular genetic studies have revealed inherited defects of intracellular calcium handling by the cardiac myocytes. Electrical instability due to triggered activity with polymorphic VT and syncope occur during physical activity or emotional stress. There may be a family history of syncope or sudden death in young relatives related to similar triggers. The resting ECG is normal and there is a prominent U wave. The QTc is normal.

The diagnosis is based on finding reproducible ventricular arrhythmias during exercise testing. The complexity of these arrhythmias often increases with increasing work load, starting with ventricular premature beats, and ending with bidirectional ventricular tachycardia with beat-to-beat alternating frontal plane axis that rotates 180° (which is very typical and resembles the classic bidirectional VT of digitalis toxicity), to polymorphic ventricular tachycardia and ventricular fibrillation. The arrhythmias tend to appear at a rate of 110–130 bpm, and disappear when the exercise is stopped.

Idiopathic Ventricular Tachycardia

Idiopathic VT that occurs in the absence of structural heart disease, genetic conditions such as long QT syndrome, or metabolic/electrolyte abnormalities is referred to as idiopathic VT. Idiopathic forms of VT are rarely life-threatening but may be associated with hemodynamic compromise and syncope when rapid and sustained. Idiopathic VTs tend to originate from a few specific anatomic locations within the heart and manifest specific ECG patterns that may help to identify their site of origin.

Most idiopathic VTs originate from the right ventricular outflow tract (RVOT) and present with a left bundle branch block (LBBB) morphology and an inferiorly directed axis (note that the VT in arrhythmogenic RV dysplasia also shows a LBBB pattern usually with a superior axis, however, the RV dysplasia is associated with a number of ECG abnormalities not present in RVOT VT). Idiopathic RVOT tachycardia originates from a triggered activity and is adenosine sensitive. Most originate from the right side of the outflow tract region and about 10% originate from the left ventricular outflow tract. A LV site is suggested by an R wave transition in V1 or V2. Then, if there are no S waves in V5 and V6 the site is supravalvular (aortic cusp). These VTs may be sustained (exercise-induced) or may present as repetitive runs of nonsustained VTs, referred to as repetitive monomorphic VTs.

A less common form of idiopathic VT results from microreentry involving the fascicles of the left bundle branch, leading to VT with a right bundle branch block (RBBB) configuration. Exit of the VT from the posterior fascicle (of the left bundle branch) produces a pattern of RBBB with left anterior hemiblock which accounts for 90–95% of the cases. Exit from the left anterior fascicle produces a pattern of RBBB with right axis deviation. A third type is upper septal VT (rare) with a normal QRS duration and axis. Interestingly, this tachycardia is sensitive to verapamil.

A third form of idiopathic VT is propranolol sensitive and rare. It is neither initiated nor terminated by programmed stimulation, does not terminate with verapamil, and is consistent with an automatic mechanism. Isoproterenol induces VT while betablockers are effective.

Newly recognized entities of idiopathic VTs are those originating in the papillary muscles and in the atrioventricular annular regions.

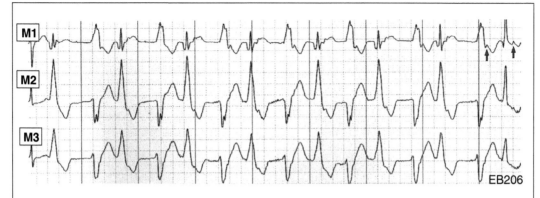

Irregular bidirectional VT in a patient with catecholaminergic VT at a rate of about 110 bpm. The arrows point towards retrograde P waves.

M1, M2, M3 are monitor leads corresponding more or less to leads I, II and III. Caution is needed since nurses could place the electrodes elsewhere to obtain a high amplitude R wave and a good P wave.

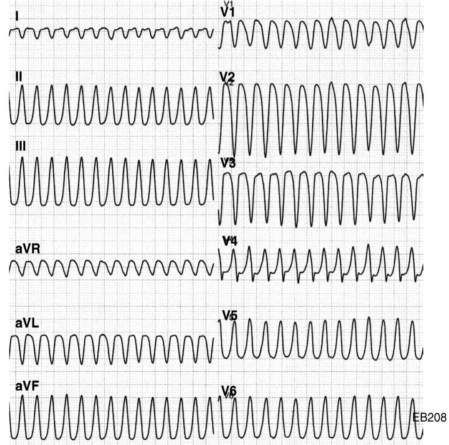

Idiopathic VT arising from the right ventricular outflow tract. Rate = 230 bpm. The VT shows a LBBB configuration with an inferior axis (right axis) in the frontal plane. The negative QRS complex in lead I suggests an origin from the septal side. A positive QRS in lead I suggests an origin from the lateral part of the RVOT. This VT was eliminated by catheter ablation.

VENTRICULAR TACHYCARDIA 9

Arrhythmogenic right ventricular dysplasia

Arrhythmogenic right ventricular dysplasia (ARVD) is a genetic nonischemic progressive condition in which the right ventricular (RV) myocardium is replaced by fat and fibrosis. It is a cardiomyopathy that involves primarily the RV causing arrhythmias originating from the RV. The RV is dilated and contracts poorly. Sudden cardiac death can be the first sign of ARVD. The symptoms of ARVD typically first occur during the late teens or young adulthood. It accounts for up to one-fifth of sudden cardiac deaths in people less than 35 years of age and 3–4% of sudden cardiac deaths that occur during exercise or playing sports.

The most common arrhythmia is monomorphic ventricular tachycardia (VT) which has a LBBB morphology and is caused by reentry. The frontal plane axis during LBBB-shaped VT may be superior in contrast to idiopathic VT arising from the right ventricular outflow tract (RVOT) where the axis is inferior. The VT may occasionally display an inferior axis mimicking the VT from the RVOT. Some patients have several VTs with different morphologies. Holter recordings may show a large number of VPCs with a LBBB configuration. Cardiac MRI is a powerful diagnostic tool because of its unique tissue characterizing capacity and potential to identify myocardial fibro-fatty infiltration and replacement.

The ECG findings are highly variable with depolarization and repolarization abnormalities. It may show incomplete or complete RBBB, inverted T waves in the anterior precordial leads (in the absence of RBBB) which in patients older than 14 years of age is the most suggestive indicator of ARVD. There may be localized prolongation of the QRS complex in leads V1 to V3 compared to V6 (> 25 ms parietal block so that the QRS in leads V1 to V3 is > 110 ms) or a QRS duration in V1 + V2 +V3 that is longer than that in leads V4 + V5 + V6 by a ratio > than 1.2. The latter is called localized right precordial QRS prolongation. The ECG may also exhibit epsilon waves visible as small, sharp discrete deflections at the terminal portion of the QRS complex in the anterior precordial leads indicative of delayed RV activation (post-excitation).

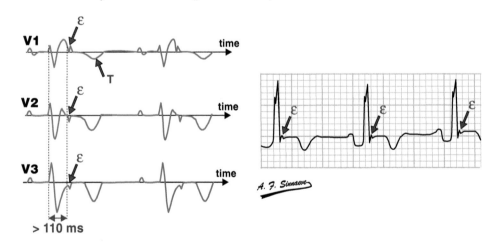

A prolonged S wave upstroke in V1 to V3 > 55 ms is found in 95% of ARVD patients. The sensitivity to detect these ECG abnormalities is enhanced by careful skin preparation to eliminate artifacts and by recording the ECG at double speed (50 mm/s) and double the usual amplitude.

Bundle Branch Reentry

Bundle branch reentry tachycardia (BBRT) is an uncommon form of monomorphic ventricular tachycardia (VT) incorporating both bundle branches into the reentry circuit. It is special because the mechanism involves abnormal conduction through structures that are normally present - the bundle of His and the bundle branches. The right bundle is responsible for the anterograde limb of the circuit in a majority of cases, with retrograde activation via one of the fascicles of the left bundle branch. This results in a typical LBBB pattern on the surface ECG during VT.

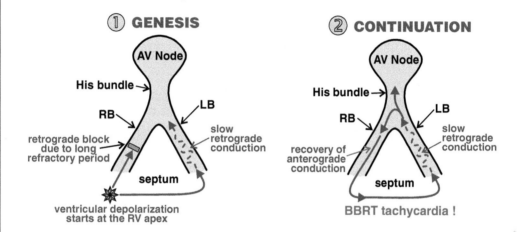

The rate is usually fast (> 200 bpm). The arrhythmia is usually seen in patients with an acquired heart disease, especially nonischemic dilated cardiomyopathy, and significant system impairment, although patients with structurally normal heart have been rarely described. Surface ECG in sinus rhythm (SR) characteristically shows intraventricular conduction defects. Patients typically present with presyncope, syncope or sudden death because of VT with fast rates frequently above 200 bpm. The QRS morphology during VT is a typical bundle branch block pattern, usually left bundle branch block, and may be identical to that in SR.

Less commonly, the circuit may travel in the opposite direction causing VT with a right bundle branch block configuration. On occasion, reentry may involve only the left anterior and posterior fascicles.

> * **BBRT responds poorly to pharmacologic therapy and has a high rate of recurrency**
> * **BBRT can account for syncope, sudden death and frequent defibrillator therapies**
> * BBRT can be eliminated by catheter ablation

DIAGNOSTIC FEATURES OF BBRT
1. Tachycardia morphology is a typical LBBB (rarely RBBB)
2. Induction of the tachycardia depends upon His-Purkinje conduction delay
3. The tachycardia terminates with a block within the His-Purkinje system
4. During BBRT, a His potential precedes each QRS complex
5. Variations in the V-V intervals are preceded by similar changes in the H-H intervals

VENTRICULAR TACHYCARDIA 10

Long QT syndrome

CATEGORIES
1. **Congenital LQTS** due to hereditary defects of ion channels responsible for the repolarization process.
2. **Acquired LQTS** as a result of electrolyte disturbances or QT-prolonging drugs impairing the repolarization process.

Long QT syndrome (LQTS) is a congenital familial disorder known to be caused by mutations of the genes for cardiac potassium channels or less commonly sodium ion channels resulting in malfunction of these channels influencing ventricular repolarization. There are at least 10 types of channelopathies but the first three, LQTS 1 to 3, are the most prevalent and most studied. LQTS1 occurs in 30–35% (K channel), LQTS2 in 25-30% (K channel), LQTS3 in 5–10% (Na channel) of patients and comprise about 95% of the congenital LQTS.

LQTS is characterized by prologation of the QT interval on ECG and a propensity to ventricular tachyarrhythmias (polymorphic ventricular tachycardia – torsades de pointes or twisting of the points), which may lead to syncope, seizures, cardiac arrest, or sudden death. Torsades may either revert spontaneously back to sinus rhythm causing syncope or degenerate into ventricular fibrillation causing sudden death.

ST segment and T wave in hereditary LQTS

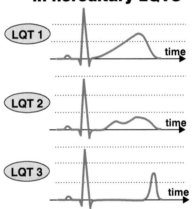

Unfortunately, a normal resting QTc does not reliably exclude LQTS, although exercise testing may provoke prolongation of the QTc and the greatest diagnostic yield occurs in the recovery phase of exercise. LQTS may also be acquired due to drugs or metabolic abnormalities. It is likely that many of those with acquired LQTS have a genetic basis.

Because the QT interval varies with heart rate (lengthening with bradycardia and shortening with tachycardia), the QT interval is corrected (QTc) for heart rate using Bazett's formula: QTc = QT divided by the square root of the RR interval in seconds. The QT which represents the duration of activation and recovery of the ventricular myocardium is measured from the beginning of the QRS complex to the end of the T wave and is normally between 0.30 and 0.44s. Any QTc interval > 0.44 s is considered prolonged. Do not rely on computer measurements. Use values from 5 RR intervals. The normal QTc can be more prolonged in females (up to 0.46 s). When marked variation is present in the RR interval (atrial fibrillation, ectopy), correction of the QT interval is difficult to define precisely. Marked variability of the QTc may occur in serial ECGs. In normal people this variation may be 50–75 ms over a 24 hr period.

LQTS1 shows broad-based T waves. LQTS2 shows low amplitude and notched T waves. LQTS3 generates a long ST segment with a late-appearing T wave. Exercise testing and 24 hr Holter may help the diagnosis. An epinephrine challenge test is sometimes useful. The diagnosis is made using a point scoring system and genetic testing though a negative genetic testing does not rule out LQTS. T wave alternans signals a poor prognosis. Finally ECGs should be done in parents and siblings.

EARLY AFTERDEPOLARIZATIONS (EAD)

* EADs originate during the phase 2 (plateau) or phase 3 (final repolarization) of the action potential.
* EADs are frequently found with prolonged action potential durations (as with LQTS) when Ca channels can partly be reactivated (note that Ca currents are depolarizing).
* EADs often occur with slow heart rates and usually following an extrasystole (i.e. after a compensatory pause).

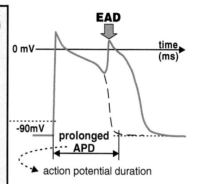

DISPERSION

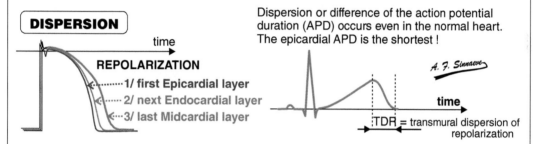

time

REPOLARIZATION
1/ first Epicardial layer
2/ next Endocardial layer
3/ last Midcardial layer

Dispersion or difference of the action potential duration (APD) occurs even in the normal heart. The epicardial APD is the shortest !

A. F. Sinnaeve

TDR = transmural dispersion of repolarization

Prolonged recovery from electrical excitation increases the likelihood of dispersing refractoriness, when some parts of myocardium might be refractory to subsequent depolarization. The interval from Tpeak to Tend (Tp-e) represents the transmural dispersion of repolarization (TDR). In long QT syndrome (LQTS), TDR increases and creates a functional substrate for transmural reentry. In LQTS, QT prolongation can lead to polymorphic ventricular tachycardia, or torsades de pointes, which itself may lead to ventricular fibrillation and sudden death.

LQTS has been recognized as mainly Romano-Ward syndrome (i.e. familial occurrence with autosomal dominant inheritance, QT prolongation, and ventricular tachyarrhythmias) or as Jervell and Lang-Nielsen (JLN) syndrome (i.e. familial occurrence with autosomal recessive inheritance, congenital deafness, QT prolongation, and ventricular arrhythmias). Two other syndromes are described, namely Andersen syndrome and Timothy syndrome, though some centers debate on whether they should be included in LQTS.

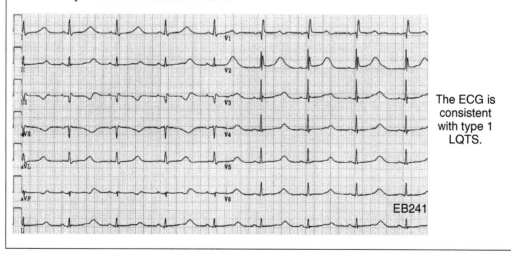

The ECG is consistent with type 1 LQTS.

EB241

VENTRICULAR TACHYCARDIA 11

Torsades de pointes

Torsades de pointes (TdP) is a form of polymorphic ventricular tachycardia (VT) that occurs in acquired or congenital QT interval prolongation. In the specific case of TdP, these variations take the form of a progressive, sinusoidal, cyclic alteration of the QRS axis with rotation of the heart's electrical axis by at least 180°. The peaks of the QRS complexes appear to "twist" around the isoelectric line of the recording. Twisting of the peak of the QRS complex occurs every 5-20 beats. Hence the name of torsades de pointes or "twisting of the points". Typical features of TdP include a ventricular rate of 160 to 250 bpm, irregular RR intervals, and a cycling of the QRS axis every 5 to 20 beats. The arrhythmia is preceded by long and short RR intervals and triggered by an early premature ventricular complex (R on T PVC). TdP is usually short-lived and terminates spontaneously. However, most patients experience multiple episodes of the arrhythmia, and episodes can occur in rapid succession with potential degeneration to ventricular fibrillation and sudden cardiac death (SCD).

Acquired LQTS usually results from drug therapy, hypokalemia, or hypomagnesemia. More than 50 medications, many of them common, can lengthen the QT interval in otherwise healthy people and cause a form of acquired long QT syndrome known as drug-induced LQTS. They include certain antibiotics, antidepressants, antihistamines, diuretics, heart medications, cholesterol-lowering drugs, diabetes medications, as well as some antifungal and antipsychotic drugs. The list is obtainable from the internet. Hypokalemia, hypomagnesemia, and bradycardia can increase the risk of drug-induced LQTS. In addition, some patients with acquired LQTS may have some subtle genetic defects, making them more susceptible to disruptions in cardiac rhythm from taking drugs that can cause prolonged QT intervals ("forme fruste" of congenital LQTS).

There is a characteristic initiating sequence before the onset of TdP, particularly in the acquired form with pause dependency. TdP are favored by bradycardia. The first ventricular complex of the sequence is usually a ventricular ectopic beat or the last beat of a salvo of ventricular premature beats. This is then followed by a compensatory pause terminated by a sinus beat. The sinus beat frequently has a very prolonged QT interval and an exaggerated U wave. A ventricular extrasystole then falls on the exaggerated U wave of the sinus beat and precipitates the onset of TdP. Alternation of the QT interval may precede the arrhythmia.

> **There is often a long-short interval before the onset of a tachycardia with "Torsades de Pointes".**

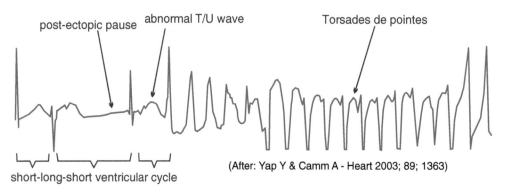

post-ectopic pause   abnormal T/U wave   Torsades de pointes

short-long-short ventricular cycle   (After: Yap Y & Camm A - Heart 2003; 89; 1363)

Rhythm strip in a patient with drug-induced TdP. Typical short-long-short ventricular cycle, pause dependent QT prolongation, and abnormal TU wave leading to classical TdP.

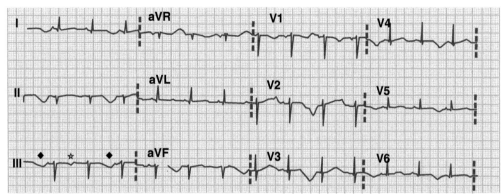

Obvious T wave alternans in a LQTS patient. This pattern is associated with a poor prognosis.
(♦ equal T waves)

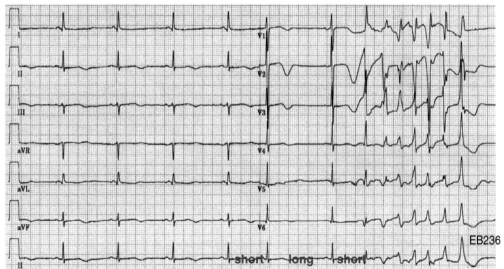

Acquired LQTS in a patient taking sotalol and hydroxychloroquine (an old antirheumatic drug).
TdP starts after a short-long-short sequence.

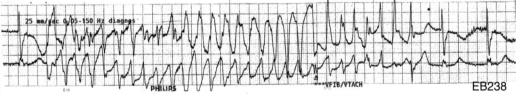

Typical Torsades de Pointes in a patient with acquired Long QT Syndrome.

VENTRICULAR TACHYCARDIA 12

Short QT syndrome

Short QT syndrome (SQTS) is an inherited cardiac channelopathy characterized by an abnormally short QT interval and an increased risk of atrial and ventricular fibrillation. SQTS diagnosis is based on the evaluation of symptoms, patient's family history and 12-lead ECG. It is essential to question the patient about the presence of key symptoms (syncope and palpitations) and family history of syncope, sudden cardiac death or atrial fibrillation at a young age. Secondary causes of short QT must also be excluded; these causes include hyperthermia, hyperkalemia, hypercalcemia, acidosis and alteration of autonomic tone. The ECG shows tall and sharp T waves and virtual absence of the ST segment. The ECG looks like an ECG of hyperkalemia. When evaluating the ECG three main aspects need to be considered: the duration of the QT interval, the morphology of the T wave and the behavior of both of them with the heart rate. A QTc < 330 ms in males and QTc < 340 ms in females makes the diagnosis.

Hypercalcemia as cause of short QT must be ruled out. Patients with SQTS show constant QT values and a lack of adaptation to heart rate with failure to prolong adequately at lower heart rates, showing none or minimal prolongation with decrease in heart rate. There is abnormal shortening during acceleration (pseudo-normalization of the QT interval at rapid rates).

Thus, an ECG taken during a higher heart rate as in a Holter recording may not show the short QT because the QT interval in these patients will often be normal during tachycardia. Therefore in order to make the diagnosis it is mandatory that the QT interval be measured at a heart rate close to 60 bpm and not corrected for heart rate.

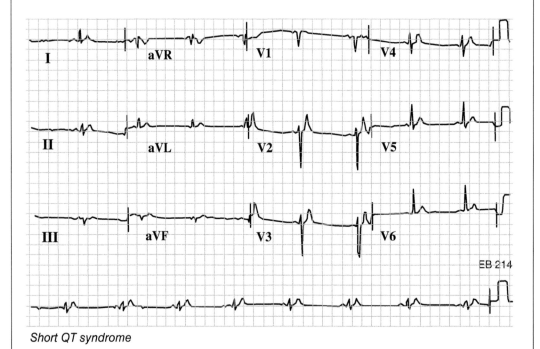

Short QT syndrome

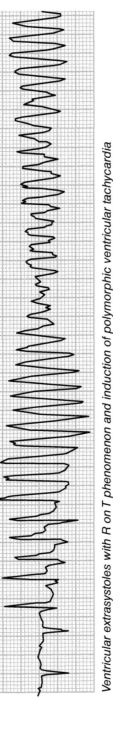

Ventricular extrasystoles with R on T phenomenon and induction of polymorphic ventricular tachycardia

Polymorphic ventricular tachycardia and cardiac ischemia

Ventricular tachycardia (VT) is classified as polymorphic when QRS complexes during tachycardia vary in appearance from beat to beat, suggesting a variable electrical activation sequence. Torsades de pointes (TdP) is the most common form of polymorphic VT and is associated with a prolonged QT interval. Acute coronary ischemia is a cause of polymorphic VT or ventricular fibrillation (VF) mostly with a normal QT interval, and is probably the most common cause of out-of-hospital sudden death. The polymorphic VT often occurs in patients without a prior history of heart disease, with normal left ventricular function and no prior myocardial infarction. This arrhythmia eventually leads to VF but it can be controlled with revascularization.

During acute ischemia, the leakage of potassium increases extracellular potassium that depolarizes myocytes in the ischemic border zone. This depolarization causes a substrate for reentry for polymorphic VT and/or VF from electrical heterogeneity of conduction and refractoriness.

In contrast, the most common setting for monomorphic VT is coronary artery disease in which myocardial scar tissue forms the substrate for electrical reentry. This type of VT can be seen in other conditions that create myocardial scarring. Scar-related monomorphic VT is not due to ischemia and usually does not lead to VF.

Short-coupled variant of Torsades de Pointes

The short-coupled variant of torsades de pointes (TdP) is a rare cause of torsades-like polymorphic VT without QT prolongation and without structural heart disease. It occurs in young patients often with a positive family history for sudden cardiac death. The most common first symptom is syncope. There is a high incidence of sudden death. The ECG displays typical TdP with a remarkably short coupling interval (always less than 300 ms) of the first TdP beat. Also, all the ventricular premature beats display this short interval. A short-long-short sequence of RR intervals is not present. The diagnosis may be missed unless the initiation of a VT is documented with an extremely short coupling interval of the first beat or of the isolated premature beats.

Further Reading

Baranchuk A, Nguyen T, Ryu MH, Femenía F, Zareba W, Wilde AA, Shimizu W, Brugada P, Pérez-Riera AR. Brugada phenocopy: new terminology and proposed classification. Ann Noninvasive Electrocardiol. 2012;17:299-314.

Barold SS. Bedside diagnosis of wide QRS tachycardia. Pacing Clin Electrophysiol. 1995;18:2109-15.

Cerrone M, Cummings S, Alansari T, Priori SG. A clinical approach to inherited diovasc Genet. 2012;5:581-90.

Kaufman ES. Mechanisms and clinical management of inherited channelopathies: long QT syndrome, Brugada syndrome, catecholaminergic polymorphic ventricular tachycardia, and short QT syndrome. Heart Rhythm. 2009;6(8 Suppl):S51-5.

Latif S, Dixit S, Callans DJ. Ventricular arrhythmias in normal hearts. Cardiol Clin. 2008;26:367-80.

Miller JM, Das MK, Yadav AV, Bhakta D, Nair G, Alberte C. Value of the 12-lead ECG in wide QRS tachycardia. Cardiol Clin. 2006;24:439-51.

Mizusawa Y, Wilde AA. Brugada syndrome. Circ Arrhythm Electrophysiol. 2012;5:606-16.

Roden DM. A practical approach to torsade de pointes. Clin Cardiol. 1997;20:285-90.

Vereckei A. Current algorithms for the diagnosis of wide QRS complex tachycardias. Curr Cardiol Rev. 2014;10:262-76.

Wellens HJ. Electrophysiology: Ventricular tachycardia: diagnosis of broad QRS complex tachycardia. Heart. 2001;86:579-85.

CHAPTER 16

VENTRICULAR FIBRILLATION AND VENTRICULAR FLUTTER

* Ventricular fibrillation
* Ventricular flutter
* Termination of ventricular fibrillation by a shock from an implanted defibrillator

ECG from Basics to Essentials: Step by Step. First Edition. Roland X. Stroobandt, S. Serge Barold and Alfons F. Sinnaeve.
Published 2016 © 2016 by John Wiley & Sons, Ltd. Companion Website: www.wiley.com/go/stroobandt/ecg

VENTRICULAR FIBRILLATION

Ventricular fibrillation (VF) consists of uncoordinated ineffectual contraction of the ventricles whereby they quiver uncontrollablly rather than contract properly. VF appears due to multiple reentry loops in the ventricles. Organized ventricular activity disappears and is replaced by rapid irregular electrical impulses at a rate of 350–450 bpm. VF is the most commonly identified arrhythmia of cardiac arrest (pulseless situation). The most common cause of VF is an acute myocardial infarction. VF is the final common pathway of many heart diseases. If this arrhythmia continues for more than 1–2 minutes, it will degenerate further into asystole (flat line) and death. Death often occurs if normal sinus rhythm is not restored within 90 seconds of the onset of VF, especially if it has degenerated further into asystole. The ECG is bizarre with a wandering baseline and shows QRS complexes of varying morphology and height so that no QRS complex looks like another. The QRS cannot be distinguished from the ST segment. There are no discernible P or T waves. VF can also be described as an undulating baseline. It may sometimes be difficult to differentiate VF from polymorphic VT. The totally disorganized ECG must be differentiated from artifact.

In about 5% of survivors of cardiac arrest no cardiac abnormality can be identified. Autopsy data confirm that in a similar percentage of victims of sudden death no structural heart disease can be identified. Occurrence of cardiac arrest in the absence of a substrate is defined as idiopathic VF. Idiopathic VF occurs in young adults who present with syncope or cardiac arrest due to polymorphic ventricular tachyarrhythmias in the absence of structural heart disease or identifiable channelopathies. The spontaneous arrhythmias are not related to stress and are invariably triggered by narrow complex ventricular extrasystoles with very short coupling intervals. Idiopathic VF is often caused by premature ventricular complexes (PVCs) arising from the right ventricular outflow tract (RVOT) or the Purkinje system in the absence of structural heart disease. Recurrent life-threatening arrhythmias may occur in approximately 25–40% of patients within 2 years. Radiofrequency catheter ablation of the trigger PVCs arising from the RVOT or Purkinje system may be effective in prevention.

J wave and early repolarization are generally considered as benign manifestations on the ECG. However recent observations suggest that they have the potential to cause cardiac arrhythmias. A higher incidence of arrhythmias was observed in patients with idiopathic VF associated with J wave and early repolarization on the ECG compared with those without such abnormalities. The association between J waves and idiopathic VF is a new finding but as yet we do not know how to distinguish "arrhythmogenic" from "normal" J waves. At present there are insufficient data to allow risk stratification in asymptomatic patients with J point elevation.

VENTRICULAR FLUTTER

Ventricular flutter is a rapid VT believed to be due to reentry. The rate is traditionally close to 300 bpm though it is sometimes described in terms of much slower rates. The ECG reveals a sinusoidal pattern and P waves, QRS complexes and T waves cannot be distinguished. Thus the ECG looks the same when it is visualized upside down. The arrhythmia may be considered an extreme form of VT and it is associated with rapid and profound hemodynamic compromise.

Ventricular flutter often deteriorates into VF

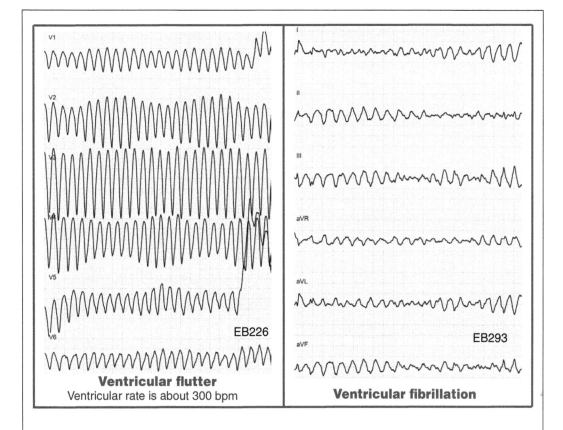

Ventricular flutter
Ventricular rate is about 300 bpm

EB226

Ventricular fibrillation

EB293

Ventricular tachycardia / ventricular fibrillation with structurally normal heart
* Right (or less commonly left ventricular) outflow tachycardia * Fascicular VT * Catecholaminergic VT * Brugada syndrome * Long QT syndrome * Short QT syndrome * Closely coupled torsades * Propranolol sensitive VT * Idiopathic ventricular fibrillation with J point abnormality * Idiopathic ventricular fibrillation

Progress in the knowledge of ventricular arrhythmias has revealed new forms of VT. A form of idiopathic VT may be propranolol sensitive and rare. It is neither initiated nor terminated by programmed stimulation, does not terminate with verapamil, and is consistent with an automatic mechanism. Isoprotenerol induces VT. Betablockers are effective. Newly recognized entities of idiopathic VTs include those originating in the papillary muscles and in the atrioventricular annular regions.

VENTRICULAR FIBRILLATION

Ventricular flutter often deteriorates into VF

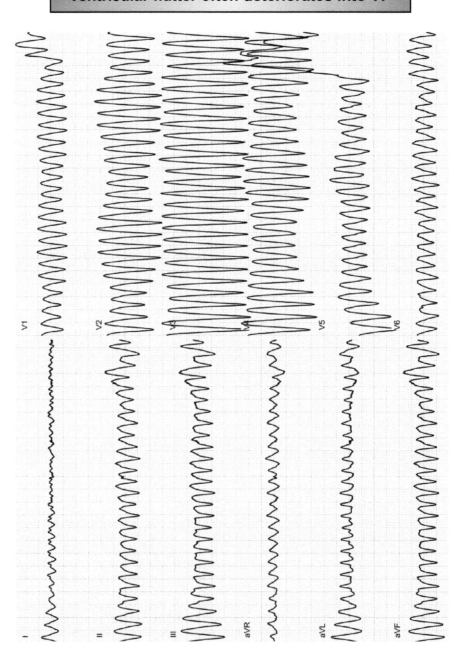

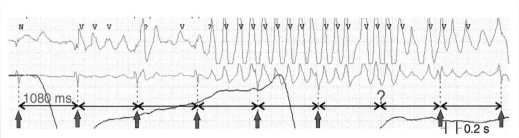

Artifact mimicking a ventircular tachycardia.
Typical peaking of the QRS complex within the artefactual recording.

Termination of ventricular fibrillation by a shock from an implanted defibrillator

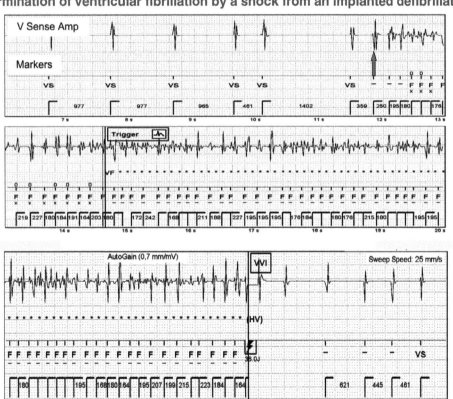

The ventricular intracardiac recordings (electrograms on top) were recorded by a single chamber implantable cardioverter (ICD-VR) programmed to deliver a shock when the heart rate exceeds 222 bpm (i.e. a cycle length of 270 ms). A ventricular premature beat (arrow) starts ventricular fibrillation (VF). The device makes the diagnosis of VF at the point labeled by the "Trigger" marker. Then, the capacitor of the ICD begins charging to a high voltage as shown by the small solid circles below the ventricular electrogram. The cycle length detected by the ICD is shown at the foot of the recording. Twelve seconds after the onset of VF the ICD delivers a 36 joule shock which immediately terminates VF. VS = sensed ventricular event with a cycle length longer than the required duration to activate the ICD. HV = high voltage.

Further Reading

Borne RT, Varosy PD, Masoudi FA. Implantable cardioverter-defibrillator shocks: epidemiology, outcomes, and therapeutic approaches. JAMA Intern Med. 2013;173:859-65.

Estes NA 3rd. Predicting and preventing sudden cardiac death. Circulation. 2011;124:651-6.

Srivathsan K, Ng DW, Mookadam F. Ventricular tachycardia and ventricular fibrillation. Expert Rev Cardiovasc Ther. 2009;7:801-9.

Surawicz B. Ventricular fibrillation. J Am Coll Cardiol. 1985;5(6 Suppl):43B-5.

Tabereaux PB, Dosdall DJ, Ideker RE. Mechanisms of VF maintenance: wandering wavelets, mother rotors, or foci. Heart Rhythm. 2009;6:405-15.

CHAPTER 17

PREEXCITATION AND WOLFF-PARKINSON-WHITE SYNDROME (WPW)

* Accessory pathways and delta waves
* ECG manifestations
* Features of the WPW syndrome
* Location of accessory pathways
* WPW is a great mimic
* Arrhythmias
* Characteristics of benign accessory pathways
* Preexcitation variants – atriofascicular, atriohisian and fasciculoventricular bypass

ECG from Basics to Essentials: Step by Step. First Edition. Roland X. Stroobandt, S. Serge Barold and Alfons F. Sinnaeve.
Published 2016 © 2016 by John Wiley & Sons, Ltd. Companion Website: www.wiley.com/go/stroobandt/ecg

PREEXCITATION AND WPW SYNDROME 1

In 1930, Wolff, Parkinson, and White (WPW) described a series of young patients who had a bundle branch block pattern on the ECG, a short PR interval, and paroxysms of tachycardia. Preexcitation was defined by Durrer et al. in 1970 with the following statement: "Preexcitation exists, if in relation to atrial events, when the whole or some part of the ventricular muscle is activated earlier by the impulse originating from the atrium than would be expected if the impulse reached the ventricles by way of the normal specific conduction system only". There are many other bypass tracts (that do not belong to the WPW syndrome) also associated with preexcitation, including atriofascicular, fasciculoventricular, nodofascicular, or nodoventricular. By far the commonest bypass tract is an accessory AV pathway of the WPW syndrome.

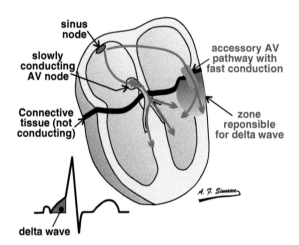

Conduction over an accessory pathway (AP) circumvents conduction delay occurring within the atrioventricular node (AVN), which leads to early eccentric activation of the ventricles and fusion complexes.

MECHANISM

WPW syndrome strictly refers to patients with symptoms. Those without symptoms strictly have a WPW pattern. However the terms are used loosely in the literature. WPW is currently defined as a congenital abnormality involving the presence of abnormal conductive tissue between the atria and the ventricles. The abnormal pathway connects directly and bypasses the AV node. The normal sinus impulse can travel down the normal pathway through the AV node, as well as the more rapidly conducting extra electrical accessory pathway. This results in ventricular depolarization starting earlier, or "preexcitation". It also produces eccentric myocardial activation. The WPW beat is a fusion beat. The presence of two pathways (the normal and the accessory one) between the atria and ventricles poses a risk of developing a "short circuit" which can result in an arrhythmia.

ECG MANIFESTATIONS

Classic ECG findings (see following figure) that are associated with WPW syndrome include the following:

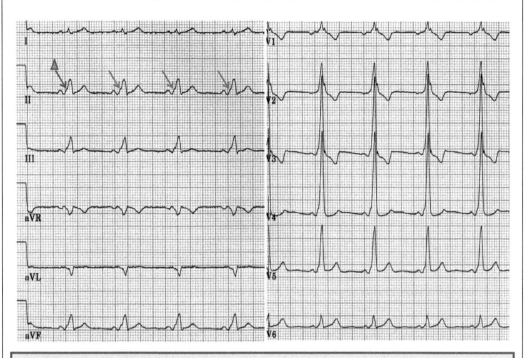

Some accessory pathways cannot conduct retrogradely under ordinary circumstances but retrograde VA conduction may sometimes become evident in high catecholamine (adrenergic) situations. Others have a concealed bypass tract with absent anterograde conduction. Although such connections are accessory pathways, they cannot conduct anterogradely. Therefore the ECG of patients with a concealed accessory pathway does not show the classic ECG abnormalities of WPW syndrome. However, these concealed bypass tracts can conduct retrogradely and can participate in orthodromic supraventricular tachycardia. About 25% of WPW patients with anterograde pathway conduction show absent retrograde conduction. Such patients are incapable of developing atrioventricular reentry tachycardia (AVRT) but are at risk of developing atrial fibrillation with rapid ventricular rates if the refractory period of the accessory pathway is short. Bystander accessory pathways may not be an active participant in an arrhythmia. This has to be confirmed by an electrophysiologic study. Some bystanders during a regular supraventricular tachycardia are not benign because they may have the capability of conducting rapid ventricular rates during atrial fibrillation.

The prevalence of ventricular preexcitation is thought to be 0.1–0.3%, or 1 to 3 per 1000 people in the general population (1 in 1000 patient years) and is more prominent in young patients. Estimates of arrhythmia incidence in patients with preexcitation vary widely, ranging from 12% to 80% in several surveys. Only about 5% of the tachycardias in patients who have WPW syndrome are antidromic tachycardias; the remaining 95% are orthodromic. The presence of an antidromic tachycardia should prompt a careful search for a second bypass tract. Patients with a WPW syndrome have a second pathway in 10–15% of cases.

PREEXCITATION AND WPW SYNDROME 2

MANIFEST or OVERT
accessory pathway (AP)

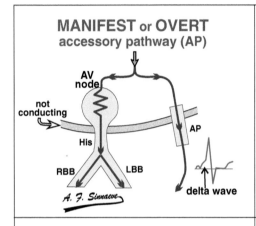

A. F. Sinnaeve

CONCEALED
accessory pathway (AP)

Retrograde conduction occurs during AVRT

LATENT AP
Nearly equal conduction times $t_1 = t_2$

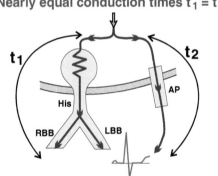

ORTHODROMIC AVRT
Atrioventricular reentry tachycardia

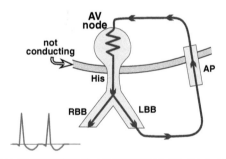

ANTIDROMIC AVRT
Atrioventricular reentry tachycardia

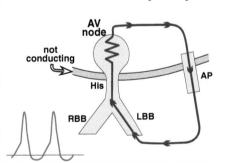

ATRIAL FIBRILLATION

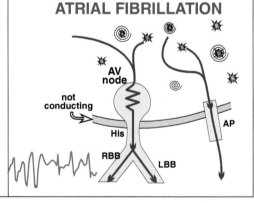

ASSOCIATED FINDINGS

1. A second accessory pathway is present in 10–15% of patients.
2. WPW patients have a higher incidence of dual AV nodal pathways.
3. The accessory pathway may not actively participate in a supraventricular tachycardia, taking the role of a bystander.

DEGREE OF PREEXCITATION

The degree of preexcitation on an ECG can be estimated by the width of the QRS complex. A wider or more preexcited QRS with a short PR interval indicates that most (or all) of the ventricular depolarization takes place via the accessory pathway rather than via the AV node. QRS width may vary with the heart rate if catecholamines permit the pathway through the AV node to contribute more to ventricular depolarization by enhancing AV nodal conduction.

The ECG pattern of WPW is absent unless a sufficient amount of ventricular myocardium is preexcited. The longest distance from the sinus node to the atrial insertion of an accessory pathway occurs with left lateral pathways. Consequently the WPW pattern may be subtle or invisible (latent WPW) with left lateral pathways. This should not be interpreted as an anterograde block in a pathway or the absence of preexcitation. Atrial pacing close to the pathway then brings out the full ECG WPW appearance.

LOCATION OF ACCESSORY PATHWAYS

The location of the APs, in descending order of frequency, is (1) 55%, the left free wall, (2) 33%, posteroseptal, (3) 9%, right free wall, and (4) 3%, anteroseptal.
The ventricular site of an accessory pathway can often be predicted with reasonable certainty by examining the vector of the delta wave portion of the QRS. The vector should point away from the area that is first activated by the accessory pathway. A general rule is that Q waves (negative delta waves) point away from the earliest site of ventricular activation, which should be the insertion point of the bypass tract.

Using the polarity of the delta wave provides a number of generalizations:
* A negative delta wave in a left-sided lead such as I and aVL indicates a left-sided AP
* A negative delta wave in a right-sided lead such as V1 predicts a right-sided AP
* An isoelectric delta wave in V1 predicts an anteroseptal AP
* A negative delta wave in the inferior leads (II, III, aVF) indicates a posteroseptal AP
* A positive delta wave in the inferior leads predicts an anteroseptal AP

P wave polarity
During orthodromic tachycardia, an inverted P wave in lead I suggests the atrial insertion in the left ventricular free wall. An inverted P wave in the inferior leads suggests a posteroseptal insertion right or left

Several algorithms are available to predict the location of the AP using the vector of the delta wave. These algorithms may not be totally accurate because maximal preexcitation is not available and because the WPW beat is a fusion between activation via the AV node and accessory pathway depolarization and because precordial lead placement, chest shape and characteristics of the heart may vary. Many complex algorithms have been published focusing on the vector of the delta wave.

PREEXCITATION AND WPW SYNDROME 3

We prefer the algorithm published by **d'Avila** in 1995 which is based on the QRS morphology in 5 ECG leads and is 92% accurate. The diagram shows 8 distinct anatomic zones. The QRS complex is described as + (positive), – (negative) and +/– (isophasic).

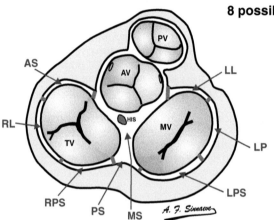

8 possible anatomic locations of the AP

(1) LL : left lateral
(2) LP : left posterior
(3) LPS : left posteroseptal
(4) PS : posteroseptal
(5) RPS : right posteroseptal
(6) RL : right lateral
(7) AS : anteroseptal
(8) MS : mid-septal

PV : pulmonary valve
AV : aortic valve
MV : mitral valve
TV : tricuspid valve

red => **lead**
blue => **location**
green => **deep Q, small r, small s
overall QRS negative**

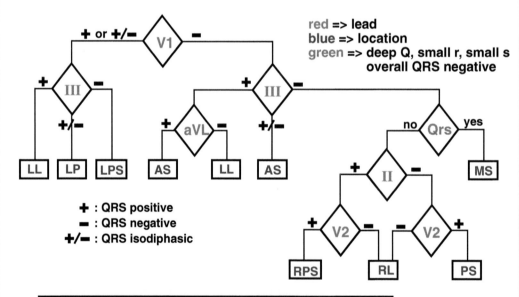

+ : QRS positive
– : QRS negative
+/– : QRS isodiphasic

ERRORS IN BYPASS LOCALIZATION
* Minimal preexcitation on the surface ECG
* Multiple pathways
* Thoracic deformities & congenital heart disease

According to the above algorithm, the previous ECG (see p.309) shows a positive QRS in V1 and a positive QRS in lead III so the accessory pathway is most probably left lateral.

The next ECG shows a WPW with a positive V1 and a negative lead III, putting the accessory pathway in the left posteroseptal region.

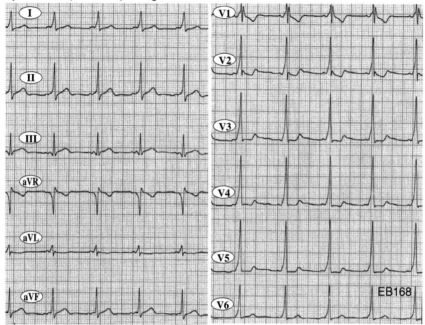

This ECG shows a WPW with negative V1, negative lead III, positive lead II and positive V2, putting the bypass tract in the right posteroseptal region.

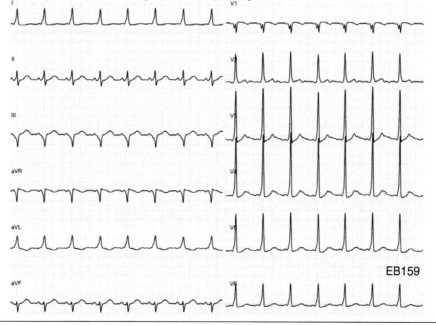

PREEXCITATION AND WPW SYNDROME 4

The following ECG is a WPW with isoelectric V1, positive lead III and negative aVL, putting the accessory pathway in the left lateral region.

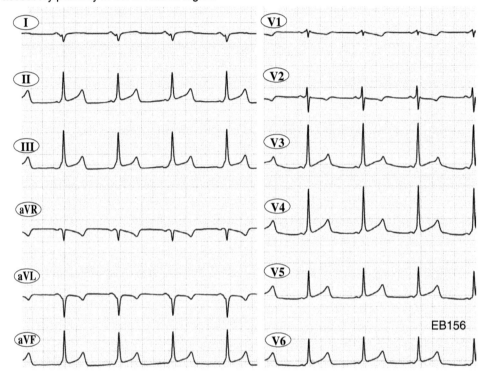

EB156

Negative delta wave in V1 → right-sided AP
Negative delta wave in II, III and aVF → posteroseptal AP

WPW is a great mimic !
* **Negative delta waves resemble MI (myocardial infarction).**
  Calling WPW Q waves in II, III and aVF (posteroseptal AP)
  an inferior MI is the commonest error.
* **Tall R waves in V1 resembles right bundle branch block.**
* **Ventricular hypertrophy.**
* **ST-T wave abnormalities may simulate cardiac ischemia.**

The next ECG shows a WPW with a negative V1, negative lead III and positive V2, putting the accessory pathway in the right posteroseptal region. This ECG is somewhat similar to the lower one in part 3; however, this ECG shows Q waves in leads II, III and aVF mimicking an inferior myocardial infarction.

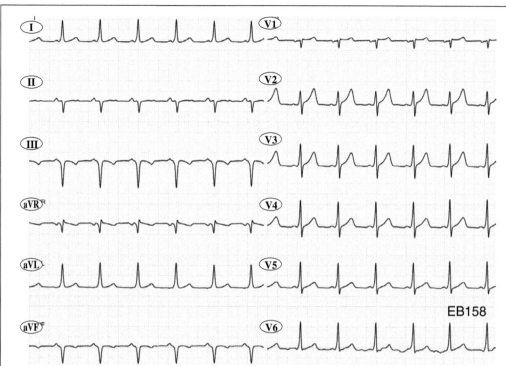

Posteroseptal accessory pathway mimicking inferior myocardial infarction with Q waves in leads III and aVF

ARRHYTHMIAS

Patients with WPW syndrome usually present with supraventricular tachycardia but they are potentially at an increased risk of dangerous ventricular arrhythmias due to extremely fast conduction across the bypass tract if they develop atrial flutter or atrial fibrillation.

About 2/3 of WPW patients have arrhythmias. Types of SVT include orthodromic tachycardia and antidromic tachycardia down the AP and retrograde conduction up the His-Purkinje system and AV node. In patients with WPW in which the AP participates in macro-reentry, 95% of SVT is due to orthodromic tachycardia and 5% is due to antidromic tachycardia. Overall 80% of the arrhythmias are AVRT and about 20% are atrial fibrillation and flutter though the latter is unusual. Conduction in an accessory pathway is generally rate-independent.

Orthodromic tachycardia
In orthodromic tachycardia (AVRT), the normal pathway is used for ventricular depolarization, and the AP is used for retrograde conduction essential for reentry. On ECG findings, the delta wave is absent, the QRS complex is normal, and P waves are typically inverted in the inferior and lateral leads.

Antidromic tachycardia
Antidromic tachycardia is regular and produces a wide QRS, reflecting an exaggeration of the delta wave during sinus rhythm. This tachycardia is difficult to differentiate from ventricular tachycardias and often has a slurred R wave upstroke with QRS duration longer than 160 ms. There are two types: (1) anterograde conduction along an accessory pathway and retrograde conduction via the AV node; (2) anterograde conduction along an accessory pathway and retrograde conduction via another accessory pathway.

PREEXCITATION AND WPW SYNDROME 5

Atrial fibrillation (AF)

For reasons that are not clear atrial fibrillation is relatively common (20%) in patients with WPW syndrome compared with the normal population. Many AF patients also have inducible AVRT that can degenerate into AF. In AF several patterns are possible bearing in mind that a rapidly conducting accessory pathway conducts faster than the AV node and therefore avoids the rate-limiting function provided by the normal conducting pathways.

Preexcitation activation of the ventricles is predominantly via a rapidly conducting accessory pathway causing an irregular rapid rhythm with wide QRS and bizarre morphology. The atria generate electrical impulses at an extremely rapid rate; those impulses can travel down the accessory pathway and stimulate the ventricles at an also extremely rapid rate, leading to a dangerous situation which may be life-threatening. The ventricular rate may be faster than 250 bpm, with some RR intervals approaching a corresponding rate of 300 bpm. Therefore AF may resemble ventricular tachycardia. However, the extreme irregularity suggests that the arrhythmia is not ventricular tachycardia. Extremely rapid ventricular rates may exceed the ability of the ventricles to follow in an organized manner resulting in disorganized ventricular activation, hypotension and eventually ventricular fibrillation.

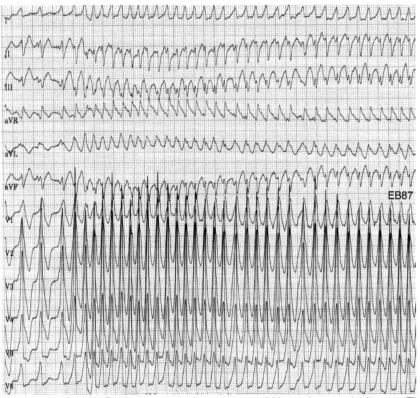

WPW syndrome with atrial fibrillation producing a very rapid irregular ventricular rate. The shortest RR interval measures 200 ms or slightly less and the ventricular rate is close to 300 bpm. The QRS is wide showing exclusive conduction via a left posteroseptal accessory pathway.

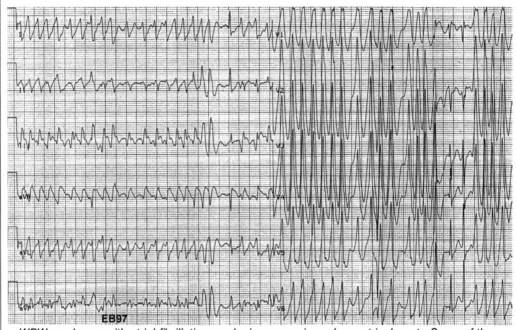

EB97

WPW syndrome with atrial fibrillation producing a very irregular ventricular rate. Some of the intervals measure 200 ms or slightly less. The QRS complexes are mostly wide because of conduction along a left accessory pathway (AP). There is competition between impulses traveling down the AV node and those traveling along the AP. This competition produces beats of varying morphology with normal QRS duration and fusion beats from ventricular activation by conduction in the 2 pathways. The change in the axis in lead II suggests the presence of 2 APs which were found in the left posteroseptal and left posterior regions. The combination of the varying QRS morphologies and irregular ventricular rate is very typical of atrial fibrillation in the presence of a rapidly conducting AP.

A malignant accessory pathway is defined by the occurrence of very fast arrhythmias during spontaneous attacks of atrial fibrillation (faster than 240–250 bpm).

In atrial fibrillation with preexcitation, activation of the ventricles is predominantly via the accessory pathway. Occasional activation of the ventricles occurs via the AV node resulting in a capture beat with a normal QRS together with a variety of fusion beats with inconsistent morphology as the ventricles are activated via both the accessory pathway and the AV node. This produces an irregular tachyarrhythmia with changing QRS morphology and shape.

Predominant or complete conduction via the AV node occurs when the accessory pathway has a long refractory period.

A broad QRS tachycardia that is irregular with a ventricular rate above 200 bpm and QRS morphology usually attributable to ventricular tachycardia should immediately arouse the suspicion of atrial fibrillation with conduction over an accessory pathway

PREEXCITATION AND WPW SYNDROME 6

Characteristics of benign accessory pathway

(1) The best indicator of low risk is the sudden disappearance of the preexcitation pattern during exercise testing. That finding indicates a long anterograde refractory period of the accessory pathway (AP). Intermittent preexcitation is present when, during sinus rhythm, some QRS complexes show preexcitation and are followed by QRS complexes showing AV conduction over the normal AV conduction pathway. One must be careful, however, to distinguish true block in the AP from diminution of the degree of preexcitation over the AP produced by sympathetic stimulation during exercise, which will shorten the trans-AV nodal conduction time. This is more likely to occur when the AP is left-sided. Therefore, several leads should be taken simultaneously. The exercise response must also be differentiated from a bigeminal ventricular rhythm with a long coupling interval.

(2) Intermittent WPW pattern on Holter registration.

(3) The accessory bundle responds to blockade by medication (especially sodium channel blockers).

About 1/3 of pathways conducting anterogradely eventually become nonfunctional with long-term follow-up.

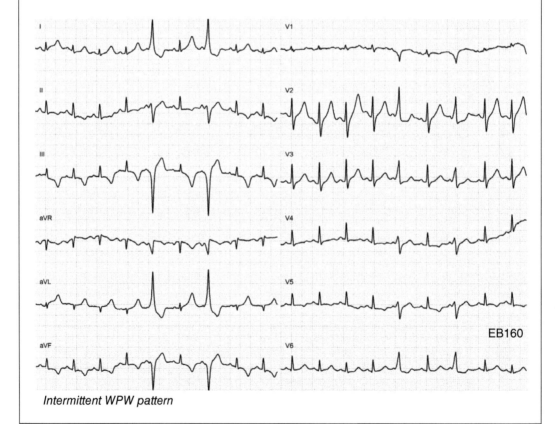

EB160

Intermittent WPW pattern

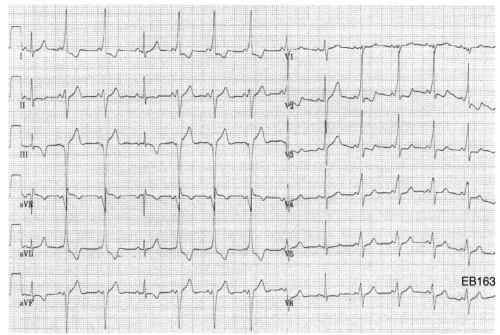

Intermittent WPW pattern

EB163

> **The location of the pathway or the degree of preexcitation do not predict the clinical course.**

Mortality

Mortality in WPW syndrome is rare and is related to sudden cardiac death (SCD). The incidence of SCD in WPW syndrome is approxmately 1 in 1000 symptomatic cases when followed for up to 15 years. Although relatively uncommon, SCD may be the initial presentation in as many as 4.5% of cases. Factors that appear to influence the risk of SCD are the presence of multiple bypass tracts, short AP refractory periods (< 240–250 ms), AF and atrial flutter (RR interval during arrhythmia < 240–250 ms) or a family history of premature sudden death.

> **If an electrophysiologic study is performed for risk stratification, the combination of inducible AVRT and a shortest preexcited RR interval in AF of less than 240–250 ms provide the most compelling indications for ablation in selected asymptomatic patients. The benefits of ablation should be weighed against the complications of the procedure.**

The management of the asymptomatic patient remains controversial. Asymptomatic patients with ventricular preexcitation may be considered for an electrophysiologic study to determine if the accessory pathway (AP) is associated with a high risk of sudden cardiac arrest and if the refractory period of the AP is short. If so, catheter ablation may be considered if their livelihood, profession, high risk occupation (bus driver, scuba diver, pilot) or professional athletes, insurability, or mental well-being may be influenced by unpredictable tachyarrhythmias or in whom such tachyarrhythmias would endanger the public safety. Patients with WPW and a family history of sudden cardiac death should also be considered for catheter ablation if noninvasive testing fails to reveal a low risk AP.

PREEXCITATION AND WPW SYNDROME 7

PREEXCITATION VARIANTS
* Atriofascicular
* Nodofascicular (most probably the same as atriofascicular)
* Nodoventricular (most probably the same as atriofascicular)
* Fasciculoventricular
* Atriohisian (James). Lown Ganong Levine syndrome?

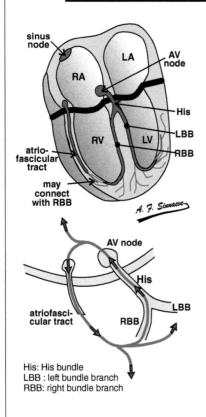

sinus node
LA
AV node
RA
His
RV LV LBB
atrio-fascicular tract RBB
may connect with RBB

A. F. Sinnaeve

AV node
His
atriofasci-cular tract LBB
RBB

His: His bundle
LBB : left bundle branch
RBB: right bundle branch

ATRIOFASCICULAR BYPASS

Atriofascicular fibers (called Mahaim bypass tracts in the past) originate in the right atrial free wall and insert into the distal part of the right bundle branch (RBB) or the adjacent ventricular myocardium. They are functionally similar to that of the AV node. Many so-called nodoventricular and nodo-fascicular bypass tracts studied in the past were actually atriofascicular tracts (like the AV node). In any case true nodoventricular and nodofascicular bypass tracts are very rare. The anterograde conduction time of atriohisian bypass tracts is rate-dependent. Approximately 6% of patients presenting with supraventricular tachycardia with a typical left bundle branch block morphology (with left axis deviation) have been found to have an atriofascicular bypass tract. In such cases, antidromic AV reentrant tachycardia results from anterograde conduction down the bypass tract and retrograde propagation via the normal conduction system. Orthodromic AVRT almost never occurs, because these bypass tracts generally do not conduct in a retrograde direction.

It is not uncommon for atriofascicular fibers to coexist with other accessory pathways which may serve as the retro-grade limb of a preexcited (typical) LBBB tachycardia. Atriofascicular bypass tracts may coexist with other supra-ventricular tachycardias that do not require an AV bypass tract for initiation and maintenance. Thus with AV nodal reentrant tachycardia, atriofascicular pathways may be present and function as a bystander.

ATRIOHISIAN BYPASS

An atriohisian bypass tract is a form of preexcitation manifested as a short PR interval shorter than 0.12 s that is the result of enhanced or rapid atrioventricular (AV) conduction. The usual cause is an accessory pathway (James bundle) which links the atrium to the ventricle and bypasses the normal AV node. As in WPW syndrome, the accessory pathway does not share the rate-slowing properties of the AV node, and may conduct electrical activity at a significantly higher rate than the AV node even up to 300 bpm (in the presence of a total AV nodal bypass) with obvious disastrous consequences. The QRS complexes in Lown Ganong Levine (LGL) are normal because ventricular activation is initiated in the normal manner. The association of a short PR interval and supra-ventricular tachycardia has been called LGL syndrome but this terminology is now rarely used.

* The QRS is normal unless there is functional aberration at rapid heart rates. The delta waves and broad complexes seen in WPW syndrome are not seen in LGL syndrome as the accessory pathway does not connect to the ventricles and so ventricular activation does not start early.
* Possible existence of intranodal or paranodal fibers that bypass all or part of the AV node. In some cases there is accelerated conduction through the normal AV node rather than along an accessory pathway. If a true accessory pathway is present, there is the potential for developing a reentrant supraventricular tachycardia (involving the node and the bypass tract) or having rapid ventricular rates during atrial fibrillation or atrial flutter.
* Patients with an isolated finding of short PR interval and no tachycardia may be characterized as having accelerated atrioventricular nodal conduction. Normal variant ?

FASCICULOVENTRICULAR BYPASS

These are rare causes of preexcitation which do not give rise to any reentrant tachycardia, appear to be only an ECG oddity (mimicking manifest WPW) and constitute an EP curiosity.

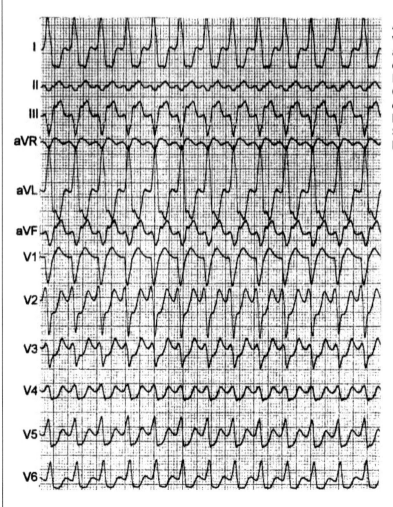

Antidromic AVRT with conduction over a right-sided atriofascicular bypass tract. Note the typical broad QRS tachycardia with complete LBBB and left axis deviation. Short RP interval and long PR interval.

Further Reading

Calkins H, Sousa J, el-Atassi R, Rosenheck S, de Buitleir M, Kou WH, Kadish AH, Langberg JJ, Morady F. Diagnosis and cure of the Wolff-Parkinson-White syndrome or paroxysmal supraventricular tachycardias during a single electrophysiologic test. N Engl J Med 1991;324:1612-18.

d'Avila A, Brugada J, Skeberis V, Andries E, Sosa E, Brugada P. A fast and reliable algorithm to localize accessory pathways based on the polarity of the QRS complex on the surface ECG during sinus rhythm. Pacing Clin Electrophysiol. 1995;18(9 Pt 1):1615-27.

Fengler BT, Brady WJ, Plautz CU. Atrial fibrillation in the Wolff-Parkinson-White syndrome: ECG recognition and treatment in the ED. Am J Emerg Med. 2007;25:576-83.

Mark DG, Brady WJ, Pines JM. Preexcitation syndromes: diagnostic consideration in the ED. Am J Emerg Med. 2009;27:878-88.

Pappone C, Vicedomini G, Manguso F, Baldi M, Pappone A, Petretta A, Vitale R, Saviano M, Ciaccio C, Giannelli L, Calovic Z, Tavazzi L, Santinelli V. Risk of malignant arrhythmias in initially symptomatic patients with Wolff-Parkinson-White syndrome: results of a prospective long-term electrophysiological follow-up study. Circulation. 2012;125:661-8.

Sethi KK, Dhall A, Chadha DS, Garg S, Malani SK, Mathew OP. WPW and preexcitation syndromes. J Assoc Physicians India. 2007;55 Suppl:10-5.

Wolff, L, Parkinson, J, White, PD. Bundle-branch block with short P-R interval in healthy young people prone to paroxysmal tachycardia. American Heart Journal. 1930/08;5:685-704.

CHAPTER 18

ELECTROLYTE ABNORMALITIES

* Hyperkalemia
* Hypokalemia
* Hypomagnesemia
* Hypermagnesemia
* Hypocalcemia
* Hypercalcemia

ECG from Basics to Essentials: Step by Step. First Edition. Roland X. Stroobandt, S. Serge Barold and Alfons F. Sinnaeve.
Published 2016 © 2016 by John Wiley & Sons, Ltd. Companion Website: www.wiley.com/go/stroobandt/ecg

ELECTROLYTE ABNORMALITIES 1

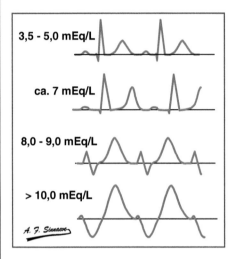

3,5 - 5,0 mEq/L

ca. 7 mEq/L

8,0 - 9,0 mEq/L

> 10,0 mEq/L

A. F. Sinnaeve

A very broad QRS > 0.20 s in an idioventricular rhythm and no visible P waves should be considered due to hyperkalemia until proven otherwise.

HYPERKALEMIA

Hyperkalemia is defined as a potassium level greater than 5.5 mEq/L. Ranges are as follows :
 * Mild : 5.5–6 mEq/L
 * Moderate : 6.1–7.0 mEq/L
 * Severe : 7.0 mEq/L and greater

Hyperkalemia causes depression of conduction with widening of the P wave and QRS complex, while the function of the sinoatrial (SA) node and the AV node are suppressed. Early changes of hyperkalemia include tall tented or peaked T waves with narrow base seen best in the precordial leads (the Eiffel tower effect). The T wave shows a steep ascent and descent in the precordial leads. There is a shortened QT interval, and ST segment depression. The T wave changes occur before changes in the QRS. These changes are followed by a widening of the QRS complex, increases in the PR interval, and decreased amplitude and widening of the P wave. This produces the appearance of a bizarre idioventricular rhythm with very wide QRS complexes (nonspecific intraventricular conduction disorder with a QRS that may be > 180 ms) without P waves. Without treatment, the P wave eventually disappears and the QRS morphology widens to resemble a sine wave.

Hyperkalemia may cause complete AV block, hemiblock, bundle branch block and an axis shift because of an intraventricular conduction delay. These abnormalities are reversible. Occasionally the ECG in severe hyperkalemia shows ST elevation in V1 and V2 resembling cardiac ischemia and infarction but these changes disappear after dialysis in patients with chronic renal failure.

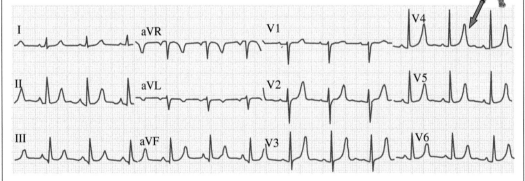

Suspect hyperkalemia when the amplitude of the T wave ≥ R wave in more than one lead.

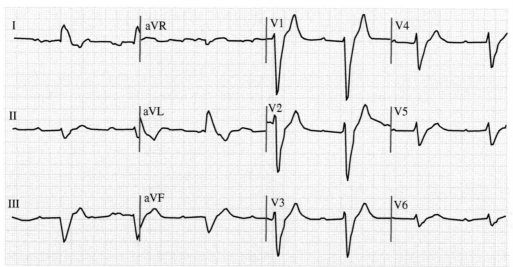

Sinus rhythm with attenuated P waves and marked first-degree AV block, intraventricular conduction delay (QRS = 0.28 s) when the potassium level was 7.3 mEq/L. The ECG showed a normal PR interval and a narrow QRS complex when the potassium level was normal.

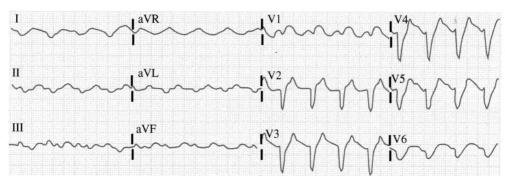

Hyperkalemia. Patient with a potassium level of 7.1 mEq/L. Probable slow ventricular tachycardia (rate = 115 bpm). P waves are not visible. Note the ST elevation in lead V1 suggesting ischemia or infarction.

Simulation of infarction

Even though the pseudoinfarction pattern of hyperkalemia (in the right precordial leads) is well known, the ST segment elevation can be so striking that it raises the possibility of coexistent acute infarction. The elevated ST segment is often downsloping, a finding that is unusual in acute myocardial infarction, which is more likely to show an ST segment that has a plateau or a shoulder or is uprising.

ELECTROLYTE ABNORMALITIES 2

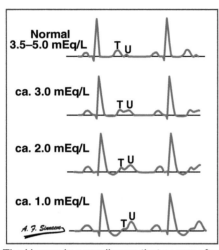

Normal
3.5–5.0 mEq/L

ca. 3.0 mEq/L

ca. 2.0 mEq/L

ca. 1.0 mEq/L

A. F. Sinnaeve

HYPOKALEMIA

Hypokalemia may been defined as a potassium level lower than 3.5 mEq/L. Moderate hypokalemia is a serum level of < 3.0 mEq/L. Severe hypokalemia is defined as a level < 2.5 mEq/L. ECG changes appear when K$^+$ falls below about 2.7 mEq/L; these changes are mainly due to a delayed ventricular repolarization. The changes normally do not correlate well with the plasma concentration and the ECG is unreliable in the diagnosis of hypokalemia. The ECG changes are not very dramatic and are rare in mild hypokalemia. The hearts of patients with hypomagnesemia or digoxin therapy are more sensitive to hypokalemia. Changes that may be noted are: prominent U wave; increased amplitude and width of the P wave; slight prolongation of the PR interval and minimal QRS prolongation; T wave flattening and inversion; mild ST depression.

The U wave is a small wave that occurs after the T wave and is usually 1/10 th the height of the T wave in the normal situation. The origin of the U wave is uncertain and is believed that it may arise from repolarization of the Purkinje fibers. U waves are not specific for hypokalemia. They also occur in bradycardia and left ventricular hypertrophy. Prominent U waves (best seen in the precordial leads as a bump) are the most common ECG abnormality of hypokalemia. The apparent prolongation of the QT interval is caused by fusion of the T and U waves as the T wave becomes smaller and the U wave larger and the U wave becomes higher than the T wave. These 2 waves may no longer be distinguished (long QU interval), while the true QT interval remains normal. With worsening hypokalemia, a potential to develop life-threatening ventricular arrhythmias exists (VT, VF, torsades de pointes). In patients on digoxin, hypokalemia may precipitate the arrhythmias of digitalis toxicity.

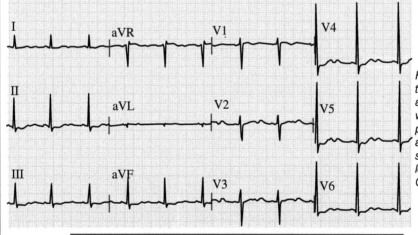

Hypokalemia. Note the ST depression and the prominent U wave. In V5 the amplitude of the T wave and the U wave are similar. There is prolongation of the QU interval.

> * A prominent U wave with a small T wave should raise suspicion of hypokalemia.
> * The end of the T wave may not be identifiable.

HYPOMAGNESEMIA

Severe hypomagnesemia occurs when the level is lower than 1.0 mEq/L. On ECG, hypomagnesemia can present with nonspecific abnormalities, prolongation of the QT and PR intervals, widening of the QRS complexes, ST segment depression, and low T waves, as well as supraventricular and ventricular tachyarrhythmias especially in patients on digoxin. Torsades de pointes may occur. Many patients will have several metabolic disorders such as hypokalemia with hypomagnesemia.

HYPERMAGNESEMIA

Magnesium levels above 10 mEq/L are defined as severe hypermagnesemia. The following changes may occur: delayed intraventricular conduction, first-degree heart block, prolongation of QT interval. Heart block progressing to complete heart block and asystole.

HYPOCALCEMIA

Hypocalcemia causes narrowing of the QRS complex and reduced PR interval. T wave flattening and inversion may occur in 50% of the patients. Occasionally with severe hypocalcemia, ST elevation mimicking an acute MI can be seen.

The ECG hallmark of hypocalcemia remains the prolongation of the QTc interval directly related to lengthening of the ST segment, which is directly proportional to the degree of hypocalcemia or, as otherwise stated, inversely proportional to the serum calcium level. The exact opposite holds true for hypercalcemia. The long ST segment is the most important diagnostic feature of hypocalcemia. With very severe hypocalcemia, AV block, torsades de pointes and ventricular fibrillation may occur. The combination of hypocalcemia and hyperkalemia is seen mostly in patients with chronic renal failure where there is prolongation of the ST segment /QT interval (there is no change in T wave duration) and tall and symmetric T waves.

The QT prolongation is in contrast to hypokalemia where it is the QU and not the QT which is prolonged.

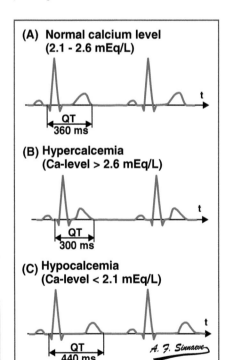

(A) Normal calcium level (2.1 - 2.6 mEq/L)

QT 360 ms

(B) Hypercalcemia (Ca-level > 2.6 mEq/L)

QT 300 ms

(C) Hypocalcemia (Ca-level < 2.1 mEq/L)

QT 440 ms

A. F. Sinnaeve

HYPERCALCEMIA

The main ECG abnormality seen with hypercalcemia is shortening of the ST segment with corresponding decrease in the QT interval.

When compared with the second half (descending limb) of the T wave, the first half (ascending limb) of the T wave is more steep. In normal subjects, the descending limb of the T wave is normally more steep than the ascending limb.

In severe hypercalcemia, ECG findings mimicking hypothermia with deflections known as Osborn waves (J waves) may be seen.

Significant hypercalcemia can cause ECG changes mimicking an acute myocardial infarction.

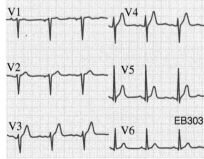

Hypercalcemia. Sinus rhythm (75 bpm) QT = about 0.24 s (240 ms); QTc = 0.268 s (268 ms)

EB303

Further Reading

Diercks DB, Shumaik GM, Harrigan RA, Brady WJ, Chan TC. Electrocardiographic manifestations: electrolyte abnormalities. J Emerg Med. 2004;27:153–60.

El-Sherif N, Turitto G. Electrolyte disorders and arrhythmogenesis. Cardiol J. 2011;18:233-45.

Medford-Davis L, Rafique Z. Derangements of potassium. Emerg Med Clin North Am. 2014;32:329-47.

Pepin J, Shields C. Advances in diagnosis and management of hypokalemic and hyperkalemic emergencies. Emerg Med Pract. 2012;14:1-17.

Webster A, Brady W, Morris F. Recognising signs of danger: EKG changes resulting from an abnormal serum potassium concentration.Emerg Med J. 2002;19:74–7.

CHAPTER 19

ELECTROPHYSIOLOGIC CONCEPTS

* Aberrant conduction
    ○ Ashman phenomenon
    ○ Phase 3 aberrancy
    ○ Bradycardia-dependent aberration
    ○ Retrograde invasion of bundle branch
* Concealed conduction
    ○ Ventricular premature beats
    ○ Atrial fibrillation and flutter
    ○ Concealed extrasystoles
* Ventricular fusion
* Overdrive suppression
* R on T phenomenon
* Atrioventricular dissociation
* Cardiac memory
* Parasystole
* Electrical alternans

ECG from Basics to Essentials: Step by Step. First Edition. Roland X. Stroobandt, S. Serge Barold and Alfons F. Sinnaeve.
Published 2016 © 2016 by John Wiley & Sons, Ltd. Companion Website: www.wiley.com/go/stroobandt/ecg

ELECTROPHYSIOLOGIC CONCEPTS 1

ABERRANT CONDUCTION 1

Aberrant ventricular conduction is defined as QRS widening due to delay or block in bundle branch or intramyocardial conduction. The alteration in the QRS contour of supraventricular beat is related to impulse transmission during periods of physiologic refractoriness, or depression of conductivity.

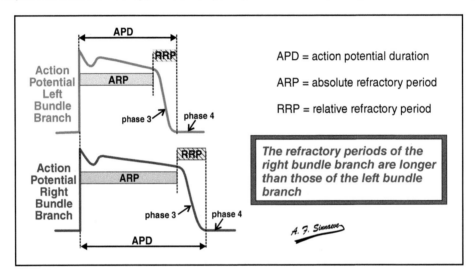

APD = action potential duration

ARP = absolute refractory period

RRP = relative refractory period

The refractory periods of the right bundle branch are longer than those of the left bundle branch

A. F. Sinnaeve

In the normal heart, a very premature impulse arriving in the ventricles may exhibit aberrant conduction or functional bundle branch block (BBB). The beat is then conducted with functional BBB (usually right BBB because the right bundle branch has a longer refractory period than the left bundle branch). Aberrant conduction may also occur with fast supraventricular tachycardias in the absence of disease of the His-Purkinje system by mechanisms outlined below.

QRS morphology is the most helpful clue in differentiating between a supraventricular and ventricular origin of wide QRS complexes. The morphologic features that favor ventricular origin of wide complexes are discussed in the VT broad QRS tachycardia sections of the book. The combination of a long RR interval followed by a short interval may lead to aberrant ventricular conduction as seen in atrial fibrillation (Ashman phenomenon).

Ashman phenomenon

The Ashman phenomenon refers to aberrant ventricular conduction due to change in QRS cycle length (rate). In 1947 Ashman reported that in atrial fibrillation (AFib), when a relatively long cycle was followed by a relatively short cycle, the beat with a short cycle length often had right bundle branch block (RBBB) morphology. This causes diagnostic confusion with ventricular premature complexes (VPCs).

The aberrant conduction depends on the relative refractory period of the components of the conduction system distal to the AV node. The refractory period depends on the heart rate. The refractory period changes with the RR interval of the preceding cycle. A longer cycle lengthens the ensuing refractory period. If a shorter cycle follows a long RR interval, the beat ending the short cycle is likely to be conducted with aberrancy. A right bundle branch block pattern is more common than a left bundle branch block pattern because of the longer refractory period of the right bundle branch.

Unfortunately the rule of bigeminy interferes with the diagnosis. The rule states that a lengthened cycle tends to precipitate a ventricular premature beat. The diagnosis of aberrancy therefore relies heavily on QRS morphology.

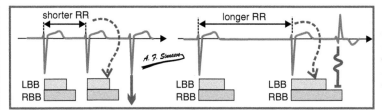

The longer the preceding RR interval, the longer the refractory periods and the greater the chance for aberrant ventricular conduction

Atrial fibrillation with irregular ventricular rate. On the left of the stated diagram the third beat (solid arrow) terminates a relatively short RR interval but its intraventricular conduction remains normal. On the right of the diagram (stated above), the last beat ends an RR interval identical to the one terminated by the 3rd beat on the left. However, this last beat is conducted with a right bundle branch block pattern.

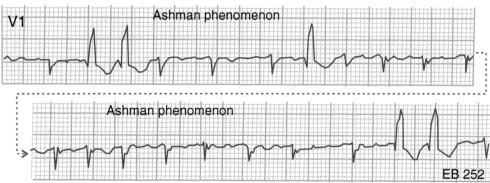

Atrial fibrillation with irregular ventricular rate. Wide complexes occur when a short cycle follows a longer one. There is a tiny r in the wide complexes so that the rsR' complex is consistent with right bundle branch block. The 2nd wide QRS (top) and the last one (bottom) probably represent continuing aberrant conduction due to retrograde invasion of the right bundle branch, a process initiated by the preceding aberrant beat according to Ashman phenomenon.

Criteria for the diagnosis of Ashman phenomenon

* A relatively long cycle immediately preceding the short cycle which terminates with aberrant QRS complex: a short-long-short interval is even more likely to initiate aberration. Aberration can be LBBB and RBBB, and both patterns may be observed even in the same patient.
* RBBB form aberrancy with normal orientation of the initial QRS vector: Concealed perpetuation of aberration is possible, such that a series of wide QRS supraventricular beats is possible.
* Irregular coupling of aberrant QRS complexes.
* Lack of a fully compensatory pause (never seen in atrial fibrillation).

Aberrancy vs. ventricular premature beats in atrial fibrillation		
	AFib with aberrant conduction	**AFib with VPCs**
QRS duration	0.12–0.15 s	0.15–0.20 s
QRS pattern*	Varying degrees of RBBB. rSR' or rR' in lead V1	Bizarre monophasic or biphasic complexes in lead V1
Coupling interval	Varying interval between the widened QRS and previous QRS	Generally fixed
Compensatory pause	No	Yes

* See section on ventricular tachycardia and broad complex tachycardia.
AFib = atrial fibrillation; VPC = ventricular premature complex

ELECTROPHYSIOLOGIC CONCEPTS 2

ABERRANT CONDUCTION 2

Phase 3 Aberrancy

This is the most common mechanism for sustained aberrancy during supraventricular tachycardia.

Tachycardia-dependent aberration

Tachycardia-dependent (phase 3) BBB is abnormal and occurs at relatively slower rates than those associated with functional aberrancy. It is due to lesion in one of the bundle branches. The abnormal bundle branch has a prolonged refractory period that allows a critical cycle length to encroach on it. The critical rate at which BBB occurs may be relatively slow or fast as a result of exercise. Normal conduction returns at a slower rate. In some cases normalization of intra-ventricular conduction occurs at a RR interval significantly longer than the RR which initiated bundle branch block. This rate discrepancy is usually due to reset of the refractory periods from retrograde invasion of the blocked bundle branch coming from the unaffected bundle branch as discussed below.

Impact of unequal refractoriness of the right bundle branch (RBB) and left bundle branch (LBB) on the intraventricular conduction of atrial extrasystoles

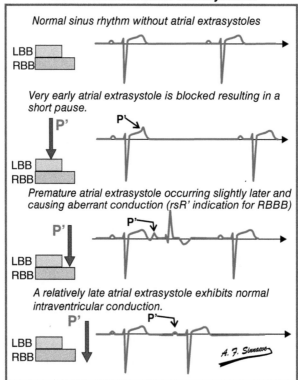

Normal sinus rhythm without atrial extrasystoles

LBB
RBB

Very early atrial extrasystole is blocked resulting in a short pause.

P'

LBB
RBB

Premature atrial extrasystole occurring slightly later and causing aberrant conduction (rsR' indication for RBBB)

P'

LBB
RBB

A relatively late atrial extrasystole exhibits normal intraventricular conduction.

P'   P'

LBB
RBB

A. J. Sinnaeve

Typical phase 3 aberrancy

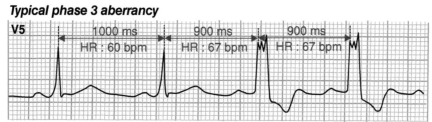

LBBB appears when the heart rate (HR) > 60 bpm and the cycle length < 1000 ms

Bradycardia-dependent aberration

Bradycardia-dependent BBB (phase 4 block) is rare and due to disease in the His-Purkinje system. Abnormal His-Purkinje cells may acquire the property of spontaneous phase 4 depolarization. During a long pause, the site of the diseased His-Purkinje abnormality continues to depolarize. As their membrane potential becomes more positive, the conduction velocity of subsequent impulses decreases and can even be blocked altogether.

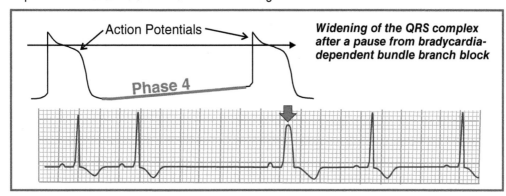

Widening of the QRS complex after a pause from bradycardia-dependent bundle branch block

Retrograde invasion of bundle branch

This occurs in tachycardia-dependent block or aberrancy during supraventricular tachycardia. The sequence of QRS widening that is often observed with phase 3 aberration in the first premature beat of supraventricular tachycardia. Assuming the block occurs in the left bundle branch, it leaves the left bundle refractory for the next complex. This next beat is conducted by the right bundle and once it reaches the apex, it is conducted retrogradely by the left bundle branch. This can continue until a new premature ventricular complex causes a compensatory pause and "resets" the system and aberrancy disappears.

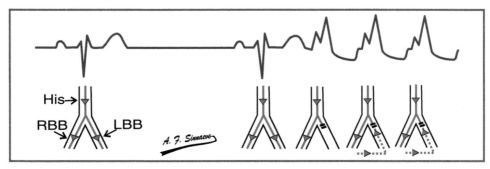

ELECTROPHYSIOLOGIC CONCEPTS 3

CONCEALED CONDUCTION

Concealed conduction is defined as the propagation of an impulse within the specialized conduction system (AV node and His-Purkinje system), which cannot be recognized on surface ECG. This impulse travels only a limited distance within the conduction tissue with incomplete anterograde or retrograde penetration. The concealed impulse can interfere with the formation or conduction of a subsequent supraventricular or ventricualr impulse. It is recognized by its after-effect on the conduction or formation of the ensuing impulse.

!! Concealed conduction is inferred only because of its influence on the subsequent cardiac cycle! !!

Ventricular premature beats

Concealed conduction commonly occurs when an interpolated ventricular premature impulse (VPC) enters the His-Purkinje system and atrioventricular (AV) node retrogradely but does not reach the atrium. Consequently the ensuing sinus impulse either does not conduct to the ventricle or conducts with a prolonged PR interval due to the increased AV nodal refractoriness initiated by retrograde conduction of the VPC. This effect on AV conduction of the next sinus impulse should not be misdiagnosed as AV block.

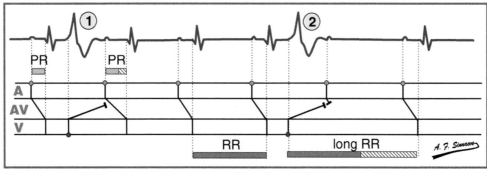

Concealed retrograde conduction of ventricular extrasystoles.
1. VPC produces partial refractoriness in AV junction and causes a prolonged PR interval of the succeeding sinus beat.
2. VPC producing complete refractoriness in the AV junction so that the next sinus impulse is not conducted.

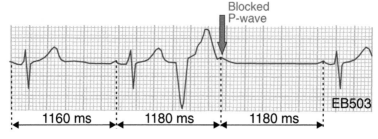

Atrial fibrillation and flutter

In atrial fibrillation the AV node is bombarded by impulses. Some impulses traverse the AV node and reach the specialized infranodal conduction system and then the ventricles. However, most atrial impulses penetrate the AV node for varying distances and then are extinguished when they encounter the refractoriness of an earlier wavefront. The irregularity of the ventricular rate associated with atrial fibrillation, therefore, indicates changes of refractoriness of the AV junctional tissues from cycle to cycle.

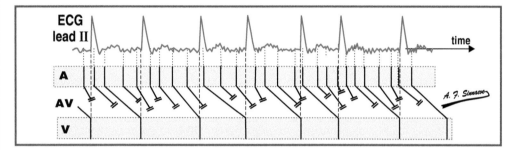

The irregular ventricular rate in atrial fibrillation is due to varying degrees of penetration of "blocked" atrial impulses into parts of the AV junction, and to the effect of such concealed conduction on the propagation of subsequent impulses.

Another example can be seen in atrial flutter. As a result of the rapid atrial rate, some of the atrial activity fails to get through the AV node in an anterograde direction but can alter the rate at which a subsequent atrial impulse is conducted. In this circumstance, an alteration in the F wave to QRS relationship is seen.

Concealed extrasystoles

Pseudo AV block is caused by concealed junctional or ventricular extrasystole. Such extrasystoles are not recorded on the surface ECG. Both the anterograde conduction and retrograde conduction are blocked and retrograde conduction may be rarely preserved. Concealed conduction of these extrasystoles affects the next beat. They may cause delay of AV conduction, the sudden appearance of a long PR interval, and cause failure of conduction (AV block) with patterns resembling type I or type II and sometimes 2:1 AV block. Many patients with concealed extrasystoles have disease of the His-Purkinje system.

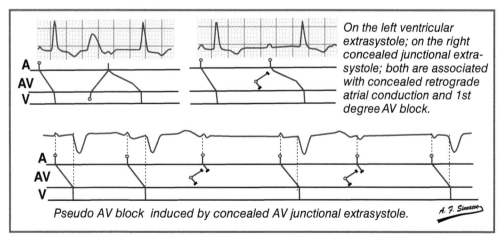

On the left ventricular extrasystole; on the right concealed junctional extrasystole; both are associated with concealed retrograde atrial conduction and 1st degree AV block.

Pseudo AV block induced by concealed AV junctional extrasystole.

ELECTROPHYSIOLOGIC CONCEPTS 4

VENTRICULAR FUSION

Fusion may occur in the atria or ventricles but only ventricular fusion beats are clinically important. Ventricular fusion beats are often seen during sustained ventricular tachycardia (VT) when the rate is relatively slow. Fusion results from partial ventricular activation by a sinus beat during a ventricular rhythm. Therefore a fusion beat has a morphology that depends on the varying contribution from the 2 ventricular depolarizing wavefronts. If sinus rhythm contributes mostly to ventricular depolarization, the QRS will resemble the sinus beat. If the ventricular rhythm contributes mostly to ventricular depolarization, the QRS will resemble the pure ventricular beat. The QRS complex of ventricular fusion can be narrow or as wide as the ventricular rhythm but it cannot be longer than the QRS of the ventricular rhythm. In VT ventricular fusion beats may coexist with ventricular capture beats (inscribing a narrow QRS like the sinus beats) when a sinus beat travels in the conduction system at a critical time to permit complete ventricular depolarization by the sinus impulse.

Causes of ventricular fusion beats

* Ventricular tachycardia (VT).
* Accelerated idioventricular rhythm (slower than VT) which often starts and terminates with a ventricular fusion beat when its rate approximates that of the sinus rhythm.
* Ventricular parasystole also generates fusion beats.
* Late ventricular premature beats.
* Escape ventricular rhythm.
* Ventricular pacing.

During AV dissociation, a ventricular fusion beat means that an atrial impulse has been able to travel in the conduction system and suggests that complete AV block is not present.

The typical QRS complex seen in Wolff-Parkinson-White syndrome represents a fused beat with early activation occurring via the accessory pathway, and activation of the ventricle slightly later via the normal His-Purkinje conduction system. The end-result is a short PR interval and fused QRS complex.

Ventricular fusion beats are common during normal ventricular pacing and must be differentiated from pseudofusion beats (see section on cardiac pacing).

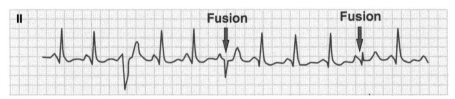

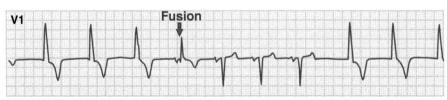

Idioventricular rhythm (60 bpm). The 4th ventricular complex is a fusion beat produced by the ectopic ventricular rhythm and normally conducted ventricular activation initiated by a sinus beat.

OVERDRIVE SUPPRESSION

In the healthy heart, AV junctional automaticity and idioventricular automaticity are not brought into play and instead are suppressed by the sinus node by virtue of its faster rate (overdrive suppression). A sudden cessation of sinus node activity or sudden AV block may be tolerated in the normal heart without significant bradycardia by the emergence of subsidiary pacemakers but in the diseased heart the same situation may result in prolonged and even fatal cardiac standstill. In the bradycardia-tachycardia form of sick sinus sydrome, an atrial tachyarrhythmia causes overdrive suppression of the diseased sinus node. After atrial arrhythmia termination, there is a variable delay before the dysfunctional sinus node (or AV junction) recovers and again generates an impulse. The period of overdrive suppression or asystole after a supraventricular tachycardia can often be correlated with the patient's symptoms. The occurrence of asystole implies additional impaired function of the lower (nonsinus) pacemakers. In addition the drugs used to prevent atrial fibrillation or control its ventricular rate are often responsible for the symptomatic bradycardia that follows cessation of an atrial tachyarrhythmia in the sick sinus syndrome.

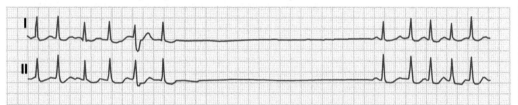

Sick sinus syndrome (SSS). Spontaneous termination of atrial fibrillation is followed by asystole of 4.2 s (overdrive suppression). The absence of AV junctional escape indicates that the AV junction is involved in the pathophysiology of the SSS. Sinus rhythm resumes for one beat followed by recurrence of atrial fibrillation.

R on T PHENOMENON

Ventricular premature contractions (VPCs) rarely have the potential to induce ventricular fibrillation (VF). If they coincide with the so-called vulnerable period near the apex of the T wave of a preceding beat VF can be initiated. This is called the R on T phenomenon. A long time ago, it was believed that this phenomenon was dangerous and a precursor of VF. It has since lost a lot of its importance. The R on T phenomenon is important with the propensity of inducing VF in only 3 specific settings: (1) Acute myocardial ischemia as in myocardial infarction; (2) Severe hypokalemia; (3) In the presence of a long QT interval. In other situations the R on T VPCs behave like other VPCs. In these situations a pacemaker stimulus can also precipitate VF.

The vulnerable period is about 0.01 s long and lies just before the peak of the T wave. A shock to convert a tachycardia may cause VF if applied during the vulnerable phase in the situations listed above. For this reason, for elective cardioversion, the shock is delivered outside the vulnerable period. This is accomplished by synchronizing the shock to the R or S wave of the QRS complex where it is sufficiently removed from the T wave. During testing of an implantable cardioverter-defibrillator VF is deliberately induced by delivery of a shock into the vulnerable phase.

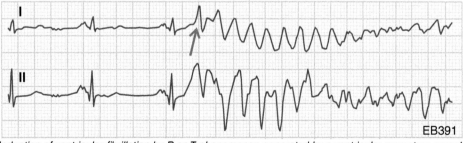

EB391

Induction of ventricular fibrillation by R on T phenomenon generated by a ventricular premature complex falling in the ventricular vulnerable period.

ELECTROPHYSIOLOGIC CONCEPTS 5

ATRIOVENTRICULAR DISSOCIATION

Atrioventricular (AV) dissociation describes a situation where there is loss of AV synchrony because the atria and ventricles function independently of each other. The atrial rate may be faster or slower than the ventricular rate. When the atrial rate is faster than the ventricular rate, complete heart block is present. Complete heart block is only one cause of AV dissociation. When the atrial rate is almost the same as the ventricular rate but the P wave does not conduct, the term "isorhythmic" AV dissociation is used ("iso" is the Greek root for "same"). Atrial and ventricular activity occur close together during the physiologic refractory period of each other so that sinus beats do not reach the ventricle during complete AV dissociation. This represents functional AV block and not true AV block. AV dissociation can be complete or incomplete. When incomplete, some of the P waves conduct and capture the ventricles and the rhythm is called interference AV dissociation. AV dissociation is a mis-understood and often misused term. AV dissociation simply means that the atria and the ventricles are under the control of separate natural pacemakers. It is not an arrhythmia; it is a symptom of an arrhythmia, just as anemia is not a disease but a symptom of a disease.

> **1. AV dissociation is not an arrhythmia but is present in conjunction with other arrhythmias; it is a result of some mechanism that causes independent beating of atria and ventricles.**
>
> **2. AV dissociation is not synonymous with 3rd degree AV block, although AV block is one of the causes of AV dissociation.**

Barring complete AV block, AV dissociation can result from (1) slowing of the dominant pacemaker (sinus node). A subsidiary escape pacemaker takes over by default (junctional or ventricular escape). Cells in the AV junction and some in the ventricles possess automaticity, but at rates slower than the sinus rate. These slower pacemakers are normally supressed by the faster sinus node. However, if the sinus node slows enough, a junctional or ventricular escape rhythm can emerge resulting in AV dissociation. (2) usurpation by acceleration of a normally slower (subsidiary) pacemaker, such as a junctional site or a ventricular site to a rate faster than sinus rhythm: takeover by usurpation. This rhythm is not associated with retrograde ventricular conduction.

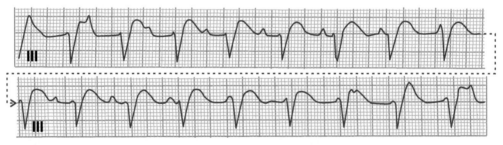

Sinus rhythm with AV dissociation from an accelerated idioventricular rhythm.

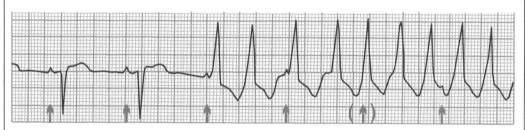

Ventricular tachycardia and atrioventricular dissociation.
In the setting of a wide QRS tachycardia, AV dissociation is diagnostic of ventricular tachycardia.

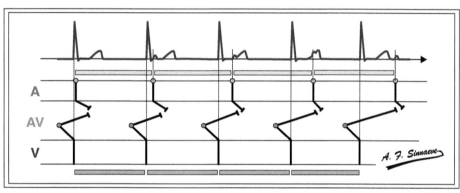

Accelerated junctional rhythm with AV dissociation by usurpation. The ventricular rhythm
is faster than the atrial rate.

Only an ignoramus states that the definition of complete AV block is AV dissociation.

SUMMARY

Categories: - Complete AV dissociation (complete AV block if A > V)
                - Incomplete AV dissociation (intermittent capture of the ventricles)
                - Isorhythmic AV dissociation (functional AV block with A = V)

Causes : - AV block
            - Slowing of dominant pacemaker (i.e. sinus node)
            - Usurpation: acceleration of subsidiary pacemaker
                (junctional or ventricular -- no retrograde conduction)

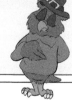

ELECTROPHYSIOLOGIC CONCEPTS 6

CARDIAC MEMORY

Cardiac memory (CM) refers to a process where the ECG does not immediately change back to baseline rhythm after a period of arrhythmia or pacing. Abnormal depolarization causes altered repolarization. CM refers to T wave abnormalities that manifest on resumption of a normal ventricular activation pattern after a period of abnormal ventricular activation, such as ventricular pacing, transient left bundle branch block, ventricular arrhythmias, or Wolff-Parkinson-White syndrome after ablation of an accessory pathway. Pacing-induced T wave inversion is usually localized to precordial and inferior leads. The direction of the T wave of the CM effect in sinus rhythm is typically in the same direction as the QRS complex during the altered depolarization. In other words, the T wave tracks the QRS vector of the abnormal impulse. CM may occur even after 1 minute of right ventricular (RV) pacing in man, with T wave abnormalities visible after 20 minutes. The marked repolarization abnormalities reach a steady state in a week with RV endocardial pacing at physiologic rates. The repolarization abnormalities related to CM persist when normal depolarization is restored, and they resolve completely in a month. The changes and their duration are proportional to the amount of delivered ventricular pacing. CM has a complex biochemical basis. The CM effect does not seem to alter long-term ventricular function.

The heart remembers

Cardiac memory can mimic ischemia or pericarditis. Knowledge of this phenomenon can help prevent unnecessary investigations.

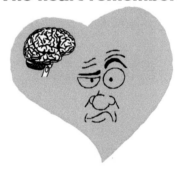

The T wave changes that occur during cardiac memory can resemble the changes that occur with cardiac ischemia or after myocardial infarction. The combination of (1) positive T waves in aVL (2) positive or isoelectric T waves in lead I, and (3) maximal precordial T wave inversion larger than the T wave inversion in lead III seems 92% sensitive and 100% specific for CM, discriminating it from ischemic precordial T wave inversion regardless of the coronary artery involved.

Electrotonic modulation of the T wave and its direction are based on the direction of the vector of the previous QRS complex during abnormal ventricular activation. In other words, the heart "learns" the pattern of ventricular depolarization during abnormal ventricular activation. Then, it retains this pattern after ventricular activation returns to normal.

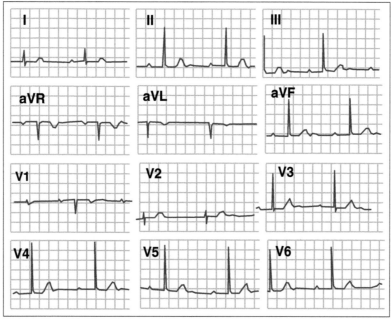

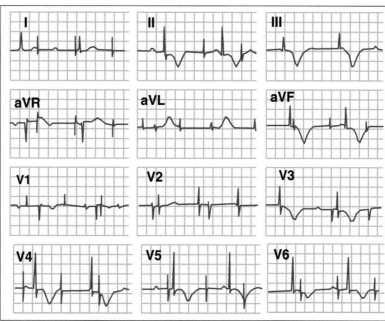

Cardiac memory effect secondary to ventricular pacing recorded in the ECG of a patient with complete heart block from a lesion in the His bundle (confirmed by His bundle recordings). Top: The tracing is normal except for the rhythm. Bottom: Chest wall stimulation (CWS) was performed to inhibit a VVI pacemaker implanted several months previously. There was no evidence of heart disease apart from AV block. Note the striking T wave inversions in leads II, III, aVF and V3 to V6. Inhibition of a pacemaker by CWS is now obsolete because of extensive device programmability. In this case CWS was delivered to external electrodes on the chest (rate 75 ppm) whereupon the stimuli were sensed by the implanted pacemaker. The chest wall stimuli produce vertical deflections not followed by ventricular capture.

ELECTROPHYSIOLOGIC CONCEPTS 7

PARASYSTOLE

Parasystole may occur anywhere in the heart in tissues that have electric properties and is most commonly manifested as a ventricular rhythm. Parasystole is a protected focus where other impulses, including sinus-related beats, cannot penetrate the focus to depolarize it (entrance block). Parasystole resembles pacing with a VOO pacemaker that captures the heart only outside the ventricular myocardial refractory period. Similarly in the transplanted heart the presence of atrial rhythms from both recipient and donor heart represents a form of parasystole. Parasystole is characterized by a regular interectopic rate and a variable interval of the parasystolic beat to the basic rhythm.

Ventricular parasystole usually has a rate of 45–55 bpm which is close to the inherent rate of ventricular rhythms and rarely up to 140 bpm. Short episodes are often mistaken as VPCs with varying coupling intervals. Diagnostic criteria of ventricular parasystole (entrance block and exit block) include:

1. Varying coupling interval from sinus to VPC.
2. Interectopic intervals are either constant or have a common denominator.
3. Ventricular fusion beats.

> **The presence of ventricular fusion beats should immediately raise the suspicion of parasystole.**

The intermittent failure of the parasystolic rhythm to become manifest is called exit block and is related to the presence of the myocardial ventricular refractory period initiated by the normal underlying rhythm. It is now clear that parasystolic foci may not be fully protected and may be modulated to some extent by the patient's normal rhythm which may be a critically timed sinus beat. Parasystole generally occurs in patients with heart disease but it may occasionally occur in normal individuals.

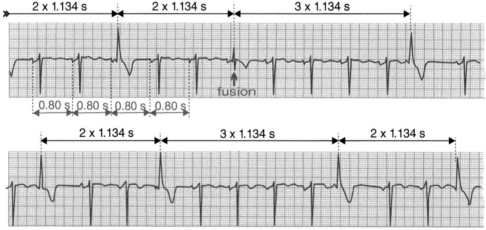

Sinus rhythm (PP intervals = 0.8 s ; atrial rate = 75 bpm) with ventricular premature complexes showing the features of ventricular parasystole. Note the varying coupling intervals, ventricular fusion and the common denominator of the interectopic intervals (common denominator = 1.134 s ; parasystolic rhythm = 53 bpm)

Characteristics of Ventricular Parasystole
1. The coupling intervals vary markedly.
2. Fusion complexes may be present.
3. Interectopic intervals are mathematically related (multiples of a common denominator).
4. It is an interesting phenomenon with no specific clinical consequences.

The presence of atrial rhythms of both recipient and donor is also a form of parasystole.

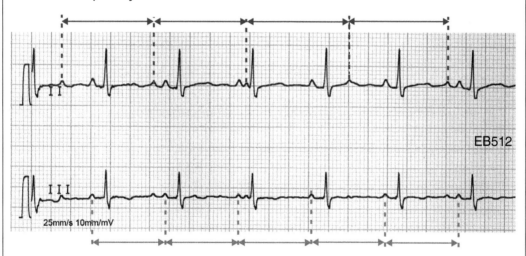

EB512

25mm/s 10mm/mV

Atrial parasystole in the transplanted heart. In patients with a transplanted heart, the recipient atrial rhythm (blue dotted vertical lines) behaves like a parasystolic focus because of complete entrance block from the donor atrium to the recipient's atrium. Sinus rhythm from the donor heart (and not the recipient's atrial rhythm) controls the rhythm (green dotted lines). Therefore there are two types of P waves (donor and recipient) occurring independently of each other. There is also complete exit block from the recipient atrium to the donor atrium.

ELECTROPHYSIOLOGIC CONCEPTS 8

ELECTRICAL ALTERNANS

Electrical alternans is a broad term that describes alternate-beat variation in the direction, amplitude, and duration of any component of the ECG waveform (i.e. P, PR, QRS, ST, U, QT). Electrical alternans must be distinguished from mechanical alternans (e.g. pulsus alternans), although both may coexist. The definition should include the presence of only one focus and regular RR intervals. This requirement rules out situations such as 2:1 bundle branch block or WPW syndrome.

The pathophysiologic mechanisms that cause electrical alternans can be divided into 3 categories: (1) repolarization alternans (S, T, U alternans), (2) conduction and refractoriness alternans (P, PR, QRS alternans) and (3) alternans due to cardiac motion. True electrical alternans is a repolarization or conduction abnormality of the Purkinje fibers or myocardium. Electrical alternans due to cardiac motion in pericardial effusion is effectively an artifact, as the heart swings in relation to the chest wall and electrodes, with a period twice that of the heart rate.

Repolarization alternans can be divided into T wave alternans and ST segment alternans.

T wave alternans is associated with rapid changes in heart rate or prolongation of the underlying QT interval. A long QT interval is associated with polymorphic ventricular tachycardia (i.e. torsades de pointes). T wave alternans has been reported with congenital long QT syndrome, electrolyte imbalances (e.g. hypocalcemia, hypokalemia, hypomagnesemia), treatment with amiodarone, cardiomyopathy and congestive heart failure. The presence of T wave alternans can be used as a predictor of ventricular tachyarrhythmic events, such as sudden cardiac death, sustained ventricular tachycardia, torsades de pointes, ventricular fibrillation, implantable cardioverter defibrillator activation for ventricular tachyarrhythmia, and cardiac arrest.

U wave alternans is very uncommon and is associated with electrolyte disorders.

ST segment alternans describes alternating levels of ST elevation, usually in the presence of myocardial ischemia. It has been reported with angina pectoris (including coronary spasm), and acute myocardial infarction. ST alternans during acute ischemia has been associated with the appearance of ventricular arrhythmias, including ventricular tachycardia and ventricular fibrillation.

Conduction QRS alternans is an alternation of impulse propagation along any of the anatomic structures involved in transmission of electrical impulses and is usually precipitated by changes in heart rate or input from nervous, humoral, or pharmacologic components. Conduction alternans may also be seen in the setting of myocardial ischemia.

Alternans of the surface QRS complex (defined as > 0.1 mV) in supraventricular tachycardia is not uncommon. It has a similar incidence in ventricular tachycardia (27–30%), best seen in leads V2 and V3. Alternans is rate-related and independent of the tachycardia mechanism. Subtle changes in QRS duration and amplitude in SVT with normal QRS duration occur mostly in AV reentrant tachycardia with retrograde conduction via an accessory pathway. The alternans may be due to changes in refractoriness in the peripheral His-Purkinje system or myocardium.

The most important cause is **massive pericardial effusion**, in which the alternating QRS voltage is produced by the mechanical swinging of the heart to-and-fro backwards and forwards within a large fluid-filled pericardium. Electrical alternans occurs because of alternation in the position of the heart in relation to recording electrodes. The combination of electrical alternans with sinus tachycardia and low voltage is a highly specific sign of cardiac tamponade, but is only modestly sensitive. As a result, its absence does not exclude pericardial tamponade. Not all pericardial effusions cause electrical alternans. The presence of total electrical alternans (P, QRS and T wave) is uncommon but considered diagnostic of pericardial effusion.

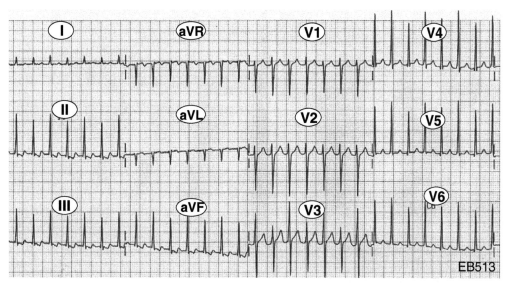

QRS alternans in a patient with AV reentrant tachycardia utilizing a concealed left posterior bypass tract.

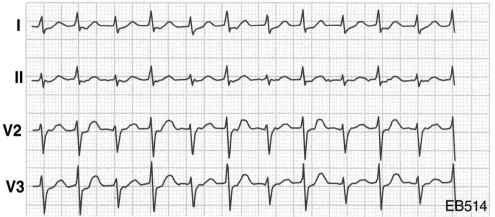

Atrial tachycardia at a rate of 160 bpm. The P waves are not discernible. Alternating atrial cycle length was documented at the time of an electrophysiologic study. The variation of the atrial cycle lengths does not explain the obvious QRS cycle alternans. There is additional QRS alternans and T wave alternans. The T wave alternans probably reflects the varying repolarization response to the marked QRS variations.

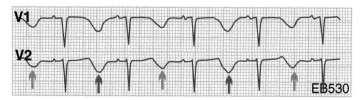

T wave alternans in a patient with congenital long QT syndrome.

Further Reading

Abrams J, Dykstra JR. Pseudo A-V block secondary to concealed junctional extrasystoles. Case report and review of the literature. Am J Med. 1977;63:434-40.

Chan AQ, Pick A. Re-entrant arrhythmias and concealed conduction. Am Heart J. 1979;97:644-62.

Chaudry II, Ramsaran EK, Spodick DH. Observations on the reliability of the Ashman phenomenon. Am Heart J. 1994;128:205-9.

Chiale PA, Etcheverry D, Pastori JD, Fernandez PA, Garro HA, González MD, Elizari MV. The multiple electrocardiographic manifestations of ventricular repolarization memory. Curr Cardiol Rev. 2014;10:190-201.

Chiladakis JA, Karapanos G, Davlouros P, Aggelopoulos G, Alexopoulos D, Manolis Significance of R-on-T phenomenon in early ventricular tachyarrhythmia susceptibility after acute myocardial infarction in the thrombolytic era. Am J Cardiol. 2000;85:289-93.

El-Menyar A, Asaad N. T-wave alternans and sudden cardiac death. Crit Pathw Cardiol. 2008;7:21-8.

El-Sherif N, Scherlag BJ, Lazzara R. Editorial: Bradycardia-dependent conduction disorders. J Electrocardiol. 1976;9:1-4.

Fisch C. Concealed conduction. Cardiol Clin. 1983;1:63-74.

Fries R, Steuer M, Schäfers HJ, Böhm M. The R-on-T phenomenon in patients with implantable cardioverter-defibrillators. Am J Cardiol. 2003;91:752-55.

Garcia Ede V. T-wave alternans: reviewing the clinical performance, understanding limitations, characterizing methodologies. Ann Noninvasive Electrocardiol. 2008;13:401-20.

Goyal M, Woods KM, Atwood JE. Electrical alternans: a sign, not a diagnosis. South Med J. 2013;106:485-9.

Huikuri HV, Raatikainen MJ, Moerch-Joergensen R, Hartikainen J, Virtanen V, Boland J, Anttonen O, Hoest N, Boersma LV, Platou ES, Messier MD, Bloch-Thomsen PE. Prediction of fatal or near-fatal cardiac arrhythmia events in patients with depressed left ventricular function after an acute myocardial infarction. Eur Heart J. 2009;30:689-98.

Jeyaraj D, Ashwath M, Rosenbaum DS. Pathophysiology and clinical implications of cardiac memory. Pacing Clin Electrophysiol. 2010;33:346-52.

Kennedy LB, Leefe W, Leslie BR. The Ashman phenomenon. J La State Med Soc. 2004;156:159-62.

Knoebel SB, Fisch C. Concealed conduction. Cardiovasc Clin. 1973;5:21-34.

Patberg KW, Shvilkin A, Plotnikov AN, Chandra P, Josephson ME, Rosen MR. Cardiac memory: mechanisms and clinical implications. Heart Rhythm. 2005;2:1376-82.

Schamroth L, Jacobs ML. A study in intracardiac conduction with special reference to the Ashman phenomenon. Heart Lung. 1982;11:381-2.

Singla V, Singh B, Singh Y, Manjunath CN. Ashman phenomenon: a physiological aberration. BMJ Case Rep. 2013 May 24.

Spurrell RA, Krikler DM, Sowton E. Retrograde invasion of the bundle branches producing aberration of the QRS complex during supraventricular tachycardia studied by programmed electrical stimulation. Circulation. 1974;50:487-95.

Statters DJ, Malik M, Redwood S, Hnatkova K, Staunton A, Camm AJ. Use of ventricular premature complexes for risk stratification after acute myocardial infarction in the thrombolytic era. Am J Cardiol. 1996;77:133-8.

Surawicz B. Contributions of cellular electrophysiology to the understanding of the electrocardiogram. Experientia. 1987;43:1061-8.

Wang K, Benditt DG. AV dissociation, an inevitable response. Ann Noninvasive Electrocardiol. 2011;16:227-31.

Wellens HJ, Durrer D. Supraventricular tachycardia with left aberrant conduction due to retrograde invasion into the left bundle branch. Circulation. 1968;38:474-9.

Zipes DP, Heger JJ, Prystowsky EN. Pathophysiology of arrhythmias: clinical electrophysiology. Am Heart J. 1983;106(4 Pt 2):812-28.

CHAPTER 20

ANTIARRHYTHMIC DRUGS

* The action potential and Vaughan-Williams classification
* Proarrhythmia
* Prolongation of the QT interval and torsades de pointes
* Overview of antiarrhythmic drugs
* Digitalis toxicity

ECG from Basics to Essentials: Step by Step. First Edition. Roland X. Stroobandt, S. Serge Barold and Alfons F. Sinnaeve.
Published 2016 © 2016 by John Wiley & Sons, Ltd. Companion Website: www.wiley.com/go/stroobandt/ecg

ANTIARRHYTHMIC DRUGS 1

The action potential

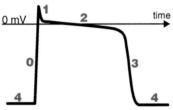

Representation of a myocardial action potential with its 4 phases

As already discussed in chapter 1, the transmembrane potential of myocardial cells is determined by the concentration of Na, K and Ca ions. The movement of these ions produces the current that forms the action potential.

The rapid depolarization called phase 0 is mediated by rapid sodium entry into cells. Phase 1 marks the inactivation of the fast sodium channels and the outflow of potassium. Phase 2 corresponds to the plateau phase that depends on the balance between slow calcium entry and potassium exit. Phase 3 is the final repolarization due to potassium efflux from the cells. Phase 4 occurs in some cells if potassium re-enters and sodium exits (e.g. by the Na-K pump).

Vaughan-Williams Classification of Antiarrhythmic Drugs

The Vaughan-Williams classification of antiarrhythmic drugs was first proposed in the 1960s and remains in clinical use despite its limitations. Amiodarone classified as a class III agent also has sodium (class I) and calcium (class IV) blocking actions as well as class II effects. Consequently amiodarone has class I, II, III, and IV actions.

Class I : Sodium channel blockers

The class I antiarrhythmic agents interfere with the Na^+ channel and reduce the rate of rise of phase 0 of the action potential, thereby decreasing conduction. Class I agents are grouped by what effect they have on the Na^+ channel, and the effect they have on the cardiac action potential.
Type I is divided into three classes (A, B, and C) with slightly different mechanisms of activity.

Class 1A agents

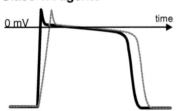

Class 1A agents decrease V_{max} (maximum upstroke velocity) and increase action potential duration

Class IA agents are active in the atria and ventricles and are the most cardiotoxic group. Class IA agents moderately slow the conduction and moderately prolong the duration of the action potential (which in turn increases refractoriness).
Class IA agents block the fast sodium channels. Blocking these channels depresses the phase 0 depolarization thereby reducing V_{max} (maximum upstroke velocity). This prolongs the action potential duration by slowing conduction.
Agents in this class also increase refractoriness. These agents also exhibit type III properties with prolongation of the action potential and the QT interval.
Examples: quinidine, procainamide, disopyramide.

Class 1B agents

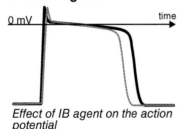

Effect of IB agent on the action potential

Class IB agents show minimal effect on the conduction and shorten the duration of the action potential. These agents have little or no effect at slower heart rates but have more effect at faster rates. These agents either do not change the action potential duration or they may decrease the action potential duration and reduce refractoriness. They decrease V_{max} in partially depolarized cells with fast response. They show the lowest potency of the type I groups.

Class 1C agents

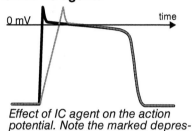

Effect of IC agent on the action potential. Note the marked depression of phase 0.

Class 1C agents markedly depress the phase 0 depolarization (decreasing V_{max}) resulting in markedly slowed conduction. They are the most potent of the 3 groups.

The QRS complex is prolonged but the QT interval remains normal.

Examples: flecainide, encainide, propafenone and moricizine.

Class II: Beta blockers

These agents affect the sinoatrial (SA) and atrioventricular (AV) nodes as well as the ventricular myocardium. These agents act indirectly on the electrophysiologic substrate by blocking adrenergic receptors. There is virtually no proarrhythmic effect.
* Slowing of AV conduction and PR prolongation
* Increase in AV nodal refractoriness
* Slowing of the SA node
* Depression of left ventricular function
* Reduction of adrenergic activity and blunting of sympathetic stimulation

Class III agents

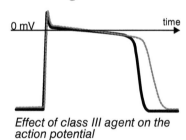

Effect of class III agent on the action potential

These agents predominantly block the potassium channels, thereby prolonging repolarization and therefore the action potential. Since these agents do not affect the sodium channels, conduction velocity is not decreased. The QRS complex is not affected. The prolongation of the action potential duration and refractoriness combined with the maintenance of normal conduction velocity prevent reentrant arrhythmias (the reentrant impulses are less likely to interact with tissue that has become refractory).

Examples: amiodarone, sotalol, dofetilide, ibutilide.

Class IV: Calcium channel blockers

These agents block the calcium current. They slow the conduction in areas of the heart that are primarily depolarized by calcium channels (SA and AV nodes). There is virtually no proarrhythmic effect. Dihydropyridines such as nifedipine have little or no effect on the SA and AV nodes.
Examples: verapamil, diltiazem.

The Vaughan-Williams classification has severe limitations but it remains popular even with the introduction of many more antiarrhythmic drugs since 1970 and still incomplete understanding of drug mechanisms. The classification system breaks down especially for the class I and III drugs. Many of these drugs have mechanisms of action that are shared with drugs found in the other classes. For example, amiodarone, a class III antiarrhythmic drug, also has sodium and calcium blocking actions. Many class I compounds also affect potassium channels.

All antiarrhythmic drugs directly or indirectly alter the movement of ions through the membrane of cells, consequently altering the physical characteriscs of cardiac action potentials. For example, some drugs are used to block fast sodium channels which determine the speed of membrane depolarization (phase 0) during an action potential. Since conduction velocity is related to how fast the membrane depolarizes, sodium channel blockers reduce conduction velocity. Decreasing conduction velocity can abolish tachyarrhythmias caused by reentry circuits.

ANTIARRHYTHMIC DRUGS 2

Other types of antiarrhythmic drugs affect potassium channels and therefore the duration of action potentials (phase 3) and especially the effective refractory period are increased. By prolonging the effective refractory period, reentry tachycardias can also be abolished. Drugs that block slow inward calcium channels are used to reduce pacemaker firing rate by slowing the rate of rise of depolarizing pacemaker potentials (phase 4). These drugs also reduce conduction velocity at the AV node, because the cells depend on the inward movement of calcium ions to depolarize.

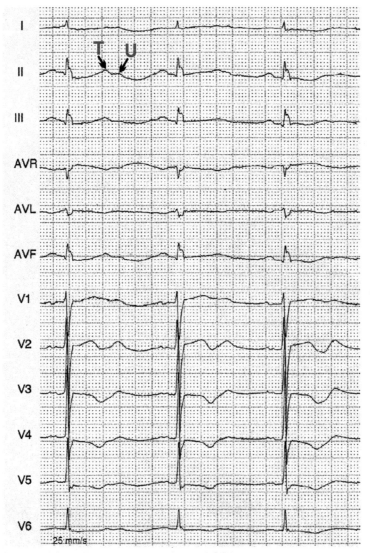

Sinus bradycardia at 44 bpm; prolonged QT interval and prominent U wave due to amiodarone

Proarrhythmia

Proarrhythmia is the exacerbation or aggravation of the arrhythmia being treated with anti-arrhythmic drugs. In other words it is the worsening or change of a preexisting arrhythmia or the development of a new arrhythmia or the occurrence of a bradyarrhythmia resulting from a drug-induced depression of sinus node function or atrioventricular nodal conduction. Whether the aggravation, change or induction of an arrhythmia is due to the direct effect of an antiarrhythmic agent may be difficult to determine. The change in the characteristics of an arrhythmia may be related to the natural history of the pathophysiologic substrate or to random variability. Proarrhythmia is also probable if a major change of the arrhythmia occurs relatively soon after initiation of drug therapy or a change in dose. However, "late" proarrhythmia may occur !

Ventricular proarrhythmia
* Torsades de pointes (type IA and type III drugs).
* Sustained monomorphic ventricular tachycardia (usually type IC drugs), incessant ventricular tachycardia (VT) or increase in the rate of VT being treated.
* Sustained polymorphic ventricular tachycardia or ventricular fibrillation without long QT (types IA, IC, and III drugs).

Abnormalities of conduction or impulse formation
* Sinus node dysfunction, atrioventricular block (almost all drugs).
* Accelerated conduction over accessory pathway (digoxin, intravenous verapamil, diltiazem).
* Acceleration of ventricular rate during atrial fibrillation (type IA and type IC drugs).

Atrial proarrhythmia
Atrial arrhythmias are not spared but atrial proarrhythmias are not as common or important as the above ventricular types. It may occur during the administration of antiarrhythmic drugs in atrial fibrillation (which drug therapy may convert to atrial flutter) or atrial flutter without the use of concomitant AV nodal blocking drugs. Proarrhythmia occurs because the rate of atrial flutter (for example slowing to 200 bpm) permits 1:1 AV conduction to the ventricles at a faster rate than the original ventricular rate of the arrhythmia being treated (atrial fibrillation or flutter with 2:1 AV block).

Class IC drugs
Proarrhythmia may be provoked by increased heart rate.
Exercise stress test after loading is needed.
Proarrhythmia can occur a long time after initiation of therapy.

Prolongation of the QT interval and torsades de pointes
Prominent U waves should be included in the measurement if they merge into the T wave. QT should be assessed during peak plasma concentration of QT prolonging substances.
* *Class IA drugs*
  Dose independent, occurring at normal levels.
  Follow QT interval.
* *Class III drugs*
  The occurrence of torsades de pointes (TdP) may be dose-related with selective class III drugs such as sotalol and dofetilide.

During the initiation of therapy, monitor the patient for several days. Assess the change in QT interval, the presence of bradycardia and follow the K level closely.
Proarrhythmias due to drug-induced QT prolongation are the second most common cause for drug withdrawal. The prolongation of repolarization and the QT interval are rate-related, being more pronounced at slower heart rates and decreasing at faster heart rates. This is known as "reverse use-dependent" effects on repolarization. TdP is relatively rare with amiodarone, despite long QT prolongation in contrast to other class III drugs.

ANTIARRHYTHMIC DRUGS 3

Increased risk of proarrhythmia manifested by torsades des pointes
(Reduced repolarization reserve).

* Presence of structural (advanced) heart disease with left ventricular systolic dysfunction
* Left ventricular hypertrophy
* Cardiac ischemia
* Bradyarrhythmias
* Hypokalemia
* Severe hypomagnesemia
* Recent conversion from atrial fibrillation especially with QT prolonging drugs
* Increased age
* Female gender
* Concomitant administration of drugs that prolong the QT interval
* Baseline QT prolongation

The QT interval is an imperfect marker for proarrhythmia risk. It is not clear whether the development of arrhythmias is more closely related to an increase in the absolute QT interval or in the corrected interval QTc, but most drugs that have caused torsades de pointes (TdP) clearly increase both the absolute QT interval and the corrected QTc interval. An absolute uncorrected QT interval > 500 ms is generally regarded as conferring an increased risk of proarrhythmia with TdP. In practice it is probably wise to monitor both the QT and the QTc intervals. An increase of 30 ms is a potential cause for concern. An increase of 60 ms is a definite cause for concern! Proarrhythmia usually occurs early in the course of therapy (first week). TdP with class IA drugs may occur with therapeutic or subtherapeutic doses. Amiodarone is the exception because the QT interval routinely prolongs to > 500 ms, yet it is a rare cause of TdP. The risk of TdP with amiodarone predominantly occurs in patients with other concomitant risk factors, such as hypokalemia or bradycardia. Amiodarone rarely causes TdP even in patients who developed TdP as a complication of other QT prolonging drugs.

OVERVIEW OF ANTIARRHYTHMIC DRUGS

VW Class	Site of action	Level of efficiency	End-organ toxicity	Proarrhythmia potential
IA	A, V	++	+++	++
IB	V	+	+	+
IC	A, V	+++	+	+++
II	AVN, V	+	+	0
III	A, V	++ (Amio++++)	+ (Amio ++++)	++ (Amio +)
IV	AVN	+	+	0

VW = Vaughan-Williams ; A = atrium ; V = ventricle ; AVN = AV node ; Amio = amiodarone

DIGITALIS TOXICITY

Cardiac glycoside toxicity continues to be a problem because of the wide availability of digoxin (a preparation of digitalis) and a narrow therapeutic window. Digitalis is a plant-derived glycoside commonly used in the treatment of systolic heart failure, atrial fibrillation, and reentrant supraventricular tachycardia. Digitalis toxicity should be suspected when there is evidence of increased automaticity and depressed conduction.

In addition to these effects, the direct effect of digitalis on repolarization often is reflected in the ECG by ST segment and T wave forces opposite in direction to the major QRS forces. Decrease in T wave amplitude, shortening of the QT interval and increase in U wave amplitude may occur. Digitalis toxicity is exacerbated by hypokalemia, hypomagnesemia, hypercalcemia, renal insufficiency and hypoxia. Certain drugs such as amiodarone and verapamil (and some antibiotics) may precipitate digitalis toxicity by increasing the serum digoxin level.

Depression of normal conduction: the atrial pacemakers, resulting in SA arrest, sinus bradycardia, type I second-degree AV block, high grade AV nodal block are commonly seen.

Ectopic rhythms: frequent and multiform premature ventricular contractions, accelerated junctional rhythm, nonparoxysmal junctional tachycardia, nonparoxysmal atrial tachycardia with AV block, fascicular ventricular tachycardia, bidirectional ventricular tachycardia are due to enhanced automaticity, reentry, or both. Bidirectional ventricular tachycardia is particularly characteristic of severe digitalis toxicity. Atrial fibrillation with a regular rhythm should be considered to be digitalis toxicity until proven otherwise. The causes of a regular rhythm in atrial fibrillation with digitalis toxicity include: complete AV nodal block with junctional tachycardia (70–140 bpm) or fascicular ventricular tachycardia. A typical rhythm in digitalis toxicity is junctional rhythm which exhibits group beating from a Wenckebach form of exit block.

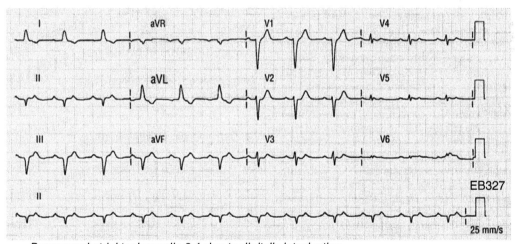

EB327

25 mm/s

Paroxysmal atrial tachycardia 2:1 due to digitalis intoxication.
The rhythm strip shows T waves with unusual sharp peaks which represent the deformity produced by the "hidden" P waves inside the T wave.

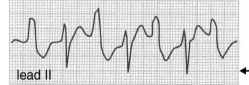

lead II

Bidirectional VT in a patient with manifest digitalis toxicity

Further Reading

Behr ER, Roden D. Drug-induced arrhythmia: pharmacogenomic prescribing? Eur Heart J. 2013;34:89-95.

Kannankeril P, Roden DM, Darbar D. Drug-induced long QT syndrome. Pharmacol Rev. 2010;62:760-81.

Ma G, Brady WJ, Pollack M, Chan TC. Electrocardiographic manifestations:digitalis toxicity. J Emerg Med. 2001;20:145-52.

Podrid PJ. Proarrhythmia, a serious complication of antiarrhythmic drugs. Curr Cardiol Rep. 1999;1:289-96.

CHAPTER 21

PACEMAKERS AND THEIR ECGs

* Introduction – rate or interval?
* Pacing nomenclature
* Sensing – undersensing and oversensing
* Ventricular fusion and pseudofusion
* Timing cycles of the DDD mode of pacing
* Refractory periods and upper rate behavior
* Ventricular safety pacing
* Wenckebach upper rate response
* Pacemaker-mediated tachycardia
* Repetitive nonreentrant ventriculoatrial synchrony
* Automatic mode switching
* Patterns of depolarization during ventricular pacing
* Cardiac resynchronization with biventricular pacing
* Electrical complications during ventricular pacing
* Algorithms to minimize right ventricular pacing

ECG from Basics to Essentials: Step by Step. First Edition. Roland X. Stroobandt, S. Serge Barold and Alfons F. Sinnaeve.
Published 2016 © 2016 by John Wiley & Sons, Ltd. Companion Website: www.wiley.com/go/stroobandt/ecg

PACEMAKERS AND THEIR ECGs 1

Introduction

There are 2 types of pacemaker leads: bipolar with the 2 electrodes both embedded inside the heart and unipolar leads with only one electrode inside the heart and the other electrode on the pacemaker can. New lead technology and design have eliminated the previous advantage of unipolar leads. In practice, the long-term performance of unipolar and bipolar systems is similar but their sensing function is different.

> **The pacing lead functions as a "two-way street" for the transmission of electricity to the heart for pacing and in the other direction from the heart to the pacemaker by sensing of spontaneous electric activity.**

The lithium-iodine battery is the gold standard of pacemaker power sources. Battery depletion requiring pacemaker replacement can be determined quite simply by measuring the pacemaker rate on an ECG because slowing of the rate occurs with battery depletion. However, a more accurate method involves a direct electronic measurement of battery voltage.

Contemporary digital ECG recorders distort the pacemaker stimulus on the ECG, so it may become larger and show striking changes in amplitude and polarity. Digital recorders can also miss some of the pacemaker stimuli because of sampling characteristics. Diagnostic evaluation of the pacemaker stimulus is only possible with analog machines which are now rarely in use.

Rate or interval?

The pacemaker itself, design engineers, and most health care workers all "think" in terms of intervals rather than rate. Rate is a relatively simple designation during continuous pacing or continuous inhibition but is of little value and confusing if pacing and sensing alternate. Yet, for ease of programming, manufacturers have expressed parameters in terms of rate (i.e. in pulses per minute - ppm) rather than interval (in milliseconds - ms).

$$\text{Heart Rate in ppm} = \frac{60{,}000}{\text{Interval in ms}}$$

A pacemaker rate of 70 ppm gives an interval of 857 ms.

Pacing nomenclature

A four-letter code describes the basic function of the various pacing systems. The first position represents the chamber or chambers where stimulation occurs. "A" refers to the atrium, "V" to the ventricle and "D" stands for dual chamber (both atrium and ventricle). The second position stands for the chamber or chambers where sensing occurs: "A", "V", and "D" are the same as those for the first position, while "O" means no sensing. The third position refers to the response of the pacemaker to a sensed event. "I" indicates that the sensed event inhibits the output pulse of the pacemaker; the pacemaker then restarts the timer controlling the lower rate interval. "T" indicates that the sensed event triggers an output pulse. The triggered stimulus may or may not be delayed. In a dual chamber pacemaker a sensed atrial event inhibits the atrial stimulus but may trigger a ventricular stimulus after a delay (akin to an electronic PR interval) to provide AV synchrony. "D" denotes both I and T functions in the third position. If the second position is "O", the third position must also be "O". The fourth position of the code indicates with the letter "R" the presence of a non-atrial sensor to control the pacing rate independently of intrinsic atrial activity.

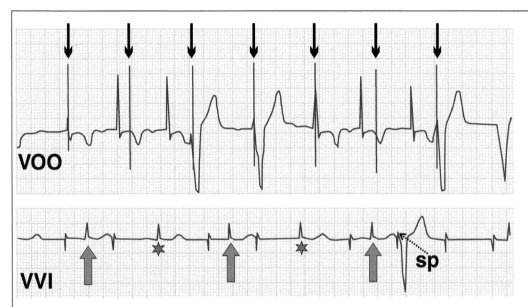

Fig. 1 *Failure of ventricular capture by ventricular pacemaker.*
Top panel: VOO pacing with functional noncapture. The pacemaker competes with the spontaneous rhythm. Pacemaker stimuli capture the ventricle only beyond the ventricular myocardial refractory period. This response is physiologic. The arrows point to the pacemaker stimuli.
Bottom panel: VVI pacing showing supernormal phase of excitability (sp). The stimuli from the VVI pacemaker are ineffectual beyond the ventricular myocardial period. The high pacing threshold was close to the output of the pacemaker. The third last stimulus captures the ventricle in the supernormal phase when the pacing threshold is at its lowest level in the cardiac cycle. The pacemaker senses the QRS complex only when it falls beyond the sensing refractory period of the pacemaker (350 ms) initiated by a ventricular stimulus (stars). QRS complexes within the 350 ms sensing refractory period are not sensed, and therefore do not initiate a new lower rate interval (blue arrows).

VOO pacing

A VOO pacemaker generates stimuli with no relationship to the spontaneous rhythm. The VOO mode is often labeled "fixed-rate" or "asynchronous", and functions like a parasystolic focus. The competitive stimuli will capture the ventricle only when they fall outside the absolute refractory period of the ventricle that follows spontaneous beats (Fig. 1). The VOO mode is now only used for testing purposes by applying a magnet over the pacemaker. Ventricular fibrillation induced by a competitive pacemaker stimulus falling in the ventricular vulnerable period (the R on T phenomenon) is quite rare outside of circumstances such as myocardial ischemia or infarction, electrolyte abnormalities or autonomic imbalance.

> **VOO pacing behaves like parasystole**

VVI pacing

A VVI pacemaker senses the intracardiac ventricular depolarization or electrogram by measuring the potential difference (voltage) between the two electrodes used for pacing. A VVI pacemaker has a lower rate timing cycle that begins with a sensed or paced event.

> **A VVI pacemaker senses the intracardiac ventricular electrogram**

PACEMAKERS AND THEIR ECGs 2

In a VVI device a sensed ventricular event inhibits the pacemaker and resets the timing clock so that the lower rate interval returns to baseline. A new pacing cycle is reinitiated and if the device senses no ventricular event, the timing cycle ends with the release of a ventricular stimulus according to the lower rate interval. The sensing function prevents competition between pacemaker and intrinsic rhythm. During continuous VVI pacing the atrium may exhibit sinus rhythm with AV dissociation, an atrial tachyarrhythmia or retrograde ventriculoatrial (VA) conduction. The latter may be regular on a 1:1 basis or irregular (such as 2:1 etc). (Fig. 2)

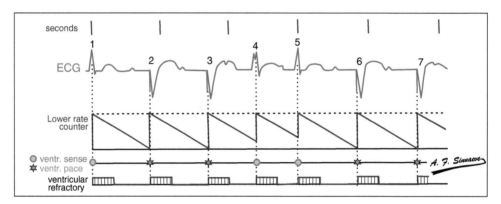

Fig. 2 *Diagrammatic representation of the VVI mode of pacing (rate = 80 ppm). The QRS marked 1 is sensed by the pacemaker. Beats 2 and 3 are paced complexes. A ventricular extrasystole (4) and a normal QRS (5) are then sensed. The sixth and seventh beats are paced. The pacemaker refractory period (300 ms) is shown by a rectangle. Complexes 4 and 5 reset and restart the lower rate counter before zero level has been reached (shown by the straight line at the bottom), i.e. before completion of the ventricular escape interval of the device (equal to the automatic interval). The pacemaker emits its stimulus only from zero level of the lower rate counter.*

When a patient with a pacemaker presents with an ECG showing no pacemaker stimuli, the pacing function should be tested by the application of a special magnet, which eliminates sensing and converts any pacemaker to the fixed-rate or asynchronous mode (VVI to VOO or DDD to DOO). One should refrain from producing bradycardia by performing carotid sinus massage to challenge the pacemaker.

Interval terminology of a VVI pacemaker

The stimulus-to-stimulus interval is called the *automatic interval* and is usually equal to the *escape interval* which is measured electronically from the time of intracardiac sensing to the succeeding stimulus. In practice, the (ventricular) escape interval is measured from the onset of the sensed QRS complex in the surface ECG. The escape interval measured in this way must necessarily be longer than the electronic escape interval because intracardiac sensing takes place a finite time after the onset of the surface QRS complex depending on the temporal relationship of the intracardiac electrogram and the surface ECG. In *hysteresis* the electronic escape interval is longer than the automatic interval. Its purpose is to maintain sinus rhythm and AV synchrony for as long as possible at a spontaneous rate lower (e.g. 50 bpm - the hysteresis rate at which the pacemaker will be inhibited) than the automatic rate of the pacemaker (e.g. 70 bpm) (Fig. 3).

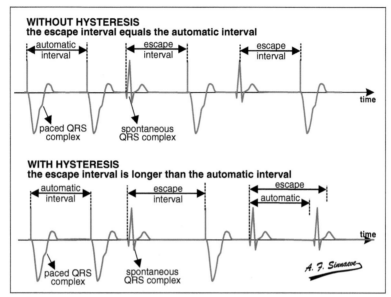

Fig. 3 *In a VVI pacemaker after a sensed ventricular event, the pacemaker only delivers a stimulus to the ventricle at the end of the escape interval. A spontaneous QRS complex beyond the automatic interval but before termination of the escape interval will be detected and inhibit the stimulus. Hysteresis allows the intrinsic rate to be lower than the basic pacing rate, but if pacing occurs it will happen at that basic pacing rate.*

Sensing

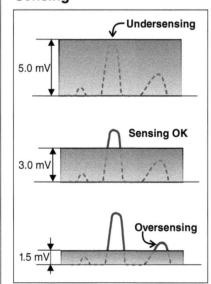

A VVI pacemaker senses the intracardiac ventricular electrogram which is the potential difference between the 2 electrodes used for pacing. The electrogram must exceed the ventricular *sensitivity* of the pacemaker for reliable sensing. A unipolar pacemaker senses the potential difference (or voltage) of a single intracardiac electrode (negative pole) and the pacemaker can which provides the positive pole. The sensitivity is programmed according the amplitude of the atrial or ventricular electrograms transmitted by telemetry to an external device. The ventricular signal often measures 6–15 mV, a range that exceeds the commonly programmed ventricular sensitivity of 2–3 mV (the higher the numerical value of sensitivity, the less sensitive the pacemaker becomes; Fig. 4). The intracardiac atrial signal is smaller and shoud ideally exceed 2 mV. Oversensing of extraneous activity requires a decrease in sensitivity (increase in the numerical value). Application of a magnet over the pacemaker eliminates sensing.

Fig. 4 *Ventricular sensitivity of a VVI pacemaker*

PACEMAKERS AND THEIR ECGs 3

AAI pacing

An AAI pacemaker is identical to the VVI mode except that it paces and senses in the atrium. It requires a higher sensitivity because the amplitude of the atrial electrogram is smaller than the ventricular one. An AAI pacemaker may be considered in patients with sick sinus syndrome and normal AV conduction. The subsequent development of AV block in carefully selected patients is less than 1–2% per year. The advantages of AAI pacing are related to the preservation of normal ventricular depolarization and cost-effectiveness. AAI pacing is used in Europe but rarely in the US.

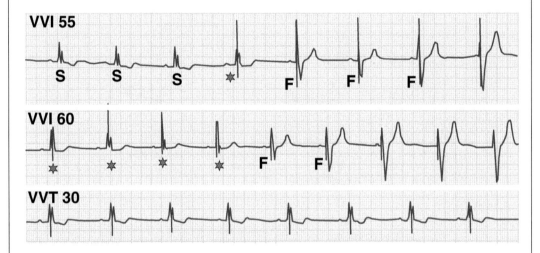

Fig. 5 *Manifestations of the VVI and VVT modes of pacing.*
Top panel: VVI pacing at 55 ppm. The first three beats are sensed by the pacemaker (S) and the fourth (star) is a ventricular pseudofusion beat. The fifth, sixth and seventh beats are ventricular fusion beats (F).
Middle panel: VVI pacing at a rate of 60 ppm. The first three beats are pseudofusion beats (stars). The fourth beat (star) appears to be a pseudofusion beat because the initial QRS vector occurs just before delivery of the stimulus. Note that the fourth beat has a T wave identical to that of previous beats, suggesting that unchanged repolarization indicates unchanged spontaneous depolarization as in the preceding pseudofusion beats. The fifth and the sixth beats are fusion beats (F) and the last three beats are pure ventricular paced beats.
Bottom panel: Same patient as the above panels. The pacemaker was programmed to the VVT (triggered) mode at a rate of 30 ppm. The pacemaker now emits (triggers) a stimulus immediately upon sensing each QRS complex. Thus, a stimulus marks the precise time of sensing in the VVT mode. This may be correlated with the stimulus in the pseudofusion beats in the middle panel where these beats are deformed by a stimulus just before the R wave begins to return to the baseline, i.e., just before sensing would have occurred as determined from the timing of the stimulus in the VVT mode.

Ventricular fusion

Fusion beats occur when the ventricles are depolarized simultaneously by spontaneous and pacemaker-induced activity. Thus, fusion occurs within the heart itself. A ventricular fusion beat can exhibit various configurations depending on the relative contributions of the 2 foci involved in ventricular activation. A ventricular fusion beat is often more narrow than a pure ventricular paced beat but obviously, it cannot be longer than a pure ventricular paced beat. Occasionally a fusion beat generates an isoelectric QRS complex in a single lead, hence the importance of recording more than one lead and preferably a 12-lead ECG for pacemaker evaluation (Fig. 5).

Ventricular pseudofusion

A ventricular pseudofusion beat consists of the superimposition of an ineffectual ventricular stimulus (in the ventricular myocardial refractory period) on a surface QRS complex originating from a single ventricular focus. A large portion of the surface QRS complex can be inscribed before the intracardiac electrogram reaches the sensing electrodes with the required voltage amplitude (according to the programmed sensitivity) to inhibit the pacemaker (Figs. 5 and 6). Thus a VVI pacemaker can deliver a ventricular stimulus (according to its electronic clock) within a spontaneous (surface) QRS complex before the arrival of the intracardiac signal at the sensing electrodes. In other words arrival of the electrogram is "delayed" as far as the surface ECG is concerned. The stimulus thus falls in the absolute refractory period of the ventricular myocardium and does not depolarize any portion of the ventricles. Pseudofusion does not indicate malfunction of the sensing circuit and is a normal manifestation of a VVI pacemaker. True sensing failure must always be excluded with long ECG recordings. Pacemaker stimuli falling beyond the surface QRS complex always indicate undersensing and a potential problem.

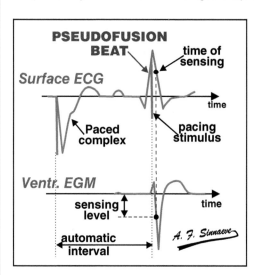

Fig. 6 *Diagrammatic representation of the mechanism of ventricular pseudofusion. The surface ECG and the ventricular electrogram are assumed to be recorded simultaneously. The ventricular electrogram generates the necessary intracardiac voltage (sensing level) to inhibit the pacemaker at a point corresponding with the descending limb of the surface QRS complex in its second half ("time of sensing" at the dotted line on the right). Consequently, it is possible for a pacemaker stimulus to occur near the apex of the surface R wave (dotted line on the left) just before the point of intracardiac sensing because the ventricular electrogram has not yet generated the required voltage (sensing level) to inhibit the pulse generator.*

DDD pacing

A DDD pacemaker may be considered to be a VVI unit with the addition of an atrial channel to provide AV synchronous pacing (Fig. 7). The pacemaker now acquires 2 new intervals. The atrioventricular (AV) interval is the electronic analog of the PR interval. The paced AV interval starts from the atrial stimulus and extends to the following ventricular stimulus. The sensed AV interval starts from the point of P wave sensing (atrial electrogram), and terminates with the release of the ventricular stimulus. The paced AV delay is usually 20–50 ms longer than the sensed AV delay to allow for the difference in interatrial conduction time between intrinsic and paced atrial events.

PACEMAKERS AND THEIR ECGs 4

The upper rate interval (corresponding to the upper rate) is the speed limit necessary to control the response of the ventricular channel to sensed atrial activity. It is the shortest allowable interval between 2 consecutive ventricular stimuli or from a sensed ventricular event to the succeeding ventricular stimulus. The atrial escape interval is often used to describe DDD function and it is the interval from a ventricular event to the succeeding atrial stimulus.

Interpretation of pacemaker function requires knowledge of TIMING CYCLES

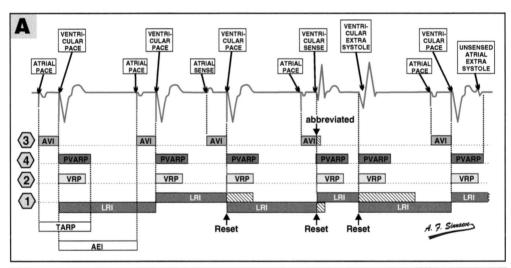

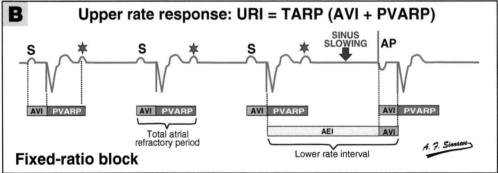

Fig. 7 Panel A: *Diagram showing the function of a simple DDD pacemaker with only four basic timing cycles. Lower rate timing is ventricular-based and controlled by ventricular events (paced or sensed). AP = atrial paced beat; AS = atrial sensed beat; VP = ventricular paced beat; VS = ventricular sensed beat.*
The four fundamental intervals (labeled 1 to 4) are: LRI = lower rate interval, VRP = ventricular refractory period, AVI = AV delay, PVARP = post ventricular atrial refractory period. There are also 2

derived intervals: the atrial escape interval (AEI = LRI − AVI) and the total atrial refractory period (TARP = AVI + PVARP). Reset refers to the termination and reinitiation of a timing cycle before it is timed out to its completion according to its programmed duration. Premature termination of the programmed AV delay (by ventricular sensing) is indicated by its abbreviation. The upper rate interval (URI) is equal to the TARP in this simple pacemaker. AS (third beat) initiates an AV interval terminating with a VP. AS also aborts the AEI initiated by the second VP. The third VP resets the LRI and starts the PVARP, VRP and URI. The fourth beat consists of AP which terminates the AEI initiated by the third VP, followed by a sensed conducted QRS complex (VS). The AV delay of the fourth beat is therefore abbreviated. VS of the fourth beat initiates the AEI, PVARP, VRP, LRI and URI. The fifth beat is a ventricular extrasystole that initiates the AEI, VRP and PVARP and resets the LRI and URI. The last beat is followed by an unsensed atrial extrasystole because it falls within the PVARP.

Panel B*: Diagrammatic representation of fixed-ratio (2:1) upper rate response in a simple DDD pacemaker with URI = TARP as in panel A. The pacemaker fails to sense every second P wave because it falls within the TARP. When sinus slowing occurs on the right, the pacemaker functions according to its LRI. S = sensed P wave; ✹ = unsensed P wave*

What are refractory periods?

The terminology is somewhat confusing because traditionally signals are "unsensed" in a refractory period and cannot start a new timing cycle. Yet, a pacemaker can detect signals in a refractory period and use them for functions other than initiating fundamental timing cycles such as a lower rate interval. Refractory periods all start with a short blanking period where no signal whatsoever can be used for any pacemaker function.

Atrial refractory periods and DDD pacemakers

It is axiomatic that the atrial channel of a DDD pacemaker must be refractory during the AV delay to prevent initiation of a new AV delay before completion of the AV delay already in progress. The postventricular atrial refractory period (PVARP) begins immediately after a paced or sensed ventricular event. An atrial signal falling within the PVARP cannot initiate a programmed AV interval. The PVARP is designed to prevent the atrial channel from sensing retrograde P waves and far-field QRS signals (a QRS voltage that can be seen by the atrial channel). The total atrial refractory period (TARP) is the sum of the AV delay and the PVARP which are individually programmable. The duration of the TARP always defines the shortest upper rate interval or fastest paced ventricular rate. The AV delay, PVARP and the upper rate interval are interrelated in a simple DDD pacemaker (as were the original devices) where the upper rate interval is controlled solely by the duration of the TARP according to the formula:

$$\text{Upper rate (in ppm)} = \frac{60{,}000}{\text{TARP (in ms)}}$$

Understanding the above concepts, one can appreciate how a DDD pacemaker can function quite well provided the ventricular channel does not sense the atrial stimulus. Sensing of the atrial stimulus (AV crosstalk) by the ventricular channel is potentially dangerous because it causes ventricular inhibition and ventricular asystole. Prevention of AV crosstalk requires the addition of a brief ventricular blanking period (about 10 to 60 ms) beginning coincidentally with the release of the atrial stimulus (Fig. 8). A second protective mechanism known as ventricular safety pacing (VSP) complements the blanking period but does not prevent crosstalk. It merely offsets the consequences. The VSP window extends from the onset of the AV delay for a duration of 100–120 ms. During this interval (beyond the blanking period), a sensed ventricular signal does not inhibit the DDD pacemaker. Rather, it immediately triggers a ventricular stimulus delivered prematurely only at the completion of the short VSP interval, producing a characteristic abbreviation of the paced AV (AP-VP) interval. In the second part of the AV delay beyond the VSP interval, a sensed ventricular signal inhibits the pacemaker in the usual fashion (Figs. 9, 10 and 11). The above crosstalk intervals occur only after a paced atrial event and not after an intrinsic atrial event because a native atrial depolarization cannot cause AV crosstalk.

PACEMAKERS AND THEIR ECGs 5

Ventricular safety pacing may produce strange ECGs when the QRS complex activates ventricular safety pacing. This should not be misinterpreted as undersensing when stimuli fall within the QRS complex or beyond the QRS complex.

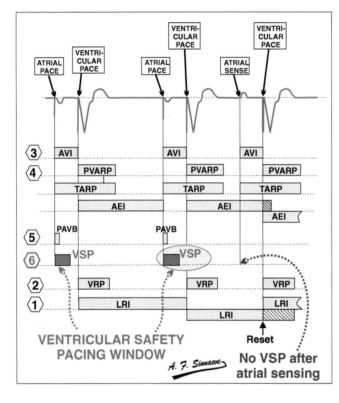

Fig. 8 *Adding 2 intervals to a DDD pacemaker for the prevention of crosstalk: postatrial ventricular blanking period (PAVB) and ventricular safety pacing interval (VSP)*

Advances in pacemaker technology have made it possible to use DDD or DDDR devices safely in patients with paroxysmal atrial arrhythmias. Dual chamber pacemakers equipped with automatic mode switching (AMS) can protect the patient from rapid ventricular pacing (related to sensing of rapid atrial rates) by automatically functioning in a non-atrial tracking mode, usually the DDI or DDIR mode. The DDI and DDIR modes avoid competitive atrial pacing by sensing atrial activity. An atrial-sensed event inhibits the release of the atrial stimulus but cannot initiate a programmed AV delay so that the pacemaker always remains at the lower rate.

DDD pacing prevents the pacemaker syndrome caused by inadequate timing of atrial and ventricular contractions. The syndrome occurs typically in patients with intermittent VVI pacing associated with retrograde VA conduction but it may also be caused by complete AV dissociation without retrograde VA conduction. The main problems are reduced cardiac output and hypotension. The symptoms may be subtle and obvious in only 10–20% of patients with VVI pacemakers.

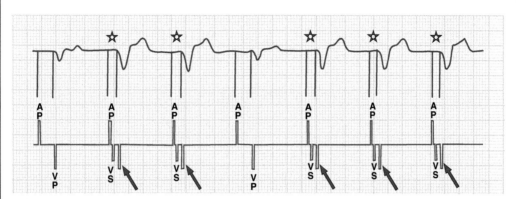

Fig. 9 *AV crosstalk and ventricular safety pacing in a DDD device (ECG and marker channel). In the absence of crosstalk the first and the fourth AV intervals are equal to the programmed value of 200 ms. Intermittent crosstalk (stars) leads to activation of the ventricular safety pacing mechanism. Thus, the AV interval of the second, third, fifth, sixth and seventh beats is abbreviated to 110 ms. The marker channel below the ECG confirms the presence of crosstalk by showing ventricular sensing (VS) of the atrial stimulus (AP) in the ventricular safety pacing period beyond the short blanking period initiated by AP. The arrows point to VP triggered at the end of the ventricular safety pacing period (110 ms starting with AP). In this device with ventricular-based lower rate timing, continual crosstalk causes an increase in the pacing rate because the AV interval is shorter while the atrial escape interval remains constant.*

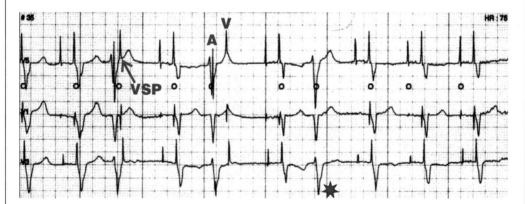

Fig. 10 *Holter recordings of DDD pacemaker showing the effect of crosstalk timing cycles during normal pacemaker function. Three ECGs were recorded simultaneously. The fifth beat is a ventricular premature complex (VPC) deformed by an atrial stimulus (A) which is followed by a ventricular stimulus (V) at the programmed AV delay. The effective ventricular electrogram of the VPC (of adequate amplitude to be sensed) occurs within the postatrial ventricular blanking period initiated by the atrial stimulus just beyond the atrial stimulus (A). The VPC is therefore unsensed by the ventricular channel of the pacemaker. The delivery of atrial stimulation within a QRS complex (capable of being sensed) is called a pseudopseudofusion beat. The seventh beat is an earlier VPC (asterisk) sensed normally by the ventricular channel. The third beat (blue arrow) is also deformed by an atrial stimulus. However, the atrial stimulus occurs earlier than in the fifth beat. This allows the pacemaker to sense the effective ventricular electrogram beyond the postatrial ventricular blanking period but still within the ventricular safety pacing period (VSP). The abbreviated AP-VP interval (110 ms) provides proof that the VPC was sensed by the ventricular channel in the VSP period.*

PACEMAKERS AND THEIR ECGs 6

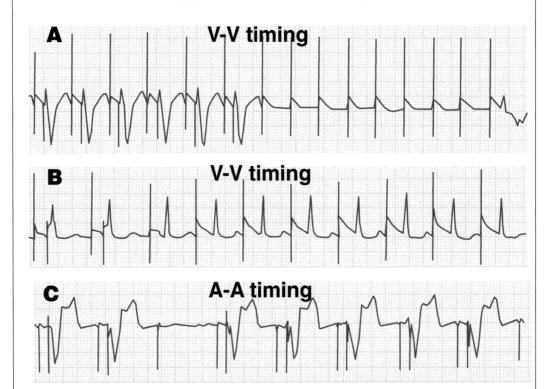

A V-V timing

B V-V timing

C A-A timing

Fig. 11 *AV crosstalk during DDD pacing without a ventricular safety pacing feature.*
Panel A : V-V lower rate timing. The lower rate of the pacemaker was increased to test for crosstalk. Lower rate interval = 580 ms; AV delay = 170 ms. During crosstalk the interval between the atrial stimuli on the right becomes shorter than the lower rate interval because the ventricular channel senses the atrial stimulus thereby initiating a new atrial escape interval (ventricular-based lower rate interval). Crosstalk therefore causes the atrial pacing rate to be faster than the programmed lower rate. Continual crosstalk causes prolonged ventricular asystole.
Panel B: Crosstalk with AV conduction. Lower rate interval = 857 ms; AV interval = 200 ms (ventricular-based lower rate interval). Crosstalk occurs with the third atrial stimulus and produces characteristic prolongation of the interval between the atrial stimulus and the succeeding conducted QRS complex to a value longer than the programmed AV interval. The rate of atrial pacing increases because the sensed atrial stimulus (by the ventricular channel) initiates a new atrial escape interval just beyond the postatrial ventricular blanking period. The atrial pacing rate is faster than the programmed lower rate (ventricular-based lower rate timing). The interval between two consecutive atrial stimuli becomes equal to atrial escape interval of 657 ms (857 – 200) plus the duration of the ventricular blanking period (50 ms) providing a total of about 700 ms. In a device with atrial-based lower rate timing, the atrial rate would not have changed, remaining equal to the programmed lower rate.
Panel C: A-A timing. ECG showing AV crosstalk in a pacemaker with atrial-based lower rate timing. An atrial stimulus causes crosstalk and inhibits release of the ventricular stimulus. The interval between consecutive atrial stimuli remains unchanged and equal to the lower rate interval.

Upper rate response of DDD pacemakers

The maximum paced ventricular rate of a DDD pacemaker (sometimes known as the maximum tracking rate) can be defined either by the duration of the total atrial refractory period (TARP) as in Fig. 12 or by a separate timing circuit (as in all pacemakers) with the capability of programming a longer upper rate interval (URI) independently of the TARP (URI > TARP). A pacemaker then provides 2 levels of upper rate response. (1) The first level defines the onset of a Wenckebach (or pseudo-Wenckebach) upper rate response (Fig. 13) and occurs when the P-P (atrial-atrial) interval is shorter than the upper rate interval but longer than the TARP. (2) The second level uses the TARP to define the onset of block when the P-P interval becomes shorter than the TARP (Fig. 12). Upper rate limitation by only the TARP is less suitable because it produces a sudden fixed-ratio block (or multiblock) such as 2:1 or 3:1 block (2:1 or 3:1 atrial sensing) with potential unfavorable hemodynamic consequences.

Fixed-ratio block

The upper rate interval is a function of TARP only (= AVI + PVARP). As the atrial rate increases, any P wave falling within the PVARP is unsensed and, in effect, blocked. The AV delay always remains constant. If the programmed upper rate is 120 ppm (TARP = 500 ms) and the lower rate is 60 ppm, a 2:1 response will occur when the atrial rate reaches 120 bpm. One P wave is blocked (or unsensed) and the other initiates an AV delay and triggers a ventricular response. An upper rate response using fixed-ratio block is inappropriate in young or physically active individuals.

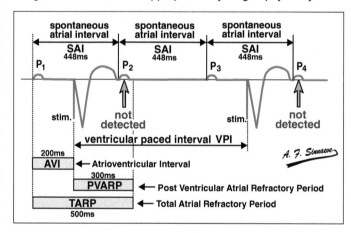

Fig. 12 *Fixed ratio block. DDD pacemaker at upper rate when the spontaneous atrial interval (SAI) is shorter than the total atrial refractory interval (TARP)*

Wenckebach upper rate response

The Wenckebach (or pseudo-Wenckebach) upper rate response requires a separately programmable upper rate interval longer than the TARP (Figs. 13 and 14).

The purpose of the Wenckebach response is to avoid a sudden reduction of the paced ventricular rate (as occurs in fixed-ratio block) and to maintain some degree of AV synchrony at faster rates. During the Wenckebach upper rate response, the pacemaker will synchronize its ventricular stimulus to sensed atrial activity. The pacemaker cannot violate its upper rate interval. Therefore upon atrial sensing, the pacemaker has to wait until the upper rate interval has timed out before it can release a ventricular stimulus. For this reason the AV delay (initiated by atrial sensing) must be extended to deliver the ventricular stimulus at the completion of the upper rate. The sensed AV delay gradually lengthens throughout the Wenckebach sequence but the ventricular rate remains absolutely constant at the programmed upper rate. Eventually a P wave will fall in the PVARP where it cannot start an AV delay so that a pause occurs. The pauses in the upper rate Wenckebach sequences create a form of group beating which should immediately suggest the diagnosis in a pacemaker patient with a fast pacing rate. With progressive shortening of the P-P interval, the Wenckebach upper rate response eventually switches to 2:1 fixed ratio block when the P-P interval becomes shorter than the TARP.

PACEMAKERS AND THEIR ECGs 7

A Wenckebach upper rate response can only occur when the upper rate interval is longer than the total atrial refractory period

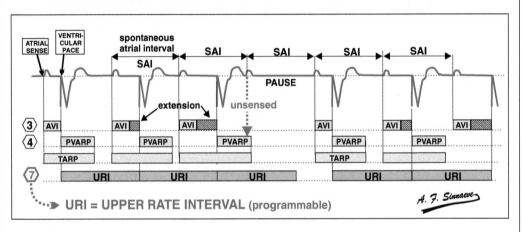

URI = UPPER RATE INTERVAL (programmable)

A. F. Sinnaeve

Fig. 13 *Diagrammatic representation of the Wenckebach upper rate response of a DDD pacemaker. The upper rate interval (URI) is longer than the total atrial refractory period (TARP) which is equal to the sum of AV interval (AVI) and the postventricular atrial refractory period (PVARP). The P-P or spontaneous atrial interval (SAI) is shorter than the URI, but longer than the programmed TARP. The sensed AVI lengthens to conform to the URI. During the Wenckebach response the pacemaker synchronizes the paced ventricular event (VP) to the sensed atrial event because the pacemaker cannot violate its (ventricular) URI. The AVI becomes progressively longer as the ventricular channel waits to deliver a VP until the URI has timed out. The maximum prolongation of the AVI represents the difference between the URI and the TARP. The AVI lengthens as long as the SAI is longer than the TARP. The fourth P wave falls in the PVARP and is unsensed, and therefore not followed by a VP. A pause occurs and the whole sequence starts again. The VP-VP intervals are constant (except when the pause occurs) and equal to the URI. When the SAI becomes shorter than the programmed TARP, Wenckebach pacemaker AV block can no longer occur and fixed ratio pacemaker AV block supervenes.*

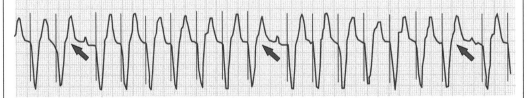

Fig. 14 *ECG lead showing Wenckebach upper rate behavior of a DDD pacemaker. Upper rate = 125 ppm (upper rate interval = 480 ms). The sinus rate is faster than the programmed upper rate but the P-P interval is longer than the total atrial refractory period. Note group beating (typical for this response) interrupted by a pause. The P waves are sensed by the pacemaker and gradually march away from the paced QRS complex. The AV (atrial sense – ventricular pace) delay lengthens*

gradually but this manifestation is masked in the ECG. Eventually a P wave coincides with the postventricular atrial refractory period where it is unsensed. This produces a pause and the sequence restarts upon sensing the next P wave. Barring the pause, the paced interval is constant and equal to the URI.

Pacemaker-mediated tachycardia

Approximately two thirds of patients with sick sinus syndrome and 20–35% of patients with AV block exhibit retrograde ventriculoatrial (VA) conduction. The VA conduction time ranges from 100 to 400 ms, rarely longer, and is influenced by autonomic factors, drugs and so on. Pacemaker-mediated tachycardia (PMT, sometimes called endless loop tachycardia) is a complication of devices that sense atrial activity. It represents a form of macro-reentry. The most common initiating mechanism is a ventricular premature complex (VPC) with retrograde VA conduction (Figs.15 and 16).

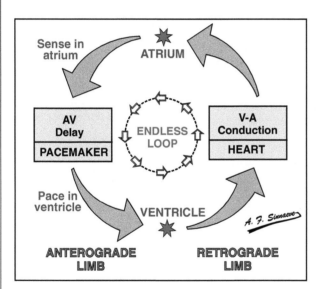

Fig.15 *Diagrammatic representation of the mechanism of endless loop tachycardia. When the atrial channel senses a retrograde P wave, the pacemaker issues a ventricular pacing stimulus at the completion of the programmed AV delay which may be longer than the programmed value to conform to the upper rate interval. The pulse generator itself provides the anterograde limb of the macro-reentrant loop because it functions as an artificial AV junction. Retrograde VA conduction following ventricular pacing provides the retrograde P wave and the process perpetuates itself. Termination of endless loop tachycardia can be accomplished by disrupting either the anterograde limb (by eliminating atrial sensing) or the retrograde limb (by eliminating retrograde conduction).*

When the atrial channel senses a retrograde P wave, a ventricular stimulus is issued at the completion of the AV delay. The pacemaker provides the anterograde loop of the reentrant mechanism. VA conduction following ventricular pacing provides the retrograde limb of the reentrant loop. The atrial channel of the pacemaker again senses the retrograde P wave and the process perpetuates itself.

The cycle length of PMT is often equal to the upper rate interval. Application of the magnet over the pacemaker immediately terminates PMT because it eliminates sensing. PMT can almost always be prevented by programming the PVARP to contain retrograde P waves. A PVARP of 300 ms offers protection against PMT in most patients. In difficult situations one can program a special function to automatically terminate PMT by automatic electronic disruption of the macro-reentrant mechanism.

PACEMAKERS AND THEIR ECGs 8

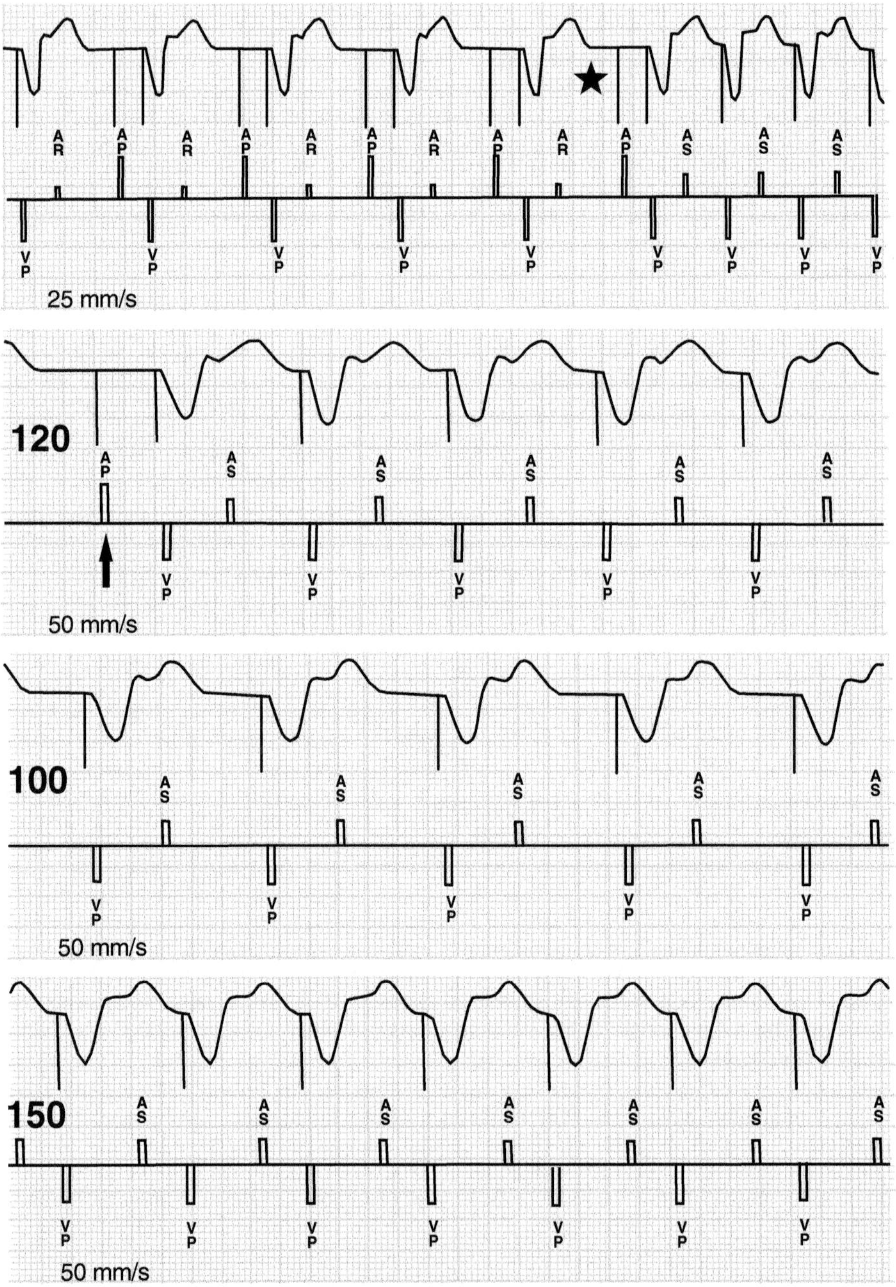

25 mm/s

120

50 mm/s

100

50 mm/s

150

50 mm/s

Fig. 16 *DDD pacing and endless loop tachycardia induced by loss of atrial capture.*

(continuation on next page)

Top panel: *ECG and marker recorded at 25 mm/s. Lower rate interval = 857 ms, AV delay = 200 ms after atrial pacing and 150 ms after atrial sensing, postventricular atrial refractory period (PVARP) = 300 ms, upper rate interval = 500 ms (120 ppm), subthreshold atrial stimulation (AP). Ventricular pacing causes retrograde VA conduction. On the left, the retrograde P waves fall within the PVARP and are depicted as AR by the marker channel. AR events cannot initiate an AV delay. The PVARP was shortened to 200 ms at the star. The pacemaker then senses the retrograde P waves (AS) and initiates endless loop tachycardia.*

Second panel: *A recording at 50 mm/s also shows the initiation of endless loop tachycardia by subthreshold atrial stimulation. The markers indicate that the VA conduction time measures approximately 240 ms (longer than the PVARP). The AS-VP interval is prolonged to conform to the upper rate interval, so that VP-VP interval = upper rate interval = 500 ms.*

Third panel: *50 mm/s. The upper rate interval was programmed to 600 ms (100 ppm). The retrograde VA conduction time during endless loop tachycardia remains constant at 240 ms, but the AS-VP interval lengthens further to conform to the upper rate interval so that VP-VP interval = 600 ms.*

Bottom pannel: *50 mm/s. The upper rate interval was programmed to 400 ms (150 ppm). The retrograde VA conduction time is now slightly longer at approximately 260 ms. The programmed AS-VP remains at 150 ms and is not extended. The tachycardia interval represents the sum of the VA conduction time and the programmed AS-VP interval, and is slightly longer (410–420 ms) than the upper rate interval (400 ms). Endless loop tachycardia was no longer induced by subthreshold atrial stimulation when the PVARP was again programmed to 300 ms as in the top panel on the left.*

Repetitive nonreentrant ventriculoatrial synchrony

Repetitive ventriculoatrial (VA) synchrony can also occur in the DDD or DDDR mode when a paced ventricular beat causes retrograde VA conduction but the retrograde P wave is unsensed because it falls within the PVARP (Figs. 17 and 18).

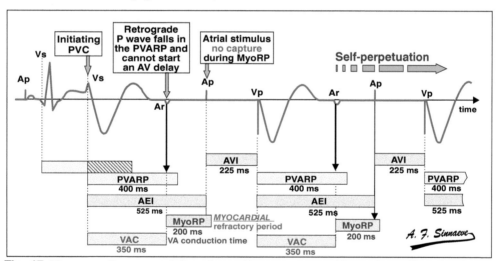

Fig. 17 *Diagrammatic representation of repetitive nonreentrant VA synchrony. There is relatively slow retrograde VA conduction (VAC) initiated by a premature ventricular complex (PVC). The retrograde P is unsensed (cannot start an AV delay) because it falls within the postventricular atrial refractory period (PVARP). At the completion of the atrial escape interval (AEI), the pacemaker delivers an atrial stimulus (Ap) that falls close to the preceding retrograde P wave (Ar = atrial event detected in the PVARP) and therefore still within the atrial myocardial refractory period (MyoRP) engendered by the previous retrograde atrial depolarization. Ap is therefore ineffectual. Barring any perturbations, this process becomes self-perpetuating. Vs = ventricular sensed event; Vp = ventricular paced event; AVI = AV interval.*

PACEMAKERS AND THEIR ECGs 9

Under certain circumstances, repetitive nonreentrant ventriculoatrial (VA) synchrony can become self-perpetuating when the pacemaker continually delivers an ineffectual atrial stimulus (despite being well above the pacing threshold under normal circumstances) in the atrial myocardial refractory period generated by the preceding retrograde P wave. The potential reentrant circuit does not close and this arrhythmia is often labeled as nonreentrant. Both pacemaker-mediated tachycardia and repetitive nonreentrant VA synchrony depend on VA conduction and are physiologically similar. Both share similar initiating and terminating mechanisms. Repetitive nonreentrant VA synchrony depends on a short atrial escape interval (relatively fast lower rate and/or a long AV delay) and a relatively long VA conduction time. Thus, it is more likely to occur during sensor-driven faster pacing rates. The arrhythmia has become more common because long AV delays may be programmed to promote AV conduction and normal ventricular activation.

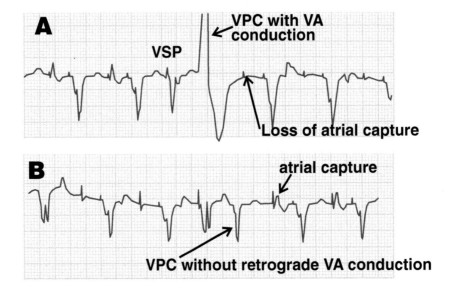

Fig. 18 *Repetitive nonreentrant VA synchrony during bipolar DDD pacing.*
Panel A: Initiation of repetitive nonreentrant VA synchrony by a ventricular premature complex (VPC). The third beat is a VPC that activates ventricular safety pacing (VSP). The fourth beat is a VPC with retrograde VA conduction (where the retrograde P wave is not seen on the ECG). The succeeding atrial stimulus is ineffectual as it falls within the atrial myocardial refractory period generated by the preceding retrograde atrial depolarization. This atrial stimulus is followed by a ventricular paced beat associated with retrograde VA conduction. Repetitive nonreentrant VA synchrony begins when the following atrial stimulus occurs in the atrial myocardial refractory period related to the retrograde P wave linked to the ventricular paced beat.
Panel B: Termination of repetitive nonreentrant VA synchrony by a VPC. Lower rate = 80 ppm, AV delay = 250 ms. The fourth beat is a VPC (with retrograde VA conduction) falling within the AV delay but beyond the VSP period. The fifth beat is a VPC which is more premature than the preceding one. This prematurely induces VA conduction block. The subsequent atrial stimulus captures the atrium because it no longer faces a refractory barrier from an atrial event in the preceding post-ventricular atrial refractory period (PVARP).

Tachycardias during DDD(R) pacing

Tachycardia (rapid ventricular pacing) during DDD pacing is relatively common and the diagnosis is often simple. Pacemaker-mediated tachycardia is terminated by magnet application. Tachycardias other than pacemaker-mediated tachycardia return upon removal of the magnet. A pacemaker Wenckebach upper rate response indicates that the atrial rate is faster than the programmed upper rate of the pacemaker but does not differentiate between supraventricular tachyarrhythmia and sinus tachycardia. Supraventricular tachyarrhythmias may induce a variety of pacemaker responses if automatic mode switching (AMS) is not programmed. A rapid and irregular ventricular rate suggests the diagnosis of atrial fibrillation or flutter. The DDI(R) mode in AMS during detected supraventricular tachycardia may generate no atrial stimuli and resembles VVI(R) pacing. Pacemaker tachycardia triggered by myopotentials sensed by the atrial channel of a unipolar DDD pacemaker can be regular or irregular with pacing cycles often at the upper rate interval. Myopotential-triggered tachycardias in the atrial channel may be associated with periods of myopotential inhibition of the ventricular channel and asynchronous pacing at the interference rate. Sensor-driven tachycardia is rare and usually related to inappropriate or overprogramming of a rate-adaptive pacemaker.

> **Pacemaker-mediated tachycardia can be prevented in almost all the patients by programming the PVARP to contain retrograde P waves.**

Automatic mode switching

Automatic mode switching (AMS) refers to the automatic change of a pacemaker mode in response to supraventricular tachycardia. The behavior of AMS varies according to the manufacturer but they all are activated by detection of an atrial tachyarrhythmia whereupon they convert a dual chamber pacemaker from an atrial tracking mode (which may cause rapid paced ventricular rates) to a nonatrial tracking mode either in the DDI(R) or VVI(R) mode. In this way, dual chamber pacing can be performed safely in patients with paroxysmal supraventricular tachycardias. Reversion to the DDD(R) mode occurs automatically upon termination of tachycardia. One must remain familiar with the behavior of the DDI(R) mode because it is used as a temporary mode during AMS (Figs. 19, 20A and 20B).

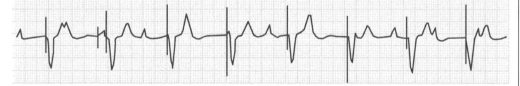

Fig. 19 *DDI pacing mode in a patient who underwent ablation of the AV junction for refractory paroxysmal atrial fibrillation, and developed pacemaker syndrome. The DDI mode functions at the programmed lower rate of 60 ppm which is slower than the prevailing sinus rate. Note that sinus P waves march through the cardiac cycle, producing AV dissociation. The P wave following the first ventricular paced beat falls in the 300 ms postventricular atrial refractory period and is unsensed, thereby allowing the release of an atrial stimulus at the end of the atrial escape interval initiated by the first ventricular paced complex (ventricular-based lower rate timing).*

The DDI and DDI(R) modes avoid competitive atrial pacing by sensing atrial activity. An atrial sensed event inhibits the release of the atrial stimulus when the atrial escape interval has timed out. The "I" in the third position of the pacemaker code indicates that only atrial and ventricular inhibition are possible. No triggered atrial function is possible. In other words, a sensed P wave cannot trigger a ventricular stimulus, i.e. DDI does not allow atrial tracking. There is no sensed AV delay. The programmed AV delay can only exist as a paced AV interval.

PACEMAKERS AND THEIR ECGs 10

The DDI(R) mode will therefore always exhibit a constant ventricular paced rate equal to the programmed lower rate or the sensor-derived lower rate. A postventricular atrial refractory period (PVARP) and crosstalk intervals are retained. It should be remembered that in the presence of complete AV block when the sinus rate is faster than the programmed lower rate the DDI mode will not provide AV synchrony (Fig. 19).

The DDI and DDIR modes and automatic mode switching

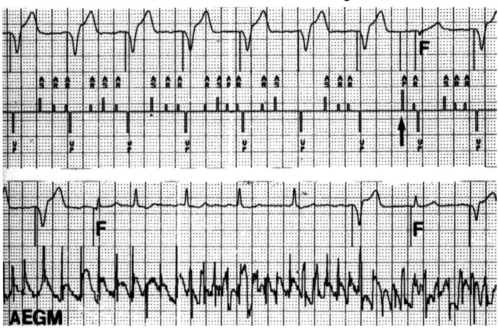

Fig. 20A *Automatic mode switching with DDI pacing during atrial fibrillation. On top the ECG was recorded simultaneously with event markers and at the bottom the ECG was recorded simultaneously with the telemetered atrial electrogram (AEGM). F = ventricular fusion beat; AS = atrial sensed event; AR = atrial event detected in the atrial refractory period; VP = ventricular paced event. Lower rate interval = 750 ms; AV interval = 200 ms; postventricular atrial refractory period = 250 ms. Sensed events in the atrial refractory period cannot inhibit the atrial channel. Although the pacemaker senses atrial events (AS) outside the atrial refractory period, it does not track them, i.e. it cannot generate an AV delay to the programmed value. Consequently ventricular pacing is forced to occur at the programmed lower rate of 80 ppm. The AS-VP intervals are always longer than the programmed AP-VP delay and display marked variability in duration which are characteristic features of the DDI mode. There is intermittent atrial undersensing of the f waves because the AEGM tends to be considerably smaller than the corresponding AEGM in sinus rhythm. The arrow points to a cycle where the pacemaker fails to sense the f waves so that AP is released at the completion of the atrial escape interval.*

> **During automatic mode switching, the ECG during DDI(R) pacing looks like the VVI(R) mode.**

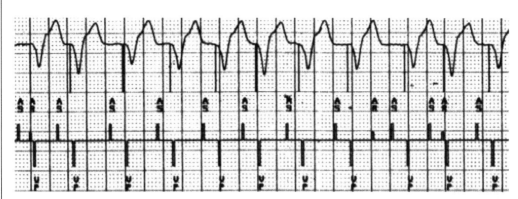

Fig. 20B *Rapid and irregular ventricular pacing during atrial fibrillation and the DDD mode. The device tracks the rapid atrial rate in the absence of automatic mode switching. AS = atrial sensed event; AR = atrial event detected during the postventricular refractory period; VP = ventricular paced event.*

Rate-adaptive pacemakers

A sensor monitors the need for faster pacing rate and attempts to mimic the rate response of the normal sinus node according to physical activity. A sensor works independently of atrial activity. A VVI pacemaker with rate-adaptive function is coded as a VVIR pacemaker and a DDD pacemaker as a DDDR device. Activity sensors (accelerometer or piezoelectric crystal) are widely used but minute ventilation, the product of respiratory rate and tidal volume, is a more physiologic sensor. Some pacemakers contain 2 sensors for improved performance.

Patterns of depolarization during ventricular pacing

Pacing from the right ventricular (RV) apex produces negative paced QRS complexes in the inferior leads with a mean frontal plane axis which is superior either in the left or the right superior quadrant (Fig. 21A). Location of the RV lead in the outflow tract or high RV septum shifts the frontal plane axis to the inferior quadrants. RV pacing, regardless of the site, produces a left bundle branch block (LBBB) pattern in the precordial leads occasionally registered as QS complexes in all the precordial leads. A dominant R wave in V1 has been called a right bundle branch block pattern of depolarization but this terminology is misleading because this pattern is often not related to RV activation delay. A dominant R wave in lead V1 occurs in approximately 8–10% of patients with uncomplicated RV apical pacing. In such a situation V1 and V2 recorded one interspace lower will usually record a negative complex. If the dominant R wave persists by this maneuver, the lead may not be in the RV. LV pacing also produces a tall R wave in V1. A tall R wave in V3 and V4 signifies that a pacemaker lead is most probably not in RV after excluding ventricular fusion from spontaneous AV conduction.

> **Right ventricular pacing produces an ECG with a left bundle branch pattern and the frontal plane axis usually points to the left superior quadrant and occasionally to the right superior quadrant.**

PACEMAKERS AND THEIR ECGs 11

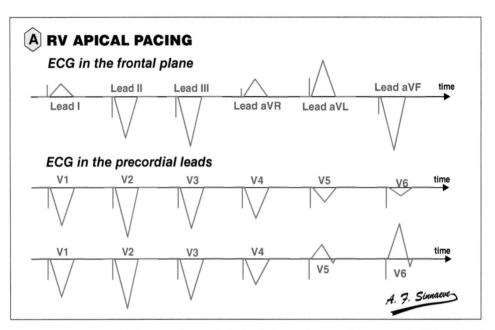

A) RV APICAL PACING

ECG in the frontal plane

ECG in the precordial leads

A. F. Sinnaeve

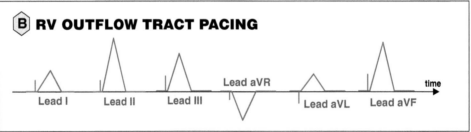

B) RV OUTFLOW TRACT PACING

Fig. 21A *ECG of right ventricular pacing.*
Upper panel: right ventricular apical pacing. The frontal plane axis is usually left superior. It may also be in the right superior quadrant where it causes leads I, II and III to be negative and lead aVR to show the largest positive deflection. Although the precordial leads normally show an LBBB pattern, the typical LBBB pattern in the left precordial leads may not be present and all leads show a QS pattern. Occasionally the left precordial leads may show a dominant R wave.
Lower panel: right ventricular outflow tract pacing. The frontal plane axis is normal, i.e. as for normally conducted beats. But as the lead moves towards the pulmonary valve, the axis becomes deviated to the right. A qR pattern can occur only in leads I and aVL. The precordial leads V1 to V6 are similar to those with RV apical pacing.

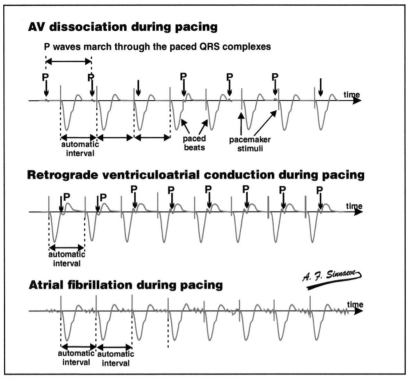

AV dissociation during pacing

P waves march through the paced QRS complexes

automatic interval

paced beats

pacemaker stimuli

time

Retrograde ventriculoatrial conduction during pacing

automatic interval

time

A. F. Sinnaeve

Atrial fibrillation during pacing

automatic interval automatic interval

time

Fig. 21B *Single chamber ventricular pacing. Patterns of atrial activity during ventricular pacing.*

Left ventricular pacing

Single chamber left ventricular (LV) pacing is sometimes used permanently for cardiac resynchronization therapy (CRT). It is frequently programmed temporarily during troubleshooting and follow-up. LV pacing from the posterior or posterolateral coronary vein (the traditional sites for CRT) almost invariably results in a right bundle branch block (RBBB) pattern in a correctly positioned lead (Fig. 22). Lead V1 is therefore positive and the frontal plane axis often shows right axis deviation. Leads V2 and V3 may or may not be positive. With apical lead position, leads V4 to V6 are usually positive. Pacing from the middle or the great (anterior) cardiac vein (unsatisfactory sites for CRT) produces a LBBB pattern of depolarization. Thus, when lead V1 during LV pacing shows a negative QRS complex, one should consider incorrect ECG lead placement.

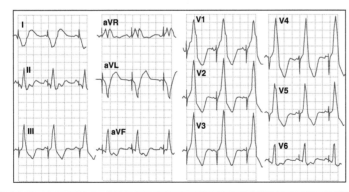

Fig. 22 *Monochamber LV pacing. QRS duration = 240 ms.*
Note the RBBB pattern with a dominant R wave in V1 and right axis deviation the frontal plane.

PACEMAKERS AND THEIR ECGs 12

Cardiac resynchronization with biventricular pacing

Biventricular pacing has emerged as beneficial therapy for patients with marked systolic left ventricular dysfunction, and heart failure associated with a wide QRS complex due to a left-sided conduction delay or block.

Biventricular pacing with a LV site in the coronary venous system and a RV apical site

Lead V1 usually shows a dominant R wave. The frontal plane QRS axis is usually in the right superior quadrant, and occasionally in the left superior quadrant (Fig. 23). A negative QRS complex in V1 may occasionally occur with uncomplicated biventricular pacing (and remains unexplained), but such a finding requires ruling out a number of abnormalities that include failure of left ventricular (LV) capture, LV lead displacement or marked LV latency (exit block or conduction delay from the stimulation site allowing the RV to overshadow the LV), ventricular fusion with the intrinsic QRS complex, and pacing via the middle cardiac vein or anterior interventricular vein. In patients with sinus rhythm and a relatively short PR interval, the ECG may show ventricular fusion with the competing native conduction during biventricular pacing. The unusual QRS in V1 is a common pitfall in follow-up and may cause misinterpretation of the ECG.

Biventricular pacing with the LV site in the coronary sinus and the RV site in the outflow tract

The paced QRS in lead V1 is often negative and the frontal plane paced QRS axis is often directed to the right inferior quadrant (right axis deviation).

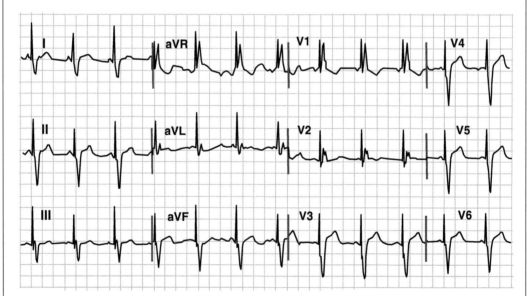

Fig. 23 *Biventricular pacing in the DDD mode with atrial sensing and ventricular pacing (left ventricular pacing was performed from the coronary venous system). The paced QRS complex is relatively narrow. There is a dominant R wave in leads V1 and V2. The frontal plane axis points to the right superior quadrant as expected when the right ventricle is paced from the apex in a biventricular system.*

Evaluation of atrial capture and sensing in dual chamber pacemakers

The presence of atrial capture can sometimes be difficult to determine from the 12-lead ECG (Fig. 24A). The presence of atrial stimuli does not mean successful atrial capture. Lack of capture can be due to unsuspected atrial fibrillation (AF). The presence of permanent AF (or atrial flutter) is often poorly recognized in a continuously paced rhythm with resultant denial of anticoagulant therapy. A 12-lead ECG at double standardization can be invaluable in bringing out a paced P wave and/or tiny bipolar stimuli.

Atrial undersensing from a small intracardiac signal is more common in the atrial than the ventricular channel of a DDD pacemaker because the atrial electrogram is much smaller than the ventricular one. P wave undersensing may also be due to other causes such as the P wave falling in the postventricular atrial refractory period (PVARP) (Fig. 24B).

> **Lack of atrial capture is often missed especially in atrial fibrillation. In questionable cases, look for atrial capture by recording the ECG at double standardization and/or doing a subxiphoid echocardiogram.**

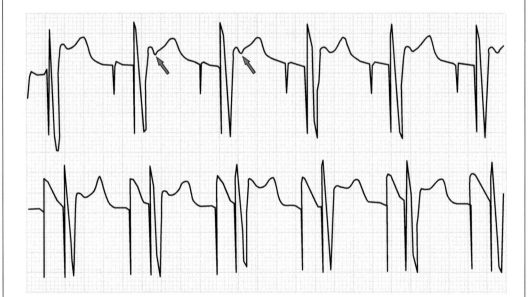

Fig. 24A *Loss of atrial capture by a DDD pacemaker.*
Top: The atrial stimulus does not give rise to visible atrial depolarization. The presence of notching on the ST segment suggests the presence of retrograde ventriculoatrial (VA) conduction indicating lack of atrial capture by the preceding atrial stimulus.
Bottom: When the atrial output was increased, retrograde VA conduction disappeared implying that there was appropriate atrial capture despite the absence of a clearly visible P wave induced by the atrial stimulus.

PACEMAKERS AND THEIR ECGs 13

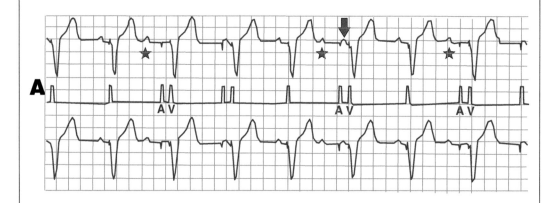

INSPIRATION

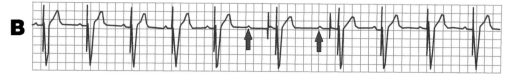

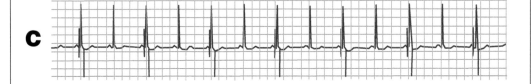

Fig. 24B *Atrial undersensing;*
Panel A: Two-lead Holter recording with special pacemaker channel showing intermittent atrial undersensing (stars). The atrial stimuli close to the unsensed P waves do not capture the atrium which is still refractory from the preceding spontaneous atrial depolarization. At the arrow atrial capture occurs just beyond the atrial myocardial refractory period generated by the preceding sinus P wave.
Panel B: ECG showing the importance of evaluating atrial sensing during deep inspiration when sensing is lost (arrows).
Panel C: Intermittent atrial sensing during DDD pacing with delivery of the atrial stimulus within the terminal portion of every second P wave. The conducted QRS complex following the atrial stimulus falls within the ventricular safety pacing period of 110 ms. The ventricular channel senses the QRS complex and triggers a ventricular stimulus after the expected abbreviation of the AV delay to 110 ms. Atrial sensing was restored and safety pacing was eliminated by programming only a higher atrial sensitivity. (Programmed paced AV delay = 200 ms)

Electrical complications during ventricular pacing

There are many causes of loss of capture by visible stimuli on the ECG and the most common causes are lead displacement or changes in the electrode-tissue interface. Artifacts may create confusion. "Triboelectric phenomena" describe high-voltage deflections generated by static electricity. Such artifactual signals are usually wider and more irregular than pacemaker stimuli and often recognizable as unrelated to a pacemaker. Occasionally, the diagnosis depends on finding subtle differences from the pacing stimulus.

Pacing failure without visible stimuli is usually due to pulse generator failure (usually the battery) or an open circuit with no current flow usually because of a electrode-lead fracture with intact insulation.

The most common cause of ventricular undersensing is a low-amplitude ventricular electrogram. Lead dislodgment is the most likely cause of undersensing soon after implantation and can often be corrected by reprogramming. The differential diagnosis includes pseudofusion beats and functional undersensing when the signal occurs in a refractory or blanking period. Pacemakers usually respond to electromagnetic interference by temporary conversion to synchronous or fixed-rate pacing.

All forms of oversensing are often associated with undersensing because an extraneous signal generates a pacemaker refractory period which may then coincide with the occurrence of a spontaneous QRS complex (functional undersensing). Oversensing of physiologic signals (P and T waves) and the pacemaker waveform itself (afterpotential) is rare. A prolonged atrial escape interval during hysteresis must not be misinterpreted as ventricular oversensing.

Abrupt changes in the resistance within a pacing system can produce large voltage changes (called false signals or voltage transients) between the two electrodes used for pacing and sensing. False signals are almost always invisible on the surface ECG so that their presence must be assumed until they are revealed by pacemaker interrogation. Such "make-break" signals may occur with loose connections, wire fracture with otherwise well apposed ends, insulation defect, or the interaction of 2 leads in the heart (one active, the other inactive) lying side by side and touching each other intermittently.

Myopotential interference

Myopotential inhibition represents oversensing of electrical activity originating from skeletal muscles. Myopotential oversensing occurs only with unipolar pulse generators (with the anode on the pacemaker can) and originates from the deltopectoral region at the implantation site. Myopotential oversensing by a unipolar ventricular pacemaker may cause device inhibition with pauses of varying duration (Fig. 25). Myopotential oversensing typically shows interference of the ECG baseline. Figure 26 shows how myopotential oversensing by the atrial channel of a dual chamber pacemaker can cause triggering of ventricular pacing. Oversensing of diaphragmatic myopotentials is rare and may occur with either unipolar or bipolar systems in contrast to the more common myopotential interference from deltopectoral muscles which only occurs with unipolar pacing.

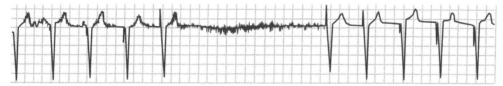

Fig. 25 *Pacemaker inhibition with ventricular asystole induced by myopotential oversensing in a patient with a unipolar VVI pacemaker programmed to a rate of 70 ppm. The baseline interference of the ECG is typical of myopotential interference.*

PACEMAKERS AND THEIR ECGs 14

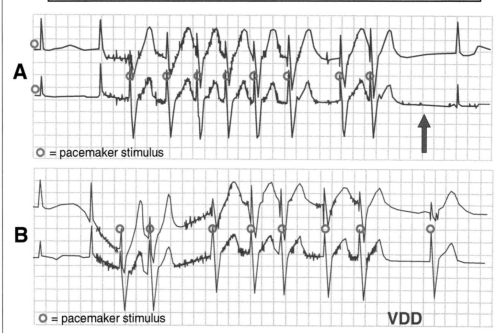

O = pacemaker stimulus

O = pacemaker stimulus   VDD

Fig. 26 *Myopotential interference of atrial and ventricular channels documented in a Holter recording in a patient with a VDD pacemaker programmed to a rate of 60 ppm. The patient had no atrial arrhythmias. Myopotential sensing by the atrial channel triggers a ventricular stimulus thereby causing an irregular increase in the ventricular pacing rate. At other times, myopotentials sensed by the ventricular channel cause pacemaker inhibition (arrow) with pauses of varying duration. Note the typical interference of the ECG baseline. The first circle in strip A suggests that a ventricular stimulus was emitted. Such a stimulus may have occurred either as a result of a ventricular fusion beat or a pseudofusion beat. The first QRS complex suggests supraventricular conduction and therefore a pseudofusion in which the ventricular stimulus was delivered during the QRS complex. Note that the ST-T wave configuration of the first beat in strip A is different from that in the last QRS complex engendered by supraventricular conduction. Altered repolarization indicates altered preceding depolarization and therefore ventricular fusion in the first beat in strip A. The tracing shows the importance of Holter recordings in the detection of pacemaker stimuli that are invisible in a standard ECG.*

Tachycardia during DDD pacing

The diagnosis of tachycardia is often simple. Pacemaker-mediated tachycardia (PMT) is terminated by magnet application. Supraventricular tachyarrhythmias may induce a variety of pacemaker responses when automatic mode switching is not programmed. A pacemaker Wenckebach upper rate response indicates that the atrial is faster than the programmed upper rate of the pacemaker but it does not differentiate between a supraventricular tachyarrhythmia and sinus tachcardia but rules out PMT. Diagnostic P, F, or f waves may not be discernible. A rapid and irregular ventricular pacing rate suggests the diagnosis of atrial fibrillation or flutter provided a defective atrial lead (with false signals) can be ruled out (Fig. 20B). Occasionally, atrial flutter or atrial fibrillation (AF) induces rapid and regular ventricular pacing at the programmed upper rate mimicking a PMT. Pacemaker tachycardia triggered by myopotentials sensed by the atrial channel of a unipolar DDD or DDDR pacemaker can be regular or irregular with pacing cycles often at the upper rate interval (Fig. 26).

Hyperkalemia

Hyperkalemia causes widening of the paced QRS complex (and paced P wave) on the basis of delayed myocardial conduction. Other common causes of a wide paced QRS complex include amiodarone therapy and severe myocardial disease. Hyperkalemia can cause reversible lack of capture with the atrial channel being more sensitive than the ventricular one. Hyperkalemia can cause prolonged latency (interval from stimulus to onset of depolarization), a condition also known as first-degree pacemaker exit block. The normal value of ventricular latency during RV pacing is 40 ms or less and is measured from the ventricular pacing stimulus to the onset of ventricular depolarization (Fig. 27).

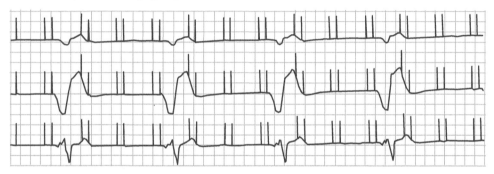

Fig. 27 *Hyperkalemia. ECG of a patient with a DDD pacemaker and hyperkalemia (K = 7.2 mEq). There is loss of atrial capture and intermittent loss of ventricular capture because of a high pacing threshold. The paced QRS complex is very wide. The atrium is more sensitive than the ventricle to the effects of hyperkalemia. Thus, atrial capture is often lost before ventricular capture.*

Algorithms to minimize right ventricular pacing

Much evidence has emerged in the last decade about the harmful effects of chronic RV pacing (mostly apical) on LV function. Minimizing RV pacing may reduce chronic changes in cellular structure, LV geometry that contribute to impaired hemodynamic performance, mitral regurgitation, and increased left atrial diameters with the aim of reducing the risk of atrial fibrillation, congestive heart failure, and death. On this basis, strategies to minimize RV pacing have become important especially in patients with sick sinus syndrome where continual RV pacing may not be necessary. There are two major algorithms that minimize RV pacing.

1. In the DDD or DDDR mode with a dynamic AV delay, the pacemaker periodically extends the AV delay (gradually or suddenly) to a programmable value aiming to search for spontaneous AV conduction. If a conducted ventricular event is sensed during this extended AV delay, the pacemaker inhibits the ventricular output and continues to function (in the functional AAI or AAIR mode) with such an extended AV delay until no ventricular sensed event is seen. The absence of a sensed ventricular event promoted pacing with the basic AV delay.

2. New pacing modes in which the algorithm maintains AAI or AAIR pacing (Fig. 28) (mode switching DDDR → AAIR → DDDR). The switch to AAIR from DDDR is achieved by periodic AV conduction checks by the device monitoring for a conducted ventricular sensed event. First- and second-degree AV block are tolerated in the AAIR mode up to a predetermined programmable limit. The permitted cycles of second-degree AV block are short but an occasional patient may become symptomatic. Supraventricular tachyarrhythmias activate automatic mode switching to the DDIR mode like other pacemakers (AAIR → DDIR or DDDR → DDIR). The AV delay is either eliminated or very prolonged. The unusual behavior of the AV delay means that the AV delay terminating with a ventricular sensed event can be very long. No ventricular pacing may occur after a long PR interval. This may cause sustained marked first-degree AV block that may be hemodynamically important and symptomatic like retrograde VA conduction (pacemaker syndrome).

PACEMAKERS AND THEIR ECGs 15

Fig. 28 MANAGED VENTRICULAR PACING (Medtronic)

Ventricular Backup:
Function of managed ventricular pacing (MVP)
Ventricular pacing only as needed in the presence of transient loss of conduction

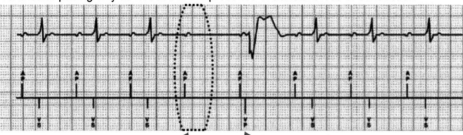

Loss of conduction —↗   ↖—Backup ventricular pace

MVP function: Loss of AV conduction induces an AP-VP beat with an abbreviated AV delay. Note the atrial pacing rate remains constant. Functional AAI(R) then continues with AV conduction and a long AV delay or PR interval. The pacemaker detects VS allowing the continuation of the AAI(R) mode.
AP = atrial paced event; VP = ventricular paced event; VS = ventricular sensed event.

AAI(R) to DDD(R) Switch: Ventricular support if loss of A-V conduction is persistent

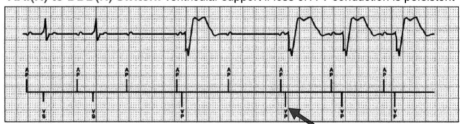

Switch to DDD(R) occurs after back-up VP; programmed
PAV/SAV are used during this mode of operation

MVP function: The functional AAI(R) mode converts to DDD(R) pacing if there is AV block in 2 out of 4 cycles. AP = atrial paced event; VP = ventricular paced event; VS = ventricular sensed beat; PAV = paced AV delay (initiated by an AP); SAV = sensed AV delay (initiated by an AS)

DDD(R) to AAI(R) Switch: If AV conduction check passes (1 beat)

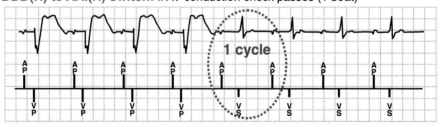

1 cycle

AV conduction check (1 beat). Scheduled every 1, 2, 4, 8 min... up to 16 hrs after a transition to DDD(R) has occurred. Temporarily uses AAI(R) timing to monitor for a conducted VS during one A-A interval. VS = ventricular sensed beat; A-A = interatrial interval.

Fig. 29

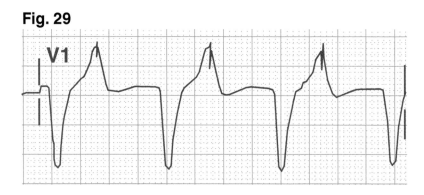

V1

The ECG shows managed ventricular pacing (MVP) with atrial pacing at a rate of 75 ppm and an AV delay = 440 ms. The atrial stimuli fall on the T wave of the conducted ventricular beats. There are no ventricular stimuli. In the MVP mode with functional AAIR pacing, atrial stimuli but no ventricular stimuli are emitted. Following an atrial sensed event (AS) or atrial paced event (AP), there is no AV delay (unlike in a dual chamber pacemaker where a ventricular stimulus terminates the programmed AV delay). If there is delayed AV conduction, the subsequent event will be a spontaneous ventricular event (VS) and not a ventricular stimulus. If VS does not occur, the subsequent event will be either AS or AP but not a ventricular stimulus. The pacemaker does not alter its timing (atrial pacing rate) in response to a VS event. However it senses it via the ventricular lead and labels the VS event as due to successful AV conduction and therefore continues the functional AAIR mode. Consequently the AS-VS or AP-VS (i.e. PR) intervals can be very long and sustained marked first-degree AV block may occur. A switch to the DDDR mode occurs when 2 out of 4 atrial intervals do not contain VS events. This arrangement is often misinterpreted as pacemaker failure and the atrial stimuli falling beyond the V event are also misinterpreted as a loss of ventricular capture and sensing.

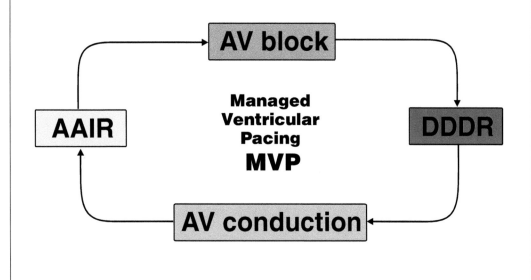

AV block

Managed
Ventricular
Pacing
MVP

AAIR

DDDR

AV conduction

Barold SS. Repetitive reentrant and non-reentrant ventriculoatrial synchrony in dual chamber pacing. Clin Cardiol. 1997;20:989-92.

Barold SS, Giudici MC, Herweg B, Curtis AB. Diagnostic value of the 12-lead electrocardiogram during conventional and biventricular pacing for cardiac resynchronization. Cardiol Clin. 2006;24:471-90.

Barold SS, Herweg B. Usefulness of the 12-lead electrocardiogram in the follow-up of patients with cardiac resynchronization devices. Part I. Cardiol J. 2011;18:476-86.

Barold SS, Herweg B. Usefulness of the 12-lead electrocardiogram in the follow-up of patients with cardiac resynchronization devices. Part II. Cardiol J. 2011;18:610-24.

Brignole M, Auricchio A, Baron-Esquivias G, Bordachar P, Boriani G, Breithardt OA, 2013 ESC Guidelines on cardiac pacing and cardiac resynchronization therapy: The Task Force oncardiac pacing and resynchronization therapy of the European Society of Cardiology (ESC). Developed in collaboration with the European Heart Rhythm Association (EHRA). Eur Heart J. 2013;34:2281-329.

Epstein AE, DiMarco JP, Ellenbogen KA, Estes NA 3rd, Freedman RA, Gettes LS, American College of Cardiology Foundation; American Heart Association Task Force on Practice Guidelines; Heart Rhythm Society. 2012 ACCF/AHA/HRS focused update incorporated into the ACCF/AHA/HRS 2008 guidelines for device-based therapy of cardiac rhythm abnormalities: a report of the American College of Cardiology Foundation/American Heart Association Task Force on Practice Guidelines and the Heart Rhythm Society. J Am Coll Cardiol. 2013;61:e6-75.

Stroobandt RX, Barold SS, Vandenbulcke FD, Willems RJ, AF Sinnaeve. A reappraisal of pacemaker timing cycles pertaining to automatic mode switching. J Interv Cardiovasc Electrophysiol. 2001;5:417-429.

Stroobandt R, Willems R, Holvoet G, Backers J, Sinnaeve A. Prediction of Wenckebach behaviour and block response in DDD pacemakers. PACE. 1986; 9: 1040-104.

Vardas PE, Simantirakis EN, Kanoupakis EM. New developments in cardiac pacemakers. Circulation. 2013;127:2343-50.

CHAPTER 22

ERRORS IN ELECTROCARDIOGRAPHY MONITORING, COMPUTERIZED ECG, OTHER SITES OF ECG RECORDING

* Inaccurate lead placement
* Superimposition of standard ECG leads with telemetry leads
* Technically unacceptable ECG recordings
* Baseline wander and wrong speed
* Electrode positioning on the torso
* Common 5-electrode system
* Right-sided precordial leads at a higher or lower intercostal space
* Lewis lead
* Esophageal recordings
* His bundle recordings

ECG from Basics to Essentials: Step by Step. First Edition. Roland X. Stroobandt, S. Serge Barold and Alfons F. Sinnaeve.
Published 2016 © 2016 by John Wiley & Sons, Ltd. Companion Website: www.wiley.com/go/stroobandt/ecg

ERRORS IN ELECTROCARDIOGRAPHY 1

Electrocardiographic diagnoses are valid only if electrodes are placed in correct locations, lead wires are attached to the appropriate electrode, and the recording is of good technical quality (proper filtering, absence of extraneous electrical noise, etc.). If comparisons of serial ECGs are required all recordings must be made using a consistent technique.

Inaccurate Lead Placement

Limb Leads

Placement of the electrodes for the limb leads (right arm, left arm, left leg) can be anywhere on the limb without substantially affecting ECG waveforms. However, clinically important misdiagnoses may occur when limb electrodes are placed on the torso, particularly if they are moved closer to the heart (e.g. arm electrodes placed closer to the sternum than the shoulders).

The change between a torso-positioned versus a standard ECG is either loss or appearance of Q waves of infarction in the inferior leads. Changes in ST-T waves may also occur which could be interpreted as acute myocardial ischemia when serial comparisons are made between standard and torso-positioned ECGs. Finally, P, R and S wave voltages may be different.

Precordial Leads

Correct placement of the lead V1 electrode is vital because the remaining 5 precordial leads are placed in relation to it. Therefore, if the V1 electrode is placed above its correct location, leads V2 to V6 may also be misplaced superiorly. High and low placement of precordial electrodes produce a change in R wave of about 1 mm per interspace, with smaller R waves when V1 and V2 are placed superior to the correct 4th intercostal space. Thus, superiorly displaced precordial leads may result in the misdiagnosis of "poor R wave progression" or "anterior myocardial infarction".

Inappropriate Serial Comparisons Using Different Lead Sets

Serial ECG comparisons of 12-lead ECGs using tracings from cardiac monitors may be mis-leading because the 12 ECG leads of monitors are mathematically derived from a reduced number of leads. Such derived 12-lead ECGs are useful for diagnoses important in the immediate care setting such as distinguishing ventricular tachycardia from supraventricular tachycardia with aberrant conduction, detection of new bundle branch block, and ST segment changes of acute myocardial ischemia. Derived and standard ECG serial comparisons should not be made for measurement of precise amplitudes (e.g. whenever ST segment elevations have resolved). Therefore, as in the case for torso-positioned ECGs, 12-lead ECGs derived from reduced lead sets should not be compared serially with 12-lead ECGs recorded in the standard way.

Limb Lead Wire Reversals

Right Leg – Left Leg Reversal. The error in connecting reversally the ECG cables of the RL and LL electrodes does not alter the ECG because potentials recorded from the right and left legs are practically the same. Many such lead reversals are described earlier in this book.

Left Arm–Left Leg Reversal. This error means that lead I on the ECG is actually lead II, and lead III is upside down because the positive and negative poles are reversed. In addition, leads aVL and aVF are reversed. This type of reversal may be difficult to identify because it may not appear out of the ordinary except for left axis deviation, which is common in hospitalized patients. One clue is the appearance of a P wave in "lead I" that is larger in amplitude than in "lead II" (exchanged amplitude of the P waves: P wave in lead I greater than in lead II). The "lead I" P wave actually represents the P wave of the true lead II, which typically has the largest P wave amplitude of any limb lead.

Right Arm–Left Leg Reversal. This reversal causes lead I to be the inverse of lead II, lead II to be the inverse of lead I, and lead II is upside down because the positive and negative poles are reversed.

In addition, aVR and aVF are also reversed. This situation produces highly abnormal-looking limb leads, with leads I, II, III, and aVF being negative and aVR being upright. During sinus rhythm, it is very unlikely to have a QRS axis in the bizarre right superior quadrant of −90° to 180°, which is typical of this type of lead reversal.

Superimposition of Standard ECG Leads with Telemetry Leads

Placing the telemetry electrodes on top of the ECG electrodes or vice versa is a common mistake. This may create a distortion of the ST segment that mimics ST-segment elevation or arrhythmias due to electromagnetic interference of the telemetry system on the ECG machine.

Technically Unacceptable ECG Recordings

Hospitals are filled with equipment that can be a source of electrical artifact. The most common artifacts are caused by skeletal muscle tremor, electrical interference, and electrode movement. Tremor-induced artifact may mimic supraventricular arrhythmias (atrial flutter/atrial fibrillation). If the artifact has sufficient amplitude, it can also mimic ventricular tachycardia and ventricular fibrillation. This abnormality is commonly seen in Parkinson's disease, or when a patient undergoes rewarming from hypothermia. Counting the peaks of the artifact helps determine the periodicity of the muscle tremor. The limb which is moving can be determined from the limb leads of the ECG: the left arm is involved if the artifact is seen in I and aVL; baseline artifact in aVR suggests that the right arm may be twitching.

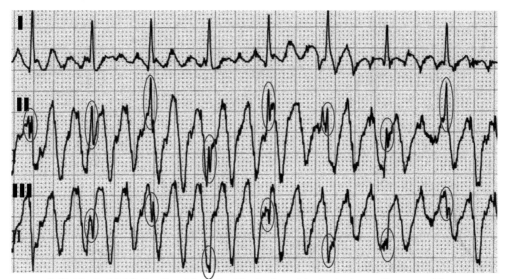

Artifactual atrial flutter (lead I) and artifactual ventricular tachycardia caused by tremor in a patient with Parkinson's disease.

The precordial leads can also show tremor artifact if the pectoral muscles, intercostal muscles, or sternocleidomastoid muscles have tremors. Misinterpretation of tremor-induced artifact may lead to serious medical errors such as the initiation of long-term use of anticoagulants for pseudo-atrial fibrillation. In patients with severe pain or tremor or other cause of an unacceptably noisy ECG signal, the filter switch on the ECG machine can be used after all attempts to eliminate the interference have failed. Temporary displacement of an electrode may cause disappearance of the ECG, simulating sinus arrest, but the finding of attenuated complexes before and after the artificial pause suggests reduced or poor contact followed by reestablishment of electrode function.

ERRORS IN ELECTROCARDIOGRAPHY 2

Baseline wander analysis shows low frequency activity (spectral content usually well below 1 Hz) in the ECG which may result in inaccurate and misleading ECG interpretation. Baseline wander may result from various noise sources including perspiration, respiration, body movements, and poor electrode contact. ST-T changes in the ECG are measured with reference to the isoelectric line. When baseline wander is present the isoelectric line is no longer well defined and hence ST analysis becomes inaccurate.

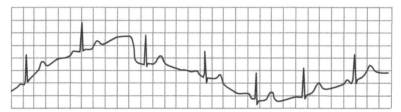

A noisy recording should be evaluated and treated according to the following steps

* Check that the electrode is not dry and contains gel (skin preparation is not needed with integrated gel electrodes which adhere well to the skin and are clean to use)

* Inspect ECG cables for proper connection and make sure they are motionless

* Inspect the cables for breaks

* Tense patients may also cause ECG artifacts

* Make sure the patient feels comfortable and is motionless

* Verify that the filter is set correctly

* Change filter setting (the clinician must ascertain whether filtering has not destroyed the subtle morphology of the ECG signal)

Wrong speed

When the ECG speed used is 50 mm/s instead of 25 mm/s, the tracing shows widened PR and QRS intervals, and the patient's heart does not tally with the ECG heart rate. One must recognize this because the tracings are nearly always unlabeled.

Illustrative example 1

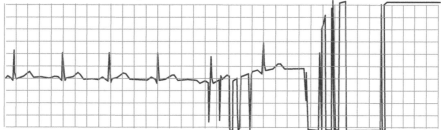

Broken cable with intermittent contact

Illustrative example 2

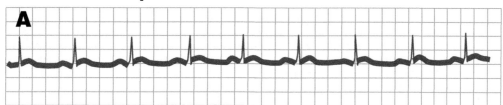

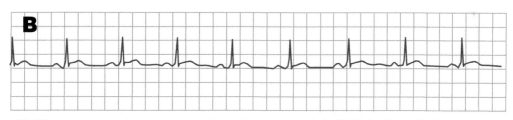

(A) Electromagnetic interference by the mains power supply (60 Hz) without filtering
(B) Same patient in the same situation when the filter was activated

Illustrative example 3

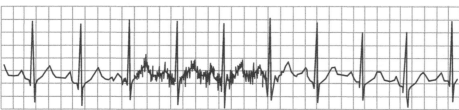

Electromyographic interference

ELECTROCARDIOGRAPHIC MONITORING

Regardless of the monitoring system used, the detection of arrhythmias or ischemia depends on high quality ECG tracings to reduce motion artifacts. Accurate placement of electrodes ensures consistent ECGs available for comparison.

ELECTRODE POSITIONING ON THE TORSO

For bedside cardiac monitoring limb electrodes are placed on the torso to reduce muscle artifact during limb movement. Therefore, the right arm (RA) electrode is placed in the infraclavicular fossa close to the right shoulder, the left arm (LA) electrode is placed in the infraclavicular fossa close to the left shoulder, and the left leg (LL) electrode is placed below the rib cage on the left side of the abdomen. The ground or reference electrode (RL) can be placed anywhere, but it is usually placed on the right side of the abdomen.

BIPOLAR LEADS

The oldest and simplest of all cardiac monitoring lead systems are bipolar leads that record the potential difference between two electrodes. A bipolar system may use leads I, II or III with an indifferent ground electrode. Lead MCL1 (modified chest lead V1) was introduced in 1968. The MCL1 lead is created by placing the positive electrode in the 4th intercostal space to the right of the sternum (left leg electrode) and the negative electrode below the left clavicle near the shoulder (left arm electrode). The ground electrode can be placed anywhere on the body. The monitor is then set to lead III which provides the difference between left leg and left arm electrodes and therefore the difference between V1 and the left arm which is MCL1.

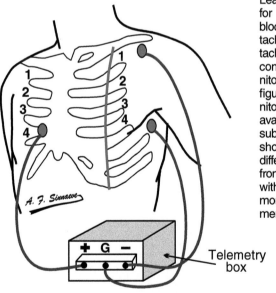

Lead V1 is considered the best bipolar lead for diagnosing right and left bundle branch block, and to distinguish ventricular tachycardia from supraventricular tachycardia with aberrant ventricular conduction. However, standard bipolar monitoring (using standard lead I, II or III configurations) is inadequate for arrhythmia monitoring because a "true" V1 lead is not available with the system. The bipolar substitute for lead V1 (i.e. MCL1) has been shown to be superior to bipolar leads and differs (by being more diagnostically useful) from bipolar recordings in 40% of patients with ventricular tachycardia. Bipolar lead monitoring also is inadequate for ST-segment monitoring.

Simple 3-electrode bipolar lead system showing electrode placement for recording single MCL1 lead. Positive electrode placed in V1 location and negative electrode placed in left infraclavicular fossa. Reference (ground) electrode shown here in V6 location; however, it can be placed in any convenient position.

COMMON 5-ELECTRODE SYSTEM: LIMB LEADS plus 1 PRECORDIAL LEAD COMBINATION

A commonly used lead system uses 5 electrodes. The 4 limb electrodes are placed in the LA, RA, LL, and RL positions on the torso (at the junction of each limb) so that any of the 6 limb leads can be obtained (leads I, II, III, aVR, aVL, aVF). This is far more convenient than applying wrist electrodes and it prevents loose or moving electrodes that add noise to the system. A fifth chest electrode can be placed in any of the standard V1 to V6 locations, but in general V1 is selected because of its value in arrhythmia monitoring. Cardiac monitors with this lead system often have 2 channels for ECG display so that 1 limb lead and 1 precordial lead can be displayed simultaneously. This 5-electrode lead system allows the recording of a true V1 lead, and prevents the inaccuracy associated with MCL1 monitoring.

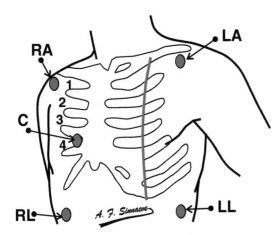

Commonly used 5-electrode lead system that allows for recording any of the 6 limb leads plus 1 precordial (V) lead. Shown here is lead placement for recording V1. A limitation of this system is that only 1 precordial lead can be recorded.

An advantage of this 5-electrode lead system is that it allows the recording of a true V1 lead, and this prevents the inaccuracy that comes from monitoring with MCL1. A limitation of this lead system is that more than one V-lead cannot be recorded simultaneously. Often, more than one V-lead is indicated. For example, although V1 is an excellent lead for diagnosing arrhythmias with a wide QRS complex (bundle branch blocks, ventricular pacemaker rhythms, and wide QRS tachycardias), it is insensitive for detecting acute myocardial ischemia.

REDUCED LEAD ECG

The use of conventional 12-lead ECG using 10 electrodes for continuous monitoring is cumbersome and impractical. Reduced lead set technology derives 12 ECG leads from a smaller number of leads/electrodes, usually 5 or 6. Several systems are commercially available. Starting with lead Is and II, the remaining 4 limb leads can be calculated accurately from these leads. A synthesized 12-lead ECG that is similar but not identical to the standard 12-lead ECG can be derived. Derived 12-lead ECG deserves serious consideration as an alternative monitoring system because of its good correlation with the standard ECG. There are few circumstances that justify the use of reduced lead 12-lead ECGs; the convenience should be weighed by the risk of misdiagnosis resulting from serial comparison of nonequivalent standard 12-lead ECGs. The lack of standardization of the available systems remains a problem.

COMPUTERIZED ELECTROCARDIOGRAPHY

Computer-based rhythm interpretation - a standard feature of most modern ECG machines - is sometimes inaccurate, and without physician intervention, such errors could lead to wrong diagnosis. The first published reports on computerized ECG analysis emerged in the early 1960s. The familiar lead configuration (I-II-III, aVR-aVL-aVF, V1-V2-V3-V4-V5-V6) was introduced in 1972. The development of signal filtering in the 1960-1970s was a crucial step in advancing computerized ECG analysis.

Computerized ECG analysis can be divided into three distinct stages: (1) signal processing, (2) measurements, and (3) interpretation. In the first stage, electrical data are acquired and converted from analog to digital signals. The signal is then filtered to eliminate noise. Data compression, transmission, and archiving are additional important aspects of digital processing. In the second stage, the processed signal undergoes wave recognition. In the final stage, the measured parameters are subjected to multiple criteria in order to arrive at the computer diagnosis.

Computerized ECG interpretation utilizes algorithms that rely on diagnostic criteria constructed by human experts. These criteria, in turn, are either met or not met, and do not allow for gradations. The inability to know the specific details of the computer algorithms represents industry-driven technology. The many logic systems for ECG interpretation have become proprietary information of manufacturers.

Although some computer programs are clearly inferior to the interpretation of cardiologists, others are comparably accurate. There is usually a disagreement rate of 10–15% when ECGs are evaluated by a computer vs. cardiologists. Of particular concern is that of the inaccurate interpretations: 25% may not be corrected by the ordering physician and 10% may receive inappropriate therapy that may include initiation of anticoagulation therapy and hospitalization.

Many junior health care workers during training are advised to fold over the computer reading at the top of the ECG tracing so it cannot influence their interpretation. Although this is done partly so that they can practice their own interpretive skills, there is also general mistrust of the computer reading. Because computerized ECG analysis is seldom reviewed during medical training, most physicians do not gain a sense of how reliable the computer reading is unless they become ECG readers.

Computerized ECG analysis should be an adjunct to, not a substitute for, physician interpretation. All computerized ECGs should be overread by an expert electrocardiographer. A certain level of interpretive skill is needed by physicians overreading the ECG if they are expected to recognize misinterpretations by the computer. A firm understanding of the strengths and limitations of computer analysis is necessary if one is to use this diagnostic tool effectively.

Strengths of computerized ECG analysis

One of the most obvious advantages of computer analysis is the automated measurement of key parameters such as heart rate, PR interval, QRS duration, and QT interval. Calculation of the corrected QT interval and axes are also performed automatically. The QT interval is the most difficult measurement because of a lack of agreement in the way T-wave offset is determined; additional errors are made if TU waves are present. For this reason, when serial QT or QTU intervals are being monitored during antiarrhythmic drug therapy, it is not sufficient to follow the computerized measurement without verifying the intervals manually in multiple ECG leads.

Computerized ECGs are useful for saving time for simple tasks such as reading normal tracings that constitute about 40% of ECGs in a hospital setting. There is also a theoretical benefit to rural physicians.

Clinical value and limitations

The more straightforward diagnoses appear to be better detected by the computer, and most time is saved when the ECGs are simple (normal) but tedious to read. Many ECG readers claim that a computer interpretation of "normal ECG" is often, but not always, correct. The computer has a high sensitivity of 99%, but somewhat lower specificity of 90% in diagnosing sinus rhythm. Because the prevalence of sinus rhythm is high, the 99% positive predictive value of a computer diagnosis of "sinus rhythm" supports the belief that a computer statement of "sinus rhythm" is generally reliable.

The most frequent errors in computer ECG interpretation are related to arrhythmias, conduction disorders, and electronic pacemakers. The computerized ECG functions poorly with an error of 30–50% in the diagnosis of non-sinus rhythms. An erroneous computer interpretation of "sinus rhythm" may occur in 10% of non-sinus rhythms. Multifocal atrial tachycardia is often misdiagnosed as atrial fibrillation. The difficulty in diagnosing atrial fibrillation is one of the most commonly encountered arrhythmia problems with computerized ECG. Lead artifacts degrade the diagnostic ability of a computerized system. The interpretation of pacemaker rhythm remains problematic. Finally and most important, the computer readout rarely gives the physician a differential diagnosis indicating the probability that certain types of heart disease are present. This is what the clinician needs.

Example of measurements needed for computer diagnosis

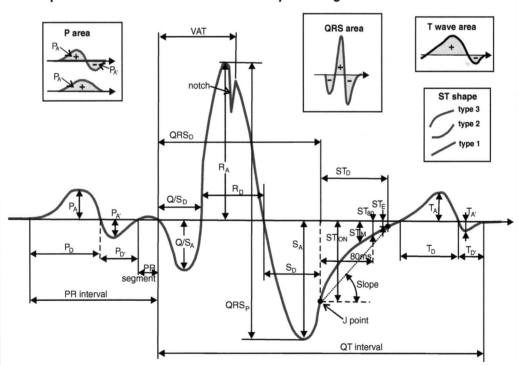

The time axis has been expanded during the QRS complex.
Meaning of the subscripts : A : amplitude ; D : duration ; P : peak-to-peak ; ON : onset ; M : midpoint ; E : endpoint.
The J point is defined as the point where the slope changes from concave to convex.
Surface areas are calculated by integration.

OTHER SITES OF ECG RECORDING 1

The standard ECG includes right precordial leads for the diagnosis of right ventricular infarction and leads V7 to V9 for the diagnosis of posterior infarction. These recording sites are part of the traditional ECG. However, recording the ECG away from the traditional sites may sometimes provide important diagnostic information.

Right-sided precordial leads at a higher or lower intercostal space

1. *Left anterior hemiblock.* Small sharp q waves that simulate an old anteroseptal myocardial infarction (ASMI) are sometimes seen in V2 and V3 at the normal level and in many cases if these leads are placed in a higher position. The q waves related to left anterior hemiblock disappear by recording V2 and V3 one interspace lower. In contrast the pattern of a true ASMI will remain. The small q waves of left anterior hemiblock correspond to the initial QRS forces directed inferiorly and to the right.

2. **Brugada syndrome.** The typical ST elevation in the right precordial leads may become evident or more obvious by displacing the right precordial leads 1 or 2 interspaces higher.

3. **Right ventricular apical pacing.** A dominant R wave in V1 placed at the correct site may occur in 10–15% cases of uncomplicated pacing. This pattern is more common if V1 is recorded 1 or 2 intercostal spaces higher. If the pacing lead is in the right ventricle, the dominant R wave in V1 will change to a negative QRS complex when V1 is recorded one interspace lower (5th intercostal space).

Lewis lead

The Lewis lead configuration can help to detect atrial activity and its relationship to ventricular activity. A Lewis lead is a special bipolar chest lead with the right arm electrode applied to the right side of the sternum at the second intercostal space and the left arm electrode applied to the fourth intercostal space adjacent to the sternum. The recording can be seen in lead I. The arrangement is roughly perpendicular to the wave of atrial depolarization. Calibration should be adjusted to 1 mV = 20 mm. This technique was described by Sir Thomas Lewis (1881–1945) to magnify atrial deflections originally focusing on atrial fibrillation. The Lewis lead is simple to use and is useful in the diagnosis of atrial flutter and complex or wide QRS tachycardias by enhancing atrial activity.

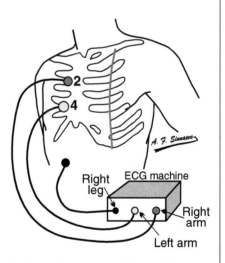

Esophageal recordings

The concept of esophageal ECG is not new; numerous studies have demonstrated its usefulness in the diagnosis of complex arrhythmias. The close proximity of the esophageal electrodes to the posterior atrium and the left ventricle provides larger signals, resulting in larger P waves as well as an amplified QRS complex. Because the atrium is behind the ventricles relative to the chest wall, P waves are often obscured by ventricular electrical activity in surface ECG recordings. Esophageal ECG monitoring helps the diagnosis of cardiac arrhythmias for which a clearly identifiable P wave is essential. To observe a bipolar esophageal ECG, the electrodes are connected to the right and left arm terminals of the monitor and lead I is selected. A prominent P wave is usually displayed in the presence of atrial depolarization, and its relation to the ventricular electrical activity can be examined. A variety of electrode catheters are available as well as a pill or capsule electrode to swallow.

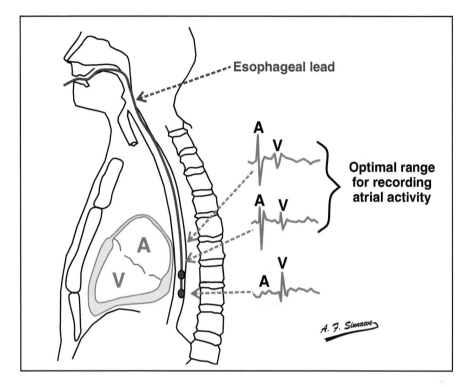

Esophageal lead

A V

Optimal range for recording atrial activity

A V

A V

A. F. Sinnaeve

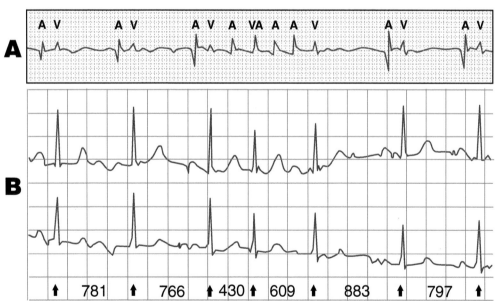

A   A V   A V   A V   A V A A A A V   A V   A V

B   ↑   781   ↑   766   ↑ 430 ↑ 609 ↑   883   ↑   797   ↑

(A): Esophageal ECG with atrial and ventricular activity
A = atrial deflection; V = QRS complex
(B): Synchronized surface ECG in same patient as (A)
Vertical arrows point to the QRS complexes
Note the run of 4 atrial beats which is not seen on the surface ECG.

OTHER SITES OF ECG RECORDING 2

His bundle recordings

The diagram represents the atrioventricular conduction system. The bundle branch system consists of a three-pronged system (2 on the left side and 1 on the right side). At the right side, the surface ECG is depicted simultaneously with a His bundle electrogram (HBE). The HBE is recorded near the septal leaflet of the tricuspid valve. A : reflects depolarization of the low atrium ; H : depolarization of the His bundle ; and V : depolarization of the upper ventricular septum. The AH interval reflects AV nodal conduction (normally 40–140 ms in adults), and the HV interval reflects conduction within the His-Purkinje system. The normal HV interval is 35–55 ms. A prolonged HV interval indicates delayed conduction in all three prongs of the conduction system and/or the His bundle. With His-Purkinje disease the HV interval (but not the surface QRS complex) can either be normal or prolonged as long as one of the three prongs conducts normally.

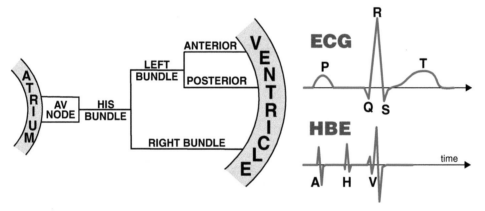

A recording catheter is inserted percutaneously into the right femoral vein and advanced fluoroscopically into the right atrium. The catheter is then manipulated to the area of the septal leaflet of the tricuspid valve where His bundle depolarization can be recorded. Right atrial pacing results in progressive lengthening of the AH interval with increasing frequency but the HV interval remains constant at all rates. The His bundle deflection is validated by showing an increase in the AH interval with an increasing rate of atrial pacing. The technique is simple, reliable and reproducible. The His bundle potential is recorded at a speed of 100 mm/s and simultaneously with 3 surface ECG leads. The "V" point represents the earliest ventricular activation from the surface or intracardiac leads. The recording of His bundle activation of the surface ECG is possible but technically difficult (signal averaging) so that the noninvasive approach is not used clinically.

The introduction of His bundle recordings has revolutionized the field of cardiac arrhythmias and clinical electrophysiology. It is now possible to ablate (destroy) the His bundle by the same approach using radiofrequency energy. Such a procedure is used to induce complete AV block in patients with atrial fibrillation and rapid ventricular rates unresponsive to drug therapy. The AV block is then treated with a permanent pacemaker. More recently pacing techniques have been developed to permanently pace the His bundle or the adjacent parahisian sites with the aim of providing a more physiologic left ventricular activation than standard right ventricular pacing.

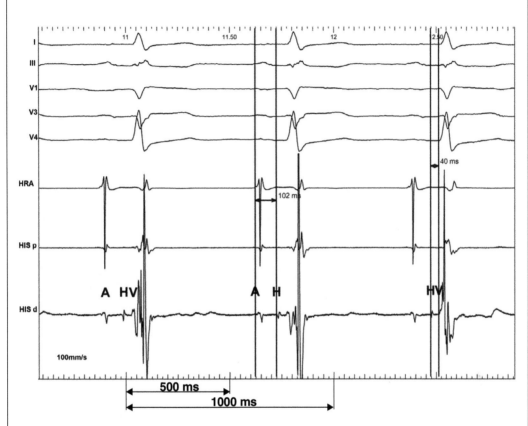

His bundle recording.
Surface ECG leads : I, III, V1, V3, V4.
Intracardiac recordings : HRA = high right atrium recording; HISp = proximal His recording;
HISd = distal His recording.
A = atrial deflection; H = His bundle deflection; V = ventricular deflection; AH interval = 102
ms; HV interval = 40 ms.
His bundle recordings permit a breakdown of the surface PR interval into its 3 components:
(1) The PA interval : the interval from the onset of the P wave in the surface electrocardiogram
to the first atrial deflection (A wave) in the His bundle electrogram. It represents the intra-
atrial conduction time and has little clinical value.
(2) The AV nodal conduction time (AH interval).
(3) The His-Purkinje system conduction time (HV interval).

Illustrative example of His bundle recording

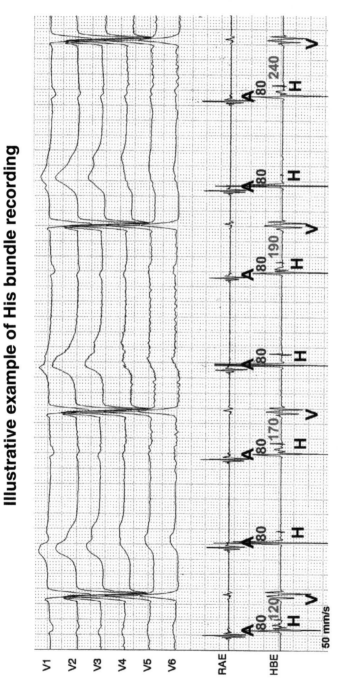

Surface ECG leads V1 to V6 and intracardiac recordings.
The atrial rate is 96 bpm while the ventricular rate is 48 bpm. The ECG shows a 2:1 AV block with a progressive prolongation of the PR intervals of the conducted beats.
*The AH interval is constant at 80 ms. Every alternate beat is blocked after inscription of a His deflection (**infra-hisian block**). There is a progressive prolongation of the HV interval in the distal Purkinje conduction system.*
Abbreviations: RAE = right atrial electrogram; HBE = His bundle electrogram; A = atrial deflection; H = His bundle deflection; V = ventricular deflection.

Baranchuk A, Kang J. Pseudo-atrial flutter: Parkinson tremor. Cardiol J. 2009;16:373-4.

Batchvarov VN, Malik M, Camm AJ. Incorrect electrode cable connection during electrocardiographic recording. Europace. 2007;9:1081-90.

García-Niebla J, Llontop-García P, Valle-Racero JI, Serra-Autonell G, Batchvarov VN, de Luna AB. Technical mistakes during the acquisition of the electrocardiogram. Ann Noninvasive Electrocardiol. 2009;14:389-403.

Hongo RH, Goldschlager N. Status of computerized electrocardiography. Cardiol Clin. 2006;24:491-504.

Kligfield P, Gettes LS, Bailey JJ, Childers R, Deal BJ, Hancock EW, van Herpen G, Kors JA, Macfarlane P, Mirvis DM, Pahlm O, Rautaharju P, Wagner GS, Josephson M, Mason JW, Okin P, Surawicz B, Wellens H; American Heart Association Electrocardiography and Arrhythmias Committee, Council on Clinical Cardiology; American College of Cardiology Foundation; Heart Rhythm Society. Recommendations for the standardization and interpretation of the electrocardiogram: part I: the electrocardiogram and its technology a scientific statement from the American Heart Association Electrocardiography and Arrhythmias Committee, Council on Clinical Cardiology; the American College of Cardiology Foundation; and the Heart Rhythm Society endorsed by the International Society for Computerized Electrocardiology. J Am Coll Cardiol. 2007;49:1109-27.

Knight BP, Pelosi F, Michaud GF, Strickberger SA, Morady F. Physician interpretation of electrocardiographic artifact that mimics ventricular tachycardia. Am J Med. 2001;110:335-8.

Mason JW, Hancock EW, Gettes LS, Bailey JJ, Childers R, Deal BJ, Josephson M, Kligfield P, Kors JA, Macfarlane P, Pahlm O, Mirvis DM, Okin P, Rautaharju P, Surawicz B, van Herpen G, Wagner GS, Wellens H; American Heart Association Electrocardiography and Arrhythmias Committee, Council on Clinical Cardiology; American College of Cardiology Foundation; Heart Rhythm Society. Recommendations for the standardization and interpretation of the electrocardiogram: part II: electrocardiography diagnostic statement list a scientific statement from the American Heart Association Electrocardiography and Arrhythmias Committee, Council on Clinical Cardiology; the American College of Cardiology Foundation; and the Heart Rhythm Society Endorsed by the International Society for Computerized Electrocardiology. J Am Coll Cardiol. 2007;49:1128-35.

Rudiger A, Hellermann JP, Mukherjee R, Follath F, Turina J. Electrocardiographic artifacts due to electrode misplacement and their frequency in different clinical settings. Am J Emerg Med. 2007;25:174-8.

CHAPTER 23

HOW TO READ
AN ECG

ECG from Basics to Essentials: Step by Step. First Edition. Roland X. Stroobandt, S. Serge Barold and Alfons F. Sinnaeve.
Published 2016 © 2016 by John Wiley & Sons, Ltd. Companion Website: www.wiley.com/go/stroobandt/ecg

HOW TO READ AN ECG 1

STEP 1: Clinical history

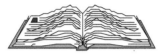

* Verify brief history
* Compare tracing with old records (if available)
* First look: "lay of the land"

STEP 2: Technical quality and calibration

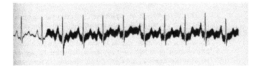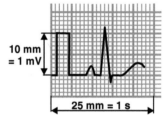

10 mm = 1 mV

25 mm = 1 s

* Check technical quality
* Check paper speed (25 mm/s ?)
* Check calibration (10 mm/mV ?)

STEP 3: Rate

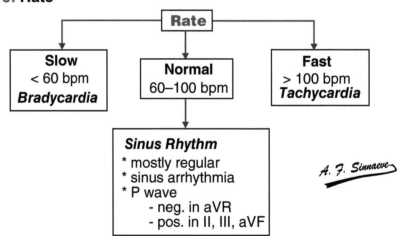

Rate

Slow
< 60 bpm
Bradycardia

Normal
60–100 bpm

Fast
> 100 bpm
Tachycardia

Sinus Rhythm
* mostly regular
* sinus arrhythmia
* P wave
  - neg. in aVR
  - pos. in II, III, aVF

A. F. Sinnaeve

if P wave is not upright in lead II consider
    * arm lead reversal (P, QRS & T wave neg. in lead I)
    * dextrocardia

STEP 4: Rhythm diagnosis

> * Rhythm regular or irregular? AFib (irregular), AFl (occasionally irregular), AV block (irregular with partial AV block)
> * P waves present or absent?
> * QRS narrow or wide?
> * rate P: rate QRS relation? (rate P = rate QRS, rate P > rate QRS, rate QRS > rate P)

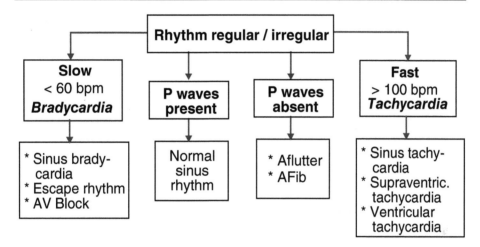

Rhythm regular / irregular

Slow
< 60 bpm
Bradycardia

P waves present

P waves absent

Fast
> 100 bpm
Tachycardia

* Sinus brady-cardia
* Escape rhythm
* AV Block

Normal sinus rhythm

* Aflutter
* AFib

* Sinus tachy-cardia
* Supraventric. tachycardia
* Ventricular tachycardia

STEP 5: Determine QRS axis in frontal plane

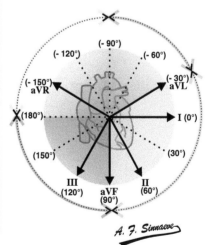

Lead I	Lead III (or aVF)	Quick and easy way	
pos.	pos.	normal axis (−30° to +90°)	
pos.	neg.	**Look at lead II**	
		lead II neg.	left axis deviation
		lead II equiphasic (R = S)	axis −30°
		lead II pos.	normal axis
neg.	pos.	right axis deviation (+90° to +180°)	
neg.	neg.	right superior "no mans land" (−90° to −180°)	

A. F. Sinnaeve

LAH : rS in Lead II and aVF and Lead III
LPH : rS in Lead I and aVL

Abbreviations: AFib: atrial fibrillation; AFl: atrial flutter; pos: positive; neg: negative; LAH: left anterior hemiblock; LPH: left posterior hemiblock

HOW TO READ AN ECG 2

STEP 6A: Measurement of PR interval

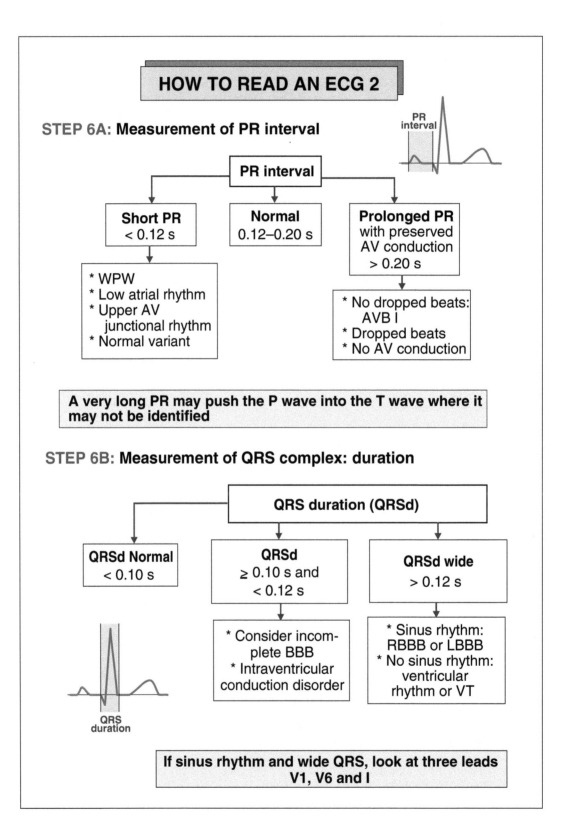

PR interval

| **Short PR** < 0.12 s | **Normal** 0.12–0.20 s | **Prolonged PR** with preserved AV conduction > 0.20 s |

Short PR < 0.12 s
* WPW
* Low atrial rhythm
* Upper AV junctional rhythm
* Normal variant

Prolonged PR with preserved AV conduction > 0.20 s
* No dropped beats: AVB I
* Dropped beats
* No AV conduction

A very long PR may push the P wave into the T wave where it may not be identified

STEP 6B: Measurement of QRS complex: duration

QRS duration (QRSd)

QRSd Normal < 0.10 s

QRSd ≥ 0.10 s and < 0.12 s
* Consider incomplete BBB
* Intraventricular conduction disorder

QRSd wide > 0.12 s
* Sinus rhythm: RBBB or LBBB
* No sinus rhythm: ventricular rhythm or VT

QRS duration

If sinus rhythm and wide QRS, look at three leads V1, V6 and I

STEP 6C: Measurement of QRS complex: voltage

QRS voltage

High QRS voltage
SV1 + RV6 > 35 mm
R in I > 15 mm
R > aVL > 11 mm

Low QRS voltage
Amplitude of all QRS complexes in limb leads < 5 mm or < 10 mm in the precordial leads

LVH

Exclude:
* Ventricular pacing (look for pacemaker stimuli)
* Hyperkalemia (if prolonged QRS)
* Look for delta wave (WPW)

The absence of LVH on ECG means nothing, if present LVH is likely.

* Pericardial effusion (triad of low voltage, tachycardia, electrical alternans)
* Pleural effusion
* Emphysema (COPD)
* Pneumothorax
* Marked obesity
* Previous massive MI
* End-stage dilated cardio-myopathy
* Hypothyroidism
* Infiltrative myocardial disease

COPD: chronic obstructive pulmonary disease; MI: myocardial infarction; LVH: left ventricular hypertrophy

Thin people, athletes, and young adults frequently show tall QRS voltage without LVH

STEP 7A: Look at R wave progression in precordial leads

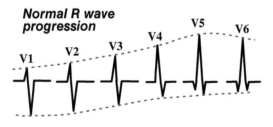

Normal R wave progression

Slow R wave progression

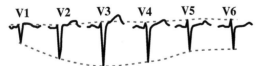

Causes of slow R wave progression:
* Anterior myocardial infarction
* Incorrect lead placement (in obese women)
* LVH, * LBBB, * WPW
* Dextrocardia
* Tension pneumothorax with mediastinal shift
* Congenital heart disease

LVH: left ventricular hypertrophy; LBBB: left bundle branch block; WPW: Wolff-Parkinson-White

HOW TO READ AN ECG 3

STEP 7B: Look at R wave progression in precordial leads

Reversed R wave progression

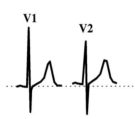

This describes abnormal R waves in lead V1 that progressively decrease in amplitude if the QRS is narrow. This pattern may occur with a number of conditions, including RVH, posterior (or posterolateral) MI, dextrocardia (in concert with a limb lead reversal pattern), misplaced leads and rarely as a normal variant. If the QRS is wide, a dominant R wave in V1 may be caused by RBBB or WPW.

MI: myocardial infarction; RBBB: right bundle branch block; WPW: Wolff-Parkinson-White syndrome; RVH: right ventricular hypertrophy;

STEP 8: QT Interval

QTc = corrected QT interval

$$QTc\ (s) = \frac{QT\ interval\ (s)}{\sqrt{RR\ interval\ (s)}}$$

Normal QTc ≤ 440 ms

slightly larger values are acceptable in women

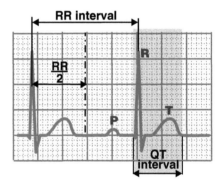

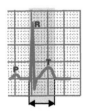

Short QTc ≤ 330 ms
Increased risk of AF & VF

Long QTc ≥ 460 ms
If QTc ≥ 500 ms : high risk for EAD & TdP (after short-long-short sequence)

Causes
* Congenital (requires family history)
* Acquired
    - drug toxicity
    - electrolyte imbalance

Abbreviations
EAD = early afterdepolarization
TdP = torsades de pointes
AF = atrial fibrillation
VF = ventricular fibrillation

The QT interval is a measure of ventricular action potential duration. It decreases when the heart rate increases.

STEP 9: U wave

* small deflection (0.5 mm), immediately following the T wave
* usually same polarity as T wave
* possibly originating from Purkinje network
* best seen in lead V2 and V3 and during slow rate

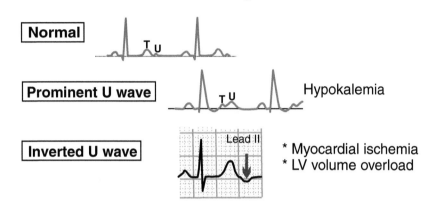

| Normal |

| Prominent U wave | Hypokalemia

| Inverted U wave | Lead II
* Myocardial ischemia
* LV volume overload

STEP 10: P wave

P waves are best seen in lead II and V1

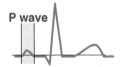
P wave

Normal P wave * lead II ≤ 0.12 s and < 2.5 mm
* lead V1 biphasic

P wave too wide
Lead II ≥ 0.12 s & notched
Prominent negative terminal forces in lead V1

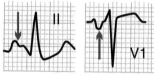
LA abnormality

P wave too tall
P peaked in lead II
P > 2.5 mm in inferior leads
P > 1.5 mm in lead V1

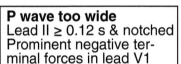
RA abnormality

P wave negative
in inferior leads
(II, III, aVF)

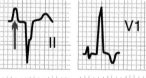
Retrograde P wave ?
Ectopic beat ?

A. F. Sinnaeve

P wave funny

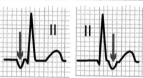
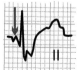
Ectopic beat ?

HOW TO READ AN ECG 4

STEP 11: T wave

Normal T wave
* T wave same polarity as main QRS deflection
* T wave is upright in I, II, V3 to V6
* T wave always inverted in aVR

T wave inversion in V1 to V3
* Common finding in children and adolescents
* Infrequently found in healthy adults
    Is not associated with adverse outcome if T waves are normal in other leads

High amplitude T waves		* Hyperacute T wave - *may be seen 5–30 min after onset of MI* - *broad-based T wave* - *round summit*
		* Hyperkalemia (best seen in precordial leads) - *narrow-based T wave* - *tenting of T wave*

Abnormal T waves

Inverted T waves    **Biphasic T waves**    **Flattened T waves**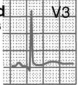

Camel hump T waves

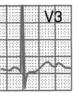

Severe hypokalemia

prominent U wave fused to end of the T wave

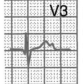

Hidden P waves
embedded in T wave
- *sinus tachycardia*
- *various types of heart block*

STEP 12: ST segment

* *The typical ST segment duration is usually around 0.08 s (80 ms).*
* *Usually flat and isoelectric and should essentially level with PR and TP segments.*
* *The ventricles remain depolarized during the ST segment.*
* *It is usually difficult to determine exactly where the ST segment ends and the T wave begins. Therefore the relationship between ST segment and T wave should be evaluated together.*

QRS complex

ST segment

T wave

Junction or "J" point

0 mV

Action potential

- 90 mV

depolarization

repolarization

A. J. Sinnaeve

The most important cause of ST segment abnormality (elevation or depression) is myocardial ischemia or infarction.

> The diagnosis of AMI and severe ischemia depend on the careful assessment of the ST segment.

AMI: acute myocardial infarction

ST segment depression

* Ischemia (**most common**)
* Subendocardial infarction
* Reciprocal changes associated with AMI
* Drug effects

ischemia or early MI   **digitalis effects**

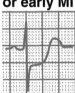

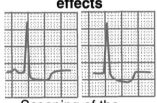

Scooping of the ST segment

ST segment elevation

* AMI (*convex ST segment elevation*)
* Transmural ischemia
* Ventricular aneurysm (*ST elevation does not subside after AMI*)
* Pericarditis

AMI   **pericarditis**

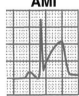

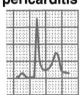

Abbreviations
  MI : myocardial infarction
  AMI: acute myocardial infarction

HOW TO READ AN ECG 5

STEP 13: ST elevation MI (STEMI)

ECG diagnosis of STEMI
* Limb leads: ST segment elevation ≥ 1 mm (0.1 mV)
* Precordial leads: ST segment elevation ≥ 2 mm (0.2 mV)
* Elevations must be present in anatomically contiguous leads

Inferior	Lateral	Septal	Anterior
II, III, aVF	I, aVL, V5, V6	V1, V2	V3, V4

* An approximation of the infarction size can be assessed from the extent of ST elevation.
* *Of note: Over 90% of healthy men have at least 1 mm (0.1 mV) of ST segment elevation in at least one precordial lead.*

Look for reciprocal changes of ST depression in leads opposite the area undergoing injury

---

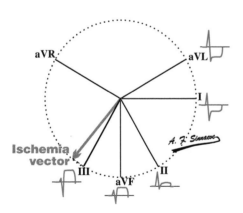

For example in acute transmural inferior ischemia, the direction of the ST vector faces the injured area (resulting in a ST elevation in leads II, III, aVF) while the tail of the ST vector faces anatomically opposite sites where it causes ST segment depression (lead aVL and lead I).

The significance of these reciprocal changes or mirror-images is unclear but they are useful diagnostically by providing confirmatory evidence for the diagnosis of STEMI.

Mirror-image changes do not occur in pericarditis

An acute STEMI can present with upwardly concave ST elevation, so the mere fact that ST elevation is upwardly concave does NOT mean that a condition other than ischemia is present.

ST elevation due to ischemia or infarction: Focus on contiguous leads and those showing reciprocal changes!

One must be well versed in recognizing the so-called ECG mimics of acute myocardial infarction. The development of reciprocal changes during STEMI helps the differentiation from the listed conditions:

ECG mimics of AMI:
* Left ventricular hypertrophy (LVH)
* Left bundle branch block (LBBB)
* Paced rhythm
* Early repolarization
* Pericarditis
* Hyperkalemia
* Ventricular aneurysm

LVH   **LVH**   **LBBB**   **Paced Rhythm**   **Ventricular aneurysm**

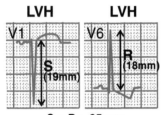

S + R > 35mm

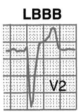

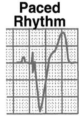

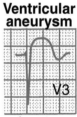

long-term changes

Evolution of STEMI

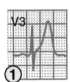

① Sometimes the earliest presentation of AMI is the hyperacute T wave, which is treated the same as ST elevation. In practice this is rarely seen

② In the first few hours the ST segments usually begin to rise

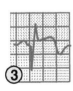

③ Pathologic Q waves may appear within hours or may take more than 24 hr. The T wave will generally become inverted in the first 24 hr, as ST elevation begins to resolve

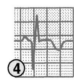

④ Long-term changes of ECG include persistent Q waves (in 90% of cases) and persistent inverted T waves

A. F. Sinnaeve

Note :  Persistent ST elevation is rare except in the presence of a ventricular aneurysm

- -

Abbreviation: *AMI: acute myocardial infarction*

HOW TO READ AN ECG 6

STEP 14: Non-ST elevation MI (NSTEMI)

* The ECG sign of non-STEMI is ST segment depression
* ST segment depression seen in subendocardial ischemia or infarction can take on different patterns. The most typical is a horizontal or downsloping depression (A, B, C). Upsloping ST depression (D) is less specific.

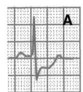 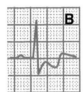 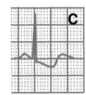 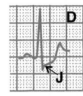 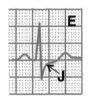

* Upsloping depression of less than 1 mm at 80 ms beyond the J point (E) is simply J point depression and not ST segment depression.

> The label of nonspecific ST-T wave abnormalities is somewhat vague but it does not mean it's not important.

* Depression is reversible if ischemia is only transient but depression persists if ischemia is severe enough to produce infarction.
* T wave inversion with or without ST segment depression is sometimes seen but not ST segment elevation or new Q waves.
* The nonspecific ST-T wave changes should be evaluated with old ECGs because myocardial ischemia is not a static process.

GUIDELINES

ECG manifestations of acute myocardial ischemia (in absence of LVH and LBBB) according to ESC/ACC/AHA (2012 definitions)
1. ST Elevation New ST elevation at the J point in 2 contiguous leads with the following cut-points: **Age and gender specific !** * ≥ 0.1 mV in all leads except leads V2-V3 in men and women * in leads V2-V3: ≥ 0.2 mV in men ≥ 40 years and   ≥ 0.25 mV in men < 40 years * in leads V2-V3: ≥ 0.15 mV in women

2. ST Depression and T wave changes
 * New horizontal or down-sloping ST segment depression
    ≥ 0.05 mV in 2 contiguous leads
 * and/or T wave inversion ≥ 0.1 mV in 2 contiguous leads with
    prominent R wave or R/S ratio > 1

STEP 15: Additional information

Early Q waves

* In the chronic phase of myocardial infarction, Q waves are regarded as a sign of irreversible necrosis.
   ° *However, about 50% of patients presenting within 1 hour of onset of ST elevation acute coronary syndrome already have Q waves in the leads with ST elevation, especially in the anterior leads.*
   ° *These Q waves may be transient and not necessarily represent irreversible damage.*
   ° *They may represent transient loss of electrical activity in the region at risk ("myocardial concussion").*
* Thus, Q waves on presentation may reflect either irreversible damage and/or a large ischemic zone.

Do not overlook RV infarction

* Request right-sided leads for the diagnosis of right ventricular (RV) myocardial infarction (MI) if ECGs show acute inferior MI, anterio-lateral and posterior MI.
* The 12-lead ECG may suggest RV MI if the magnitude of ST elevation in V1 > the magnitude of ST elevation in V2.
* The combination of ST elevation in V1 and ST depression in V2 is highly specific for right ventricular MI.

Abnormal Q waves

* In the acute phase of myocardial infarction, ST elevation is the key to the diagnosis and therapy.
* The presence of Q waves is far less important for diagnosis and treatment. Indeed, the early diagnosis does not depend on Q waves.

Definition of significant q/Q wave in myocardial infarction (MI). ECG changes associated with prior MI according to ESC/ACC and AHA (2012 definitions)

* Any Q wave in leads V2-V3 ≥ 0.02 s (20 ms) or QS complex
or
* Q wave ≥ 0.03 s (30 ms) and ≥ 0.1 mV deep
   or QS complex in leads I, II, aVL, aVF or in V4-V6
   or in any 2 contiguous lead grouping (I, aVL, V1-V6, II, III, aVF)
or
* R wave ≥ 0.04 s (40ms) in V1-V2 and R/S ≥ 1 with concordant positive T wave (in absence of conduction defect)

Abbreviations: LVH: left ventricular hypertrophy; LBBB: left bundle branch block MI: myocardial infarction

HOW TO READ AN ECG 7

STEP 16: Early repolarization

Early repolarization (ER) is defined as J point elevation with the terminal QRS showing either:
  * notching (a positive deflection on terminal QRS complex) or
  * slurring (on the downslope portion of the QRS complex)

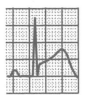 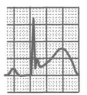 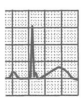 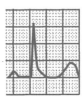

Various patterns of early repolarization

The changes tend to disappear with tachycardia.

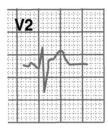

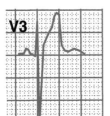

Early repolarization has recently been subject to much research because of the association of sudden death and malignant arrhythmias in patients with certain specific ECG features.

The common form of early repolarization with a high ST take-off in the right precordial leads is considered benign and common, especially in athletes.

  * There is a typical concave upward ST segment elevation (1–4 mm), prominent symmetrical T waves and absence of reciprocal ST depression.

  * These features are present in at least two conti-guous leads.

  * It is generally a benign entity commonly seen in young men. The characteristics of ER may persist for many years. It is important to discern ER from ST segment elevation due to other causes such as ischemia.

Cardiac ischemia is a dynamic process with a changing ECG while the ECG of ER generally remains stable. A changing ECG favors ischemia.

Inferolateral Early Repolarization (ER)

Inferolateral ER is characterized by a deflection in the R wave descent (slurred pattern) or a positive deflection with a secondary "r" (notching pattern) in the terminal part of the QRS complex in at least two inferior leads (II, III, aVF), in two lateral leads (I, aVL, V4 to V6) or in both.

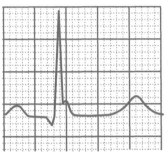

After Junttila MJ et al. European Heart Journal 2012; 33 : 2639

* A pattern of > 0.2 mV in two inferior (II, III, aVF) leads has been shown to impart a higher risk of malignant arrhythmia and sudden death.

* Early repolarization > 1 mV of horizontal or descending ST segment also carries a higher risk of sudden death.

* The management of asymptomatic patients with high risk ECG forms of early repolarization is unresolved.

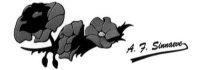

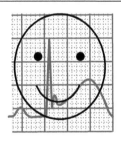

A Smiley face with concave ST segment elevation is showing a happy face because a concave form may be benign as in early repolarization.

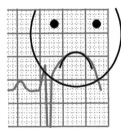

Convex ST elevation superimposed on a face as before, produces a frowny sad face because of the poor prognosis (because of acute myocardial infarction).

HOW TO READ AN ECG 8

STEP 17: Congestive heart failure

As congestive heart failure (CHF) is the outcome of many pathophysiologic disorders, the ECG may show a large variety of abnormalities. Occasionally the ECG is normal. However, CHF is unlikely if the ECG is entirely normal. In other words, a normal ECG does not rule out CHF.

The ECG abnormalities in CHF may be seen in many disorders. They consist of left ventricular hypertrophy, atrial and ventricular arrhythmias, atrioventricular and intraventricular conduction abnormalities, evidence of myocardial ischemia and infarction, right ventricular hypertrophy and atrial abnormalities.

No specific ECG feature is indicative of heart failure

Atrial fibrillation is present in 25% of patients with cardiomyopathy, especially elderly patients with severe heart failure. The prognosis is worse for patients with atrial fibrillation, ventricular tachycardia, or left bundle branch block. The presence of left bundle branch block with right axis deviation almost always indicates the presence of cardiomyopathy. Heart failure patients with implanted cardiac devices may show a paced rhythm with no diagnostic features of left ventricular function.

A prominent negative component of the P wave in lead V1 reflects elevated left ventricular end-diastolic pressure. The negativity may subside with the relatively early improvement of heart failure.

In CHF, peripheral edema may be associated with a decrease in amplitude (voltage) and duration of the QRS complex and the QT interval. These changes may hide important underlying abnormalities such as bundle branch block. The QRS and QT interval return to their baseline values when peripheral edema has subsided. The QRS abnormalities correlate with weight gain (peripheral edema). The mechanism of the attenuation of the ECG amplitude with peripheral edema is based on an increase in the electrical conductivity (i.e. decrease of resistivity) resulting in decrease of ECG voltage as per Ohm's law. Thus, QRS and even P wave changes (in V1) can be used in the follow-up of heart failure therapy.

During congestive heart failure with peripheral edema there is shortening of the QRS and QT interval.

The ECG triad suggestive of CHF is characterized by low voltage in the limb leads, and high voltage in the precordial leads, and an R/S ratio < 1 in lead V4. There is a modest sensitivity and good specificity. The absence of the ECG triad does not exclude heart failure !

ECG triad of congestive heart failure
 * Relatively low QRS voltage in all six limb leads (≤ 0.8 mV)
 * High QRS voltage in precordial leads (S in V1 or S in V2 and R in V5 or R in V6 > 3.5 mV)
 * Poor R wave progression with R/S ratio < 1 in lead V4

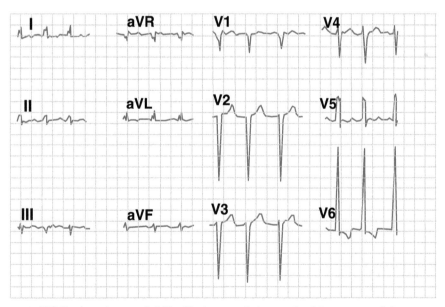

ECG showing atrial fibrillation and the typical features of the congestive heart failure triad.

El-Sherif N, Turitto G. Ambulatory electrocardiographic monitoring between artifacts and misinterpretation, management errors of commission and errors of omission. Ann Noninvasive Electrocardiol. 2014 Nov 4. doi: 10.1111/anec.12222. [Epub ahead of print] PubMed PMID: 25367291.

Glancy DL, Newman, III WP. Atrial fibrillation with QRS voltage low in the limb leads and high in the precordial leads. Proc (Bayl Univ Med Cent).2008; 21: 437–8.

Goldberger AL. A specific ECG triad associated with congestive heart failure. Pacing Clin Electrophysiol. 1982;5:593-9.

Hurst JW. The interpretation of electrocardiograms: pretense or a well-developed skill? Cardiol Clin. 2006;24:305-7.

Kataoka H, Madias JE. Changes in the amplitude of electrocardiogram QRS complexes during follow-up of heart failure patients. J Electrocardiol. 2011;44:394.e1-9.

Lopez C, Ilie CC, Glancy DL, Quintal RE. Goldberger's electrocardiographic triad in patients with echocardiographic severe left ventricular dysfunction. Am J Cardiol. 2012;109:914-18.

Lumlertgul S, Chenthanakij B, Madias JE. ECG leads I and II to evaluate diuresis of patients with congestive heart failure admitted to the hospital via the emergency department. Pacing Clin Electrophysiol. 2009;32:64-71.

Madias JE. Low QRS voltage and its causes. J Electrocardiol. 2008;41:498-500.

Madias JE. Mechanism of attenuation of the QRS voltage in heart failure: a hypothesis. Europace. 2009;11:995-1000.

Madias JE. Why recording of an electrocardiogram should be required in every inpatient and outpatient encounter of patients with heart failure. Pacing Clin Electrophysiol. 2011;34:963-7.

Madias JE, Guglin ME. Augmentation of ECG QRS complexes after fluid removal via a mechanical ultrafiltration pump in patients with congestive heart failure. Ann Noninvasive Electrocardiol. 2007;12:291-7.

Pope JH, Aufderheide TP, Ruthazer R, Woolard RH, Feldman JA, Beshansky JR, Griffith JL, Selker HP. Missed diagnoses of acute cardiac ischemia in the emergency department. N Engl J Med. 2000;342:1163-70.

Venkatachalam KL. Common pitfalls in interpreting pacemaker electrocardiograms in the emergency department. J Electrocardiol. 2011;44:616-21.

Page numbers in *italics* denote figures.

ECG from Basics to Essentials: Step by Step. First Edition. Roland X. Stroobandt, S. Serge Barold and Alfons F. Sinnaeve.
Published 2016 © 2016 by John Wiley & Sons, Ltd. Companion Website: www.wiley.com/go/stroobandt/ecg